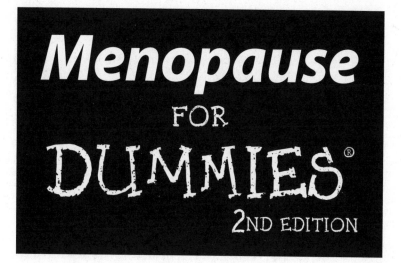

# Menopause FOR DUMMIES®
## 2ND EDITION

**by Marcia L. Jones, PhD, Theresa Eichenwald, MD, and Nancy W. Hall**

WILEY

John Wiley & Sons, Inc.

**Menopause For Dummies®, 2nd Edition**
Published by
**John Wiley & Sons, Inc.**
111 River St.
Hoboken, NJ 07030-5774
www.wiley.com

# *About the Authors*

**Nancy W. Hall, M.S., M.Phil.,** lived the menopause experience in real life as she wrote this book. In addition to delving into the most up-to-date research on perimenopause, menopause, women's health, and treatments for menopausal symptoms, she relentlessly grilled her friends and a shocking number of complete strangers about their experiences.

Nancy received her Master's degrees in psychology at Yale University. Her interest in various aspects of parenting led her to research and write about all sorts of issues pertaining to children's and women's health and work-life concerns. Nancy has been a contributing editor for both *Child* magazine and *Parents* magazine, and a frequent contributor to other parenting, women's, and health magazines and Web sites. Her books on child development, family policy, and health include *Balancing Pregnancy and Work: How to Make the Most of the Next 9 Months on the Job* (Rodale, 2004).

Nancy is the mom of a son and a daughter (both keepers). When she's not writing books and magazine articles about these and other topics, she knits, bakes artisan breads, raises bees, and studies goju ryu karate.

**Marcia L. Jones, PhD,** has life experience in fertility treatment, perimenopause, and menopause. In 1991, while attempting to start a family at the age of 38, she scoured bookstores searching for down-to-earth information on the likely problems and how to proceed. Her doctor directed her to the only information available at the time, photocopies of technical articles from medical journals and pamphlets written by pharmaceutical companies trying to sell product. Today, many women are delaying childbirth, so the issue of fertility fits nicely into a discussion of perimenopause and menopause. These experiences served as her primary motivation for writing this book. She became certain that women in their mid-thirties to late forties need current, unbiased, reliable information on perimenopause and menopause written for a layperson.

Thanks to the efforts of her doctor Jane Chihal, MD, a contributor to this book and a recognized expert on menopause and fertility, Dr. Jones was the proud mother of two girls ages 6 and 4.

Dr. Jones received her PhD from Southern Methodist University in anthropology. She led many research expeditions in the Middle East and served as an associate professor of anthropology at the University of Tulsa.

Growing weary of academia, Marcia shifted her career focus and entered the fast-paced world of software, achieving the rank of chief operating officer and co-owner of Criterion, a company that developed human-resource software for Fortune 1000 organizations. She grew Criterion from a $1.5 million company to a $10 million company and recently sold it to Peopleclick. During the past 18 years, she has written many articles on people in the workforce and taught courses in the use of human-resource technology as an adjunct professor in the Graduate School of Management at the University of Dallas.

**Theresa Eichenwald** has extensive experience caring for menopausal women as an internist at hospitals in New York, Washington D.C., Philadelphia, and, most recently, Texas. She has taught at Albert Einstein School of Medicine and Mount Sinai Medical Center in New York.

In addition to teaching and caring for patients, Dr. Eichenwald has authored a number of articles for professional journals, covering topics such as breast cancer and ovarian tumors, as well as patient education pamphlets. She is a member of the American Medical Association, the American College of Physicians, and in medical school participated in the American Medical Student Association Task Force on Aging.

# Dedication

To David, through all the ages, and to Wilson and Meg, through all the stages.

# Author's Acknowledgments

My work could not have been accomplished without the solid foundation, wit, and wisdom of the first edition's authors, the late Marcia L. Jones, PhD and Theresa Eichenwald, MD.

Special thanks to Leslie Connor and Sandi Kahn Shelton for always, always being there for me, and to Leslie, Sandi, and to Judy Theiss and the many other women with whom I spoke for graciously sharing their time and their own experiences. Thanks, too, to the hundreds of thousands of women who unselfishly participate every day in health studies and clinical trials that benefit millions of us. It's not hot in here after all, but it's nice to know it's not just me.

A huge thank you to Marilyn Allen, who put me in the right place at precisely the right time.

The terrific Wiley Publishing staff was delightful to work with. Special thanks to Michael Lewis, who brought me on board and supported my approach to the book's second edition. The wonderful support and spot-on advice of my project editor, Jennifer Connolly, didn't just make it look easy — with Jenn to light the way, it really was easy.

## Publisher's Acknowledgments

We're proud of this book; please send us your comments through our Dummies online registration form located at www.dummies.com/register/.

Some of the people who helped bring this book to market include the following:

*Acquisitions, Editorial, and Media Development*

**Project Editor:** Jennifer Connolly

**Acquisitions Editor:** Mike Lewis

**Copy Editor:** Jennifer Connolly

**Technical Editor:** Susan Kindig, MD

**Editorial Manager:** Michelle Hacker

**Editorial Supervisor:** Carmen Krikorian

**Editorial Assistants:** Erin Calligan, Joe Niesen, David Lutton

**Cover Photos:** © Moodboard_Images/iStock

**Cartoons:** Rich Tennant (www.the5thwave.com)

*Composition Services*

**Project Coordinators:** Erin Smith and Jennifer Theriot

**Layout and Graphics:** Lavonne Cook, Stephanie D. Jumper, Alicia South

**Anniversary Logo Design:** Richard Pacifico

**Proofreaders:** Laura Albert, Jessica Kramer, Tricia Liebig

**Indexer:** Beth Palmer

---

**Publishing and Editorial for Consumer Dummies**

**Kathleen Nebenhaus,** Vice President and Publisher

**David Palmer,** Associate Publisher

**Kristin Ferguson-Wagstaffe,** Product Development Director

**Publishing for Technology Dummies**

**Andy Cummings,** Vice President and Publisher

**Composition Services**

**Debbie Stailey,** Director of Composition Services

# Contents at a Glance

# Table of Contents

# Introduction

$W$e wrote this book to give women of all ages a clear view of the physical, mental, and emotional changes related to menopause. For generations, women of all ages have approached menopause without knowing specifically what it would mean for them. Oh, you probably knew that menopause and hot flashes go hand in hand, but even that information isn't always true. The truth is that you may never have a hot flash, and if you do, it will probably be years before you're menopausal. Common knowledge about menopause is still too often dominated by myth and misinformation. (The medical community didn't even officially recognize the link between estrogen and hot flashes until 1974!)

If menopause only concerned a small group of people on a desert island, this lack of information might be understandable. But over half of the world's population will become menopausal one day. Menopause has been the misfit family member of the research community for years: a collection of symptoms and a very real phenomenon, but not a disease. Even medical textbooks pay scant attention to the topic. Today, one group is paying attention to menopause. The pharmaceutical industry sees great opportunity in the field of menopause, and more research is underway. If you're looking for books to help reasonably intelligent women navigate the journey of menopause, your options are still somewhat limited to a choice between pretty, glossy pamphlets published by drug companies who may just be a tiny bit biased in their recommendations, or books that promote the natural aspects of menopause with such ferocity that you may feel guilty wishing for relief from troublesome symptoms. If you're really persistent, you will find some academic articles in medical journals, but your eyes could glaze over as you try to pick out straightforward answers to your practical questions. We hope this book can fill that void. Our goal is to help you digest the research so you can make objective and informed health decisions based on your own experience with menopause.

Menopause is not a disease — that's true. No one is going to die from menopause or its symptoms, but every day, women die from the medical effects of low estrogen levels. Your risks of certain diseases and cancers rise after menopause. Some folks may respond to that statement with one of their own, "Well, that's because women are older when they go through menopause." True again, but it's also true that estrogen plays a role in an amazing number of functions in your body, some of which protect your organs, increase your immunity, and slow degeneration. This transformation we call menopause impacts our health in very significant ways. This book helps you understand the story behind the symptoms and the diseases.

Some women choose to use hormone therapy to relieve symptoms associated with menopause and protect their body from disease. The choice of whether to take hormones or not is quite controversial because hormone therapy has its own significant set of risks. The debate goes on in the medical community and media concerning the risks of hormone therapy. If you're like many women, your confusion only grows as you read more on the subject. Each new study seems to contradict the findings of the last one. You're an intelligent person. But how can you know which study you should believe? In this book, we try to provide enough information to enable you to make informed decisions about your health.

# About This Book

We have no agenda in writing this book. We're not trying to sell you medications, alternative health strategies, or remedies. This book presents accurate and up-to-date information from the most credible sources. It contains straightforward information based on reliable medical studies without the academic lingo common to medical journals. When no clear-cut answers exist and when quality research shows mixed conclusions, we let you know.

Everyone's time is limited, so we cut to the chase. We cover the questions that are important to you during this phase of your life. If you want more detail, we provide an appendix full of resources to help with your personal research. We also try not to stray too far from the topic at hand. For example, during the years leading up to menopause, women may have difficulty getting pregnant. The same hormonal changes that cause those annoying symptoms prior to menopause also stifle fertility. Many women in their late 30s who are trying to get pregnant rely on hormone supplements. Despite the overlap in hormonal terms, fertility is not a concern for many women going through the change, so our discussion is limited.

Whether you're going through the change, have already been there, or are about to start off down that road, you'll find the information you need between these snazzy yellow and black covers. We cover all the health issues and therapy choices that confront women during the menopausal years.

# Foolish Assumptions

Every author has to make a few assumptions about her audience, and we've made a few assumptions about you:

✔ You're a woman. (But, believe it or not, your treatment choices can have implications for the guy in your life, so we'll talk just a tiny bit about his health, too.)

✔ You want to understand what's going on with your body.

✔ You're looking for straight talk for real people as opposed to scientific jargon and Medicalese (though we have a Medicalese icon to invite you into short — optional — forays into this territory).

✔ You want to evaluate your risks of disease as you pass through midlife and move into your menopausal years.

✔ You don't want a book that claims to let you diagnose yourself or figure out what medications you need. You have a medical advisor to discuss these things with.

✔ You want to be able to ask intelligent questions and discuss treatment alternatives with your healthcare providers.

✔ You want to feel more confident about the quality of your healthcare.

✔ You buy every book that has a black and yellow cover.

If any of these statements apply to you, you're in the right place.

# How This Book Is Organized

We've organized this book into five parts so you can go directly to the topic that interests you the most. Here's a brief overview of each part:

## Part 1: The Main Facts about Menopause

The journey to menopause often catches women by surprise. You may not have been expecting to take the journey, or you may have been wondering when you would begin. In this part, we give you a quick overview of what your hormones are doing before, during, and after menopause. If you haven't thought about things such as hormones and follicles for a while, don't worry; we refresh your memory. Your sixth-grade health-and-hygiene course probably never finished the story. In this part, you get the whole story from how the egg makes its journey from the ovary to the uterus to what happens when the ovary goes into retirement. We've also added a chapter to answer the special questions you may have if you're among the small group of women who (through illness, medical treatment, or some other factor) face menopause more suddenly or much earlier than most women will.

# Part II: The Effects of Menopause on Your Body and Mind

Want to know how hormones affect the health of your body and mind? You can find the answers in Part II. We devote each chapter in this part to a specific body part or health issue. In each chapter, you get an overview of how hormones function in relation to this part of your body and the types of conditions that can develop, how to recognize them, and what you can do about them.

# Part III: Treating the Effects

You may want to evaluate the pros and cons of hormone therapy (HT) from time to time during your journey through menopause. This part of the book brings you up to date on what the medical community knows about HT. We discuss the effects of HT so that you can make informed decisions. Reading these chapters provides added benefits as well: You'll probably find it easier to evaluate the news about hormone research that comes out in future years.

We also include information about non-HT drugs and alternative treatments. This will help you make informed decisions on treating menopause symptoms *and* helping to protect your health during the menopausal years without hormones. You may be one of many women for whom hormone therapy isn't medically appropriate, or you may just prefer not to take hormones, or to take them for as short a period as possible.

# Part IV: Lifestyle Issues for Menopause and Beyond

Part IV is chock full of great ways to stay healthy and enjoy a long and active life during and after menopause. Staying healthy and active is simpler than you think. We discuss healthy eating habits and simple ways to stay fit. Whether you're looking for natural ways to lower your risk of specific diseases or for ways to slow the aging process, you can find the information you need right here. We even get into the ways in which this new stage of your life can be richer and more exciting than any you've experienced yet.

# Part V: The Part of Tens

If you're a fan of *For Dummies* books, you probably recognize this part. These are short chapters with quick tips and fast facts. In Part V, we debunk ten menopause myths, review ten common medical tests you may encounter, suggest ten terrific exercise programs for menopausal women, and give you tips about ten powerhouse foods that will help keep you feeling your best — now and in the years to come.

## Part VI: The Appendixes

A glossary of menopause-related terms and a list of menopause-related resources cap the book.

# Conventions Used in This Book

We use our own brand of shorthand for some frequently used terms and icons to highlight specific information.

As you read this book, you'll discover that menopause is a process, with different stages characterized by similar symptoms. These stages are referred to as *perimenopause,* the three to ten years prior to menopause when you may experience symptoms; *menopause* itself, which you know you've reached only after you've reached it because the definition of menopause is the absence of periods for a year; and *postmenopause,* which is your life after you've stopped having periods. In this book, we use *perimenopause* to describe the premenopause condition, and we use *menopause* to refer to everything after that just because the term *postmenopause* isn't commonly used.

A major part of this book — the whole of Part III as well as sections in other chapters — talks about hormone therapy (HT), which is used to alleviate symptoms and address health concerns prompted by menopause. In literature and on Web sites, you can see hormone therapies referred to and abbreviated any number of ways, including hormone replacement therapy (HRT) and estrogen replacement therapy (ERT). But we stick pretty closely to using HT because we feel that it's the most inclusive and accurate term. Just be aware that *HT* means essentially the same thing as *HRT.*

And, speaking of hormones, a couple of the more important ones for menopausal women have several subcategories:

- ✔ Types of **estrogen** include estriol, estradiol, and estrone.
- ✔ **Progesterone** is the class of hormone; the form used in hormone therapy is often referred to as progestin.

We sometimes use these terms interchangeably and only refer to the specific hormone as necessary for clarity.

# Icons Used in This Book

In this book, we use icons as a quick way to go directly to the information you need. Look for the icons in the margin that point out specific types of information. Here's what the icons we use in this book mean.

The Tip icon points out practical, concise information that can help you take better care of yourself.

This icon points you to medical terms and jargon that can help you understand what you read or hear from professionals and enable you to ask your healthcare provider intelligent questions.

This fine piece of art flags information that's worth noting.

When you see this icon, do what it tells you to do. It accompanies info that should be discussed with an expert in the field.

The Technical Stuff icon points out material that generally can be classified as dry as a bone. Although we think that the information is interesting, it's not vital to your understanding of the issue. Skip it if you so desire.

This icon cautions you about potential problems or threats to your health.

# Where to Go from Here

*For Dummies* books are designed so that you can dip in anywhere that looks interesting and get the information you need. This is a reference book, so don't feel as though you have to read an entire chapter (or even an entire section for that matter). You won't miss anything by skipping around. So, find what interests you and jump on in!

# Part I
# The Main Facts about Menopause

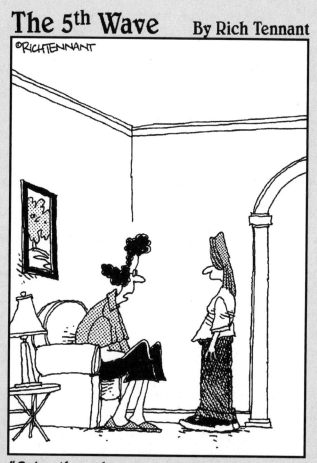

"Going through menopause is a lot like going through adolescence, but no, I'm not in love with Justin Timberlake, I don't hate your little brother, and I have no desire to dye my hair green."

## In this part . . .

The first act of *Dance of the Hormones* probably occurred three decades or so ago for you. Remember the bittersweet tale of teenage angst and joy that we call puberty? And now, intermission (the menstrual years) may be coming to a close as the hormones once again take the stage for the second act — menopause. Take your seat and get ready to peruse your program . . . uh, Part I of this book.

In Part I, we provide you with an outline to your menopausal years. We define menopause, review the biology, introduce you to the actors —your hormones — and briefly review the related symptoms and health conditions (physical, mental, and emotional). There's even a special scene with a little extra drama for those of you for whom the menopause curtain rose early. Get to it before the usher dims the lights.

# Chapter 1

# Mapping Out Menopause

. . . . . . . . . . . . . . . . . . . . . . . . . . . . . . . . . . . . . . . . . . . . . .

. . . . . . . . . . . . . . . . . . . . . . . . . . . . . . . . . . . . . . . . . . . . . .

"**Y**ou've come a long way, baby" seems like a recurring slogan for baby boomers. The phrase certainly says a lot about the women of this generation as they approach the rite of passage called menopause. As an individual, you no doubt feel like you've come a long way in your life by the time you begin to think about menopause. Society in general, and women in particular, have also come a long way in opening up the discussion about the mysteries of menopause.

The phrase "you've come a long way, baby" closes with "but you've got such a long way to go." Women today may well live 40 or 50 years after menopause. We all want to enjoy these years by visiting friends, taking care of our loved ones and ourselves, and pursuing favorite interests (old and new). In this chapter, we introduce you to menopause so you know what to expect when the time comes or what has been happening to you if you're already in transition.

## Defining Menopause

Puberty and menopause bracket the reproductive season of your life, and they share many characteristics. They're both transitions (meaning that they don't last forever); they're both triggered by hormones; they both cause physical and emotional changes (that sometimes drive you crazy); and they both close some doors and enrich your life by opening new ones.

Puberty was the time when your hormones first swung into action. It marked the beginning of your reproductive years. Remember the ride? Your hormone levels shifted wildly when you got your first menstrual period. Your emotions probably went a little haywire for a while, too. Over the course of a few years, your hormones found a comfortable level. Your unpredictable periods finally settled into a predictable pattern, and your emotional balance was more or less restored.

At the end of your reproductive years, your hormone levels go through a similar dance (this time causing the midlife mood swings), but your hormones eventually find a new, lower level of production. Your periods are erratic for a while, but they eventually wind down and stop. So do those emotional roller coaster rides. Unfortunately, this time can be just as confusing as when you experienced puberty — fortunately, we use this section to unravel the basic mystery for you.

## Getting the terminology right

Have you ever noticed how you don't really pay close attention to directions or where you're going when you're the passenger in a car? You only start to worry about every exit number and stop light when you're the one behind the wheel. Well, menopause is like that. You hear about menopause and menopausal symptoms, but you rarely pay much attention to the particulars until it's your turn.

When you do slide into the driver's seat and start paying attention, you may become frustrated by the confusing terminology associated with the whole menopause thing. Aside from the pamphlets you get from the doctor's office, most books, magazines, and articles treat menopause like a stage that starts with hot flashes and goes on for the rest of your life. But we know better. The following list gives you the lowdown on the terms associated with menopause:

✔ **Menopause:** *Menopause* actually means the end of menstruation. During the years leading up to menopause (called *perimenopause*), your periods may be so erratic that you're never sure which period will be the last one, but you aren't officially menopausal until you haven't had a period for a year.

✔ **Perimenopause:** The term *perimenopause* refers to the time leading up to the cessation of menstruation, when estrogen production is slowing down. A lot of the symptoms that folks usually label as menopausal (hot flashes, mood swings, sleeplessness, and so on) actually take place during the perimenopausal years. We're sticklers in this book about using the term *perimenopause* rather than *menopause* to describe this early phase because you're still having periods. We also use *peri-menopause* because we want to note the physiological and emotional changes you experience prior to the end of your periods and distinguish them from the changes that happen after your body has adjusted to lower levels of estrogen.

✔ **Postmenopause:** Technically, the time after your last period is called *postmenopause,* but this word has never really caught on. So, in keeping with common usage, we most often use the term *menopause* to refer to the actual event and the years after menopause and use *postmenopause* only when it helps clarify things. When we talk about *menopausal* women in this book, we're talking about women who have stopped having periods — whether they're 55 or 75.

The years leading up to and following menopause mark a pretty major transformation in a woman's life. As you make your way through this period of your life, you'll want to know where you're at within the whole grand scope of the change and what's going on inside you. Here's a brief description of the phases associated with menopause. (Don't worry: We give you a lot more detail about the various stages in Chapters 2 and 4.)

## Approaching the change: Perimenopause

*Perimenopause* is the stage during which your hormones start to shift gears. Some months, your hormones operate at the levels they've worked at for the past 30 years or so; other months, your aging ovaries don't produce estrogen when they should. Your brain responds to this lack of estrogen production by sending a signal to try to get those ovaries jumpstarted. When they receive the signal, your aging ovaries overcompensate but don't produce estrogen in the same quantities that they used to.

Your period is late because your ovaries produced less estrogen during the first part of your normal cycle, or because you may never have ovulated, making the entire cycle weird and unusual — sometimes heavy, sometimes light.

So, during perimenopause, you still have your period, but you experience symptoms that folks associate with menopause. If you go to the doctor at this stage and ask, "What's happening to me? Could this be menopause?" the doctor will often go straight to the "Could this be menopause?" part of your question. Of course you're not menopausal if you're still having periods. But the problem is that many doctors miss the first part of the question — the "What's happening to me?" part. This is the real issue you want to get to the bottom of — the cause of your weird physical and emotional conditions.

## *Menstruating no more: Menopause*

Menopause means never having to say, "Can I borrow a tampon?" again.

If you haven't had a period for a year, you've reached *menopause.* Women can become menopausal approximately anytime between the ages of 45 and 55, with the average age being 51. The definition may seem cut and dry at first glance, but here are a few situations that may leave you scratching your head.

What if you use a cyclical type of hormone therapy in which you take estrogen for several days and progestin during the last few days of your cycle? You still have a period (the progestin causes you to slough the lining of the uterus), but you don't ovulate. Are you menopausal or not? Technically, you're delaying your last period. You're taking a sufficient dosage of estrogen to rid yourself of perimenopausal symptoms, but you're no longer fertile.

Here's another tricky one: If you've had a *hysterectomy* (surgical removal of the uterus), you're considered to be "surgically menopausal." But, if you had your uterus removed but kept your ovaries, you're not "hormonally" menopausal because your ovaries still produce estrogen. By taking your blood and analyzing your hormone levels, your physician can tell you whether your hormones are officially at menopausal levels.

These tricky situations cause us to ask, "Who cares about the definition?" You know a rose is a rose. The main concern here is *what's happening with your hormones,* especially estrogen. Hormonal changes can trigger many physical and emotional health issues.

When you reach menopause, your hormone production is so low that your periods stop. Your ovaries still produce some estrogen and testosterone, but instead of producing hormones in cycles (which is why you have periods and why you're only fertile for about four or five days each month), your body now produces constant, low levels of hormones. The type of estrogen your ovaries churn out also switches from an active type to a rather inactive form.

## *Getting past menopause: Postmenopause*

*Postmenopause* is the period of your life that starts after menopause (a year after your last period) and ends when you do. This is a time when your body is living on greatly reduced levels of estrogen, testosterone, and progesterone. In this book, we simply refer to both the cessation of your period and your life afterward as menopause.

# Anticipating Menopause

When will you become menopausal? The timing varies from woman to woman. Predicting this stuff is nowhere near an exact science. Heck, you can't even use the fact that you started your period earlier than most women as a predictor that you'll stop menstruating earlier. (The same goes for starting your period later in life and ending it later in life.) Genetics and lifestyle may have some impact on the schedule, but basically, it happens when it happens. But we can give you some ballpark age ranges for these phases.

Most women become perimenopausal sometime between the ages of 35 and 50. You'll probably know it when you get there because you'll probably have some of the symptoms (check out the Cheat Sheet at the front of this book and Chapter 4) and/or some irregular periods. Women usually become menopausal sometime in their 50s.

Some events can alter these "normal" age patterns, including lifestyle habits and medical interventions. Here are a few exceptional types of menopause:

- **Premature menopause:** A term used when women go through menopause in their 30s. This timing is considered unusually early, but it may be normal for you.

- **Medical menopause:** Refers to menopause induced by chemotherapy, radiation, anorexia, or other factors. This type of menopause is sometimes reversible, though your periods may take a month, several months, or even years to return.

- **Surgical menopause:** Refers to menopause induced by surgery. Removal of both ovaries results in immediate, nonreversible menopause.

  Because your ovaries produce all types of sex hormones (estrogen, progesterone, and testosterone), surgical removal of your ovaries is fairly traumatic for your system: you'll go straight into intense menopausal symptoms such as hot flashes. (Chapter 3 is devoted to preparing for and understanding the causes and consequences of premature menopause.)

# Transitioning to Menopause

When a group of women talk about their personal experiences of puberty, menstrual cycles, and pregnancy, the stories are all over the board. Some women don't notice changes in their bodies; others recognize the moment ovulation or conception occurs. Some women have terrible problems with premenstrual syndrome (PMS); others have trouble-free cycles throughout their entire lives. Women's experiences vary with perimenopause and menopause just as much as they vary with these other changes. In this section we cover what you might experience as you begin the transition into perimenopause.

## Starting out

Most women's ovaries begin a transformation sometime between the ages of 35 and 50. If your periods end before you reach 40, you experience what's known as *premature menopause.*

Perimenopause is sometimes called a climacteric period, which simply means that it's a crucial period. Remember that your ovaries don't just shut down one day; the transition is punctuated with production peaks and valleys that cause many annoying physical and mental symptoms. Perimenopause is a time of important physiological change — when egg production along with the production of estrogen and progesterone begins slowing down.

## Identifying symptoms

We devote Chapter 4 almost exclusively to the symptoms women may experience during perimenopause. Several other chapters explain the link between your hormones and these symptoms.

Less than half of all women experience annoying symptoms such as hot flashes, heart palpitations, interrupted sleep, and mood swings during the transitional period prior to menopause. Most women who do experience these symptoms experience the symptoms while they're still menstruating on a regular schedule.

Other women recognize that they're perimenopausal because their periods, which used to be as regular as clockwork, are now irregular. Their periods may be late, they may skip a period, or their flow may be light one month and resemble a flood the next month.

Unfortunately, no objective medical test exists to determine whether you're officially perimenopausal.

## Calling in the professionals

If you're in your late 40s or 50s and you're experiencing the symptoms listed on the Cheat Sheet and in Chapter 3, you can probably assume that you're perimenopausal. But don't cancel that appointment with your medical advisor to get the symptoms checked out. (If you don't have an appointment to cancel, make one and keep it.) Many symptoms of perimenopause are the same as some of the symptoms of thyroid problems, cardiovascular disease, depression, and other serious health issues.

Your medical practitioner can help you deal with the undesirable symptoms of perimenopause and prevent serious health conditions that are more prevalent after menopause.

## Seeing it through to the end

Because you never really know when perimenopause starts, accurately defining a timeframe is difficult. Some women experience symptoms for ten years before their periods stop. The fact is that most of the symptoms you hear about are caused by the fluctuating hormone levels of perimenopause as opposed to the sustained, low levels of hormones you experience during menopause.

You're officially menopausal one year after your last period. After that, many people use the term postmenopause to mark the rest of your life (though in this book, we just keep using *menopause*).

# Treating Menopause

At the end of the perimenopause road, your ovaries (and consequently, your hormone production) finally wind down. Your body gradually adjusts to the lower hormone levels typical of life after menopause. Most of the perimenopausal symptoms disappear, but now your concerns shift to health issues associated with prolonged, lowered levels of active estrogen.

Estrogen not only plays a role in reproduction, it also helps regulate a host of other functions throughout your body. Estrogen protects your bones and cardiovascular system, among other responsibilities. Those pesky perimenopausal symptoms may make life miserable, but they aren't dangerous to your health. But the conditions associated with long periods of diminished estrogen levels are very troublesome. They include

✔ Cardiovascular disease

✔ Heart disease

✔ Hypertension (high blood pressure)

✔ Osteoporosis

✔ Stroke

So you and your doctor need to work on strategies to prevent these conditions.

Some women choose hormone therapy (HT) to help prevent disease; others choose to take medications as individual problems arise. (We cover hormone therapy in Chapters 11 through 16 and alternative and non-hormonal ways to deal with certain conditions in Chapter 17.) Whichever path or paths you choose, each strategy presents benefits and risks. Your choices depend on your medical history, your family history, and your healthcare preferences. And remember that both your experiences and medical technologies change daily, so re-evaluate your options from time to time.

# Promoting Longevity

Not long ago, 50 was about as old as we could expect to get. Today, many of us will live well into our 70s, 80s, and 90s. The fact that most women stop being fertile in their 40s doesn't mean that women are no longer productive after 40. In fact, with the whole reproduction thing out of the way, women have more time and opportunities to make new contributions to life on earth (or in space).

One of the keys to a long and happy life is good genes. Another key is taking good care of yourself and the genes you're dealt. Regular checkups can address medical issues as they arise and help prevent others. Eat healthy foods (and portions), get some exercise, and live life to its fullest.

Everyone agrees that a healthy lifestyle is the best way to reduce trouble-some perimenopausal symptoms, prevent disease, and promote a long and healthy life. It's also the least risky strategy for dealing with perimenopause and menopause. Taking up this challenge requires self-assessment and a bit of determination. Shifting to a healthy lifestyle involves eliminating unhealthy habits, getting at least a half-hour of aerobic exercise five times a week, and maintaining a healthy, balanced diet that includes at least five servings of fruit and vegetables each week. We provide some great info on diet, nutrition, and exercise in Chapters 18 and 19. In Chapter 20, we talk about how the part of your life that follows menopause can be one of the most rewarding of all.

# Chapter 2

# Talking Biology and Psychology: Your Mind and Body on Menopause

*I*f you're in your 40s, and you're like a lot of women, you've asked yourself, "What in the world is happening to me?" Maybe extra girth seemingly appeared overnight and now won't go away no matter how many crunches you do. Or maybe you notice yourself perspiring while lying in bed next to your partner just as you did when you first got together — except now it happens in the middle of the night when you're not even thinking about *that*. Does it seem as if the world has gotten dumber and that no one can do things right anymore? Maybe your irritability and mood swings aren't caused by the planets being out of alignment; maybe it's perimenopause.

In this chapter, we take a look at how your hormones work during your reproductive years and how they change as you approach and enter your nonreproductive years. Fluctuations or deviations in your hormone levels largely trigger the physiological, emotional, and mental changes you may notice during perimenopause and menopause. Getting on a first name basis with these hormones and learning about their functions won't necessarily let you control the havoc they seem to be wreaking. Knowing that your experience is normal, though, can relieve a lot of worry and uncertainty.

# Setting the Stage

Before we get started, we need to set the stage. Menopause is not a disease, deficiency, or failure. Nor is it necessarily going to be problematic for you — every woman's menopause is different. Menopause is a natural and necessary change in life. Just as infancy, toddlerhood, adolescence, and young adulthood had their challenges and their rewards, so will your menopausal years. Only this time around, you have the maturity, sophistication, and resources to learn about and deal with what's going on.

You may see and hear medical terms such as *estrogen deficiency, ovarian failure,* and *vaginal atrophy* used to describe menopause and its symptoms. You might even come across them in this book. These terms aren't meant to carry negative connotations. They're meant to describe expected conditions. Viewing menopause as a natural change — not an organ failure — is an important first step to understanding what might be in store for you and how best to deal with any symptoms you experience.

Just as women aren't put on earth for the simple purpose of bearing children, your ovaries aren't there just to supply eggs. Your ovaries live a double life — one as the holder of the seeds of life (*oocytes* that later develop into eggs), and the other as a maintenance worker. Your ovaries are a critical source of hormones for your whole body. After menopause your ovaries don't retire, they just change careers. No longer busy with developing follicles that carry eggs (which release lots of estrogen), the ovaries continue to produce hormones (though in much smaller amounts than before) to help maintain overall body functions.

Because the average life expectancy for people in the United States is about 80 years, the average woman spends a little more than half her life menstruating and being fertile. And while we live in a culture that puts a lot of emphasis on these years, the years following menopause can be — and should be — just as exciting and fruitful. It's likely that you can expect to spend a significant portion of your life just being a woman.

In some circles, the administration of hormone therapy (HT) has long had the reputation of being a part of the fix-a-failure approach to menopause. But although we know that HT can help control symptoms such as hot flashes and vaginal dryness, it's no longer being routinely recommended for the prevention of health issues such as heart disease and breast cancer. The more you know about your own body, about how natural hormones (the ones you make yourself) work, and about how replacement hormones (hormone therapy) work, the better prepared you'll be to make healthcare decisions tailored just for you.

# Making the Menstrual Cycle and Hormone Connection

Okay, admit it. You didn't find those long, boring, sterile movies that explained menstruation to you and your sixth-grade classmates very helpful. You know the ones — the health-class movies with titles such as "You're a Woman Now." (Back in those days, we didn't have interesting titles such as *Sex For Dummies*.) If you were anything like us, you had difficulty making the connection between the two-dimensional, cartoon-like illustrations of female organs and the three-dimensional, high-definition experiences of bloating and cramps.

In this section, we make the connection between your sex hormones and your menstrual cycle — hopefully more clearly and meaningfully than those old movies did.

One of the major functions of sex hormones is to prepare the body to produce life. So visiting your sex hormones at the reproduction office to watch them do their jobs as a team is a good place to start the discussion. Then we take a closer look at each individual member of Team Hormone.

The average menstrual cycle is 28 days, but a cycle that lasts anywhere from 22 to 35 days is perfectly normal. For the purpose of this discussion, we use a 28-day cycle; you can adjust the numbers as necessary to fit your personal calendar. Figure 2-1 shows hormone levels throughout a menstrual cycle.

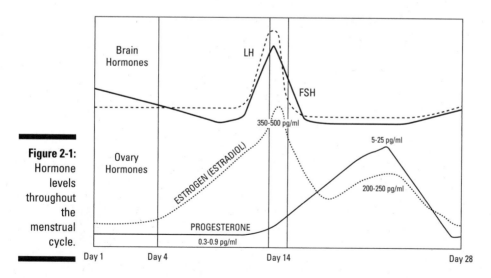

**Figure 2-1:** Hormone levels throughout the menstrual cycle.

## Days of our lives: Determining Day 1

The first day of your period is called Day 1. Simple enough, huh? Sounds pretty definitive. Well, maybe not. When it comes to your body, nothing is ever truly definitive. Here's how things can get a bit more complicated: Do you count yesterday as Day 1 because you had some light bleeding? Or do you call today Day 1 because you really started flowing today? Or maybe you should count two days ago as Day 1 because you started cramping really badly and had a bit of spotting.

How to solve this dilemma? Consistency is key. If you normally have a light day before you start your regular flow, count your light day as Day 1. But, if you're like some women who experience spotting several days before they actually begin their period, Day 1 should be the first day of your regular flow.

Day 1 of your cycle is the first day of your period (see the "Days of our lives: Determining Day 1" sidebar to find out how to determine the first day of your period). Your body begins flushing out the lining of your uterus, which isn't needed because a fertilized egg requiring nourishment and support isn't present in your uterus.

Your ovaries are filled with little seeds (eggs) surrounded by support cells (*stroma*). During the first half of your cycle (Days 1 to 14), hormones produced in your brain — *follicle-stimulating hormone* (FSH) and *luteinizing hormone* (LH) — and hormones produced in your ovaries — estrogen — work together to develop and then release an egg. (For more information on FSH and LH see the "Linking your brain and body" section later in this chapter.) During these first two weeks, your estradiol (estrogen) levels are on the rise, and your progesterone levels are very low. This particular hormone combination (high estrogen, low progesterone) is why you usually feel so good during this stretch of your cycle. You owe your energy, restful sleep, upbeat mood, sharp memory, and terrific concentration to your old friend, estrogen, which plays a role in many physical and mental systems — not just your reproductive system.

As soon as the brain senses that estrogen levels are right, it produces a surge of luteinizing hormone (LH), which triggers the release of an egg — otherwise known as *ovulation*. Ovulation usually occurs between Day 12 and Day 16 of your cycle. (You want the scoop on LH? Check out the "Linking your brain and body" section later in this chapter.)

After you've ovulated, estrogen levels drop, and progesterone production kicks in. *Progesterone*, which peaks around Day 20, is a hormone that gets the uterus ready for a baby. If the egg is fertilized, your progesterone levels stay high. If the egg isn't fertilized, progesterone and estrogen levels drop and menstruation occurs.

# Surveying the Role of Hormones

Unless you're a gynecologist, you may not be able to remember what all the hormones do (or what their various nicknames stand for). So we've included Table 2-1 as a quick review of all the specifics on the operative hormones and their functions.

| Table 2-1 | Hormones in a Nutshell | |
|---|---|---|
| *Hormone* | *Produced By* | *Main Activities* |
| Estrogens | Ovaries | Female hormones that promote breast development and cause menstrual cycles, ovulation, pregnancy, and more. |
| Estrone (E1) | | An "inactive" form of estrogen. After menopause, estrone is the dominant form of estrogen in your body. It's produced in the ovaries prior to menopause. After menopause, body fat produces estrone. High levels of estrone may be associated with breast and endometrial cancer. |
| Estradiol (E2) | | The "active" form of estrogen produced mainly in the ovaries. Services hundreds of mental and physical functions in a woman's body. Prior to menopause, it's the dominant form of estrogen in your body. |
| Estriol (E3) | | Form of estrogen only found in pregnant women. |
| Follicle-stimulating hormone (FSH) | Pituitary gland | Hormone produced in the brain that stimulates the ovaries to get follicles growing and producing estrogen. This is the hormone that kicks off the ovulation cycle. |
| Luteinizing hormone (LH) | Pituitary gland | Hormone produced in the brain that triggers the follicle to release the egg (ovulation). LH supports the production of estrogen and progesterone by the abandoned egg sac known as the *corpus luteum*. |

*(continued)*

**Table 2-1 (continued)**

| Hormone | Produced By | Main Activities |
|---|---|---|
| Progesterone | Ovaries | Prepares the womb for pregnancy and helps maintain pregnancy. Although estrogen is the dominant hormone in the first half of your menstrual cycle, progesterone is dominant in the second half. The effects of progesterone also include water retention, sweet cravings, and fatigue. High doses can work as a sedative or as a depressant. The synthetic form of progesterone is called *progestin*. |
| Testosterone | Ovaries | Considered a "male hormone" even though the bodies of both men and women produce it. In women, the ovaries produce it. During the change, testosterone levels drop. Testosterone benefits women by maintaining healthy libido, strong bones, and muscle growth. |

Quick! What's a hormone, anyway? Most of us toss this mysterious word around pretty casually in our everyday lives, and we *really* use it a lot in this book, but what does it really mean? Hormones are complex chemicals that control the release or activity of *other* chemicals. The network in your body that controls and regulates these chemicals is called the endocrine system.

## Linking your brain and body

Your brain produces the hormones that direct the production of sex hormones in your ovaries. You may say that the hormones produced by your brain act as senior management, directing operations in your ovaries. The hormones in your ovaries are the field managers, directing operations in the field, which is your entire body. The hormones produced by your brain include

- ✔ **Follicle-stimulating hormone (FSH):** When the brain senses that estrogen and progesterone levels have dropped, it shoots out some FSH to the ovaries to tell them to begin developing *follicles* (nutritious sacs that cover the eggs) and start producing estrogen.

- ✔ **Luteinizing hormone (LH):** This hormone triggers ovulation. When LH surges, the follicle releases the egg. The abandoned follicle wrapping, the *corpus luteum*, secretes progesterone and estrogen.

---

## Putting the "men" back in menopause

Do men go through menopause? Well, techni- cally, no. But men do experience a drop in testosterone levels in their 40s. The question of whether this represents an experience that might be called male menopause still divides doctors and researchers. On the other hand, the terms "andropause" and "viropause" do refer to a hypothetical male syndrome said to be characterized by weight gain, irritability, fatigue, mood swings, loss of libido, decrease in bone density, and other, remarkably familiar symp- toms. The jury's still out on whether your guy is going through the same thing you are — after all, these symptoms can all have other causes. But you might want to save him a little sympa- thy, just in case.

## Explaining estrogen

Oh how very sophisticated women are. We don't just produce estrogen; we produce three different types of estrogen:

- ✔ **Estrone (E1):** Inactive estrogen predominant after menopause
- ✔ **Estradiol (E2):** Active estrogen
- ✔ **Estriol (E3):** Estrogen produced only during pregnancy

Medical folks use a shorthand system when referring to different types of estrogen to avoid confusion (and lengthy sentences).

Throughout the book, we use the generic term *estrogen* to mean all the differ- ent types of estrogen, unless distinguishing among them is important for the discussion at hand.

### Estrone (E1)

After menopause, estrone is the predominant type of estrogen streaming through your body. Before menopause your ovaries make estrone. After menopause your body fat takes over the job of making estrone. The more body fat you have, the more estrone you have. Estrone is mainly a stored form of estrogen. Prior to menopause, your ovaries can convert estrone to the active form of estrogen, estradiol. That conversion only happens in pre- menopausal ovaries.

### Estradiol (E2)

You may hear doctors or nurses refer to estradiol by its scientific name, *17- beta estradiol,* but most folks know it as "the good stuff." Before menopause, estradiol is the predominant form of estrogen produced by your ovaries and used throughout your body. Estradiol actively helps out with hundreds of different physical and mental functions, including maintaining bone density and giving your brain feedback about levels of the sex hormones. After menopause, your ovaries stop producing estradiol, and that's when you develop many of those annoying symptoms such as hot flashes, palpitations, changes in your skin, bone, hair, and blood vessels, headaches, and so on.

Your body can convert estrone to estradiol but only with fully functioning ovaries. Your ovaries are slowing down during perimenopause and menopause, and your body doesn't get nearly as much estradiol after menopause as it used to during your reproductive years.

### Estriol (E3)

The weakest of the three estrogens is estriol, which your placenta produces only if you're pregnant. If you don't have any estriol in your body, it's okay; it just means you aren't pregnant.

## Promoting progesterone

If all these hormone names are confusing to you, here's a tip that can help you make sense of progesterone. Think of progesterone as *promoting gesta-tion*; it prepares your womb to nurture a fertilized egg.

Most of your progesterone is made after ovulation. If your egg is fertilized, the placenta takes over progesterone production during the eighth or ninth week of pregnancy. If the egg isn't fertilized, progesterone levels drop. This lack of progesterone triggers your period. Many doctors believe that symptoms of premenstrual syndrome (PMS) can be attributed to progesterone. You can thank progesterone when you crave sweets, feel fatigued, retain water, and develop acne.

Progesterone gets your body ready to support a pregnancy. How does this play out? When progesterone levels are high, you feel hungry more often. Progesterone also slows down the digestion process so that you can absorb nutrients better, but that slower digestion process can make you feel bloated or constipated.

Progesterone can cause depression and increase your cholesterol levels. Progesterone also has a sedating effect that makes some women feel calm and others feel lethargic. It's all a matter of perception, but it isn't your imagi-nation. Progesterone has been found to be eight times more potent than one of the drugs used in anesthesia!

## Looking at DHEA regulation

A technical loophole and special pleading by two U.S. senators kept DHEA from being regulated by the Food and Drug Administration under the Anabolic Steroids Act of 2004. Even so, widespread concern exists about DHEA. Because it has been used by athletes in doping (secret use of hormones to promote athletic performance), the use of DHEA has been banned by a number of athletic associations, including the International Olympic Committee, the National Collegiate Athletic Association, the National Football League, and the National Basketball Association.

# Investigating androgens

Yes, Virginia, your body does produce "male" hormones, and it's perfectly normal. Both men and (to a lesser degree) women produce a group of hormones called androgens in their adrenal glands and sex organs (testes in men, ovaries in women). The androgens affected by menopause are testosterone and DHEA (we discuss these two hormones later in this section).

As you age, your body slows its production of both female and male hormones. During the transition of menopause, estrogen and androgen levels can get a bit out of balance. Even though your androgen levels typically decrease as estrogen levels decrease, the big decrease in estrogen levels can alter the balance so that androgen has a greater relative presence than it did before menopause. This imbalance leads to changes:

✔ Fat migrates toward your waist.

✔ Hair thins on your head and starts growing on your chin or upper lip.

✔ Blood pressure rises.

✔ Total cholesterol rises.

Okay, okay. Stop cursing your androgens already. They have many positive effects on women's bodies too. Check it out:

✔ **Testosterone:** This hormone triggers sexual desire. That's right — testosterone promotes a healthy sexual desire in women. Testosterone also helps women build bone, maintain muscle mass (so you burn fat), and maintain optimal energy levels.

✔ **DHEA:** First an introduction is in order. DHEA stands for dehydroepiandrosterone (that's why we use the abbreviation). DHEA is a building block for testosterone. Your ovaries covert the DHEA from your adrenal glands into testosterone. Without DHEA you could forget about all those positives associated with testosterone.

Some news reports have called DHEA "the fountain of youth" and "the mother of all hormones," but so far there's been no real proof that using this powerful steroid hormone as a supplement to relieve the symptoms of menopause is either useful or safe. Although DHEA is widely marketed as an anti-aging supplement, women who take DHEA may experience side effects that include facial hair growth, fatigue, headaches, and deepening of their voices. We still don't know whether DHEA use is linked to an increase in breast cancer risk. Because DHEA is unregulated, you may not know how much you need or how much you're getting. The bottom line? Never take DHEA without the approval and close supervision of your healthcare provider (see "Looking at DHEA regulation").

# Understanding the Stages of Menopause

*Menopause,* the permanent pause in your periods (*menses*), is one of those things that you aren't sure has happened until long after it's over. Like the first time you met your best friend: You probably had no idea that you'd become so close. You only realized how special that occasion really was when you were able to look back on it. Okay, maybe menopause isn't a warm-and-fuzzy-greeting-card occasion, but it is a passage worth noting.

Are you or aren't you menopausal? You can answer that question only after the fact — after you've gone a year without your period. Many of the annoying symptoms assigned to menopause actually are much worse prior to menopause in the phase known as *perimenopause.* During perimenopause, you get both the annoying symptoms (hot flashes, irritability, mood swings, and so on) and your period. Lucky you.

In this section, we clarify what's happening to your body during the various stages of menopause and tell you how to recognize where you are in the great transition.

## Previewing perimenopause

For many women, perimenopause is a big case of déjà vu. Remember puberty (vaguely)? Remember the crying jags, the mood swings, and the "what's wrong with my skin!" traumas? Well, guess what? They're b-a-a-a-ck. Once again your hormones are ready to wreak havoc on your body, your emotions, and your mental faculties. This time around, however, you're a bit wiser (you bought this book, didn't you?), you have experience dealing with change, and you realize that this too shall pass.

Some doctors advise women who are still experiencing periods not to worry about "menopausal" symptoms. But you know (because you read it here) that the symptoms folks often attribute to menopause are usually felt as intensely or more intensely during perimenopause. And perimenopause can last for ten years before a woman stops menstruating altogether and becomes truly menopausal.

Your mileage may vary! We've seen lists that contain dozens of perimenopausal symptoms. Some women breeze through menopause, others have a tougher time. Don't assume that just because your mother, your sister, your best girl-friend, or the new gal on the Internet menopause message board you've been surfing describes a severe or unusual symptom that you will experience it, too.

### *Experiencing periodic periods*

During perimenopause, things change. If you welcomed your period on the same day as the full moon for 20 years, you may wake up to find the planets suddenly out of alignment.

The hormonal shift is due to changes happening in your ovaries. Your ovaries hold little *oocytes* (seeds), and each month, some of these seeds develop into *follicles* (little sacs that hold an egg). One or two lucky follicles mature and release an egg. That's when you ovulate. The oocytes in your ovaries are held together by a substance called *stroma.* The stroma produces testosterone, and the follicles produce estrogen. When you're very young, you have hundreds of thousands of these little seeds. As you age, you have fewer seeds and more stroma. As the mix of seeds and stroma in your ovaries changes, so does hormone production. Your ovaries decrease their production of estrogen but continue to produce testosterone.

Sometimes you ovulate during your cycle; sometimes you don't. Sometimes the FSH just doesn't get the follicles producing estrogen right off the bat. Estrogen levels are low at the beginning of your cycle when they should be high. Your brain responds to this lack of get-up-and-go by sending another surge of FSH (see the "Linking your brain and body" section earlier in this chapter). Finally getting the message, your ovaries become a little frantic and go into double-time production of estrogen. Right at the time when you should be ovulating and producing progesterone, your ovaries are just kicking into gear developing a follicle. That means you won't ovulate when you usually do and your period will be late.

Your menstrual cycle is all messed up. Your estrogen shoots up, and then it drops down. You get hot flashes and maybe even heart palpitations (a racing heart) when estrogen plunges. But just when you're convinced that something is seriously wrong and you need to schedule a doctor's appointment, you get your period and everything returns to normal. You wonder why you were so worried and cancel the appointment (if you made one) until the next weird thing happens.

This is all perfectly fine (maybe not with you, but with Mother Nature) — it's all part of perimenopause.

### Getting emotional

For some women, it's not the disrupted sleep, hot flashes, or palpitations that get their attention — it's the mood swings. And thank goodness for loved ones who are right there to let us know just how irritable and unpleasant we've been. Welcome to perimenopause.

### Managing mental miscues

You're already familiar with the roles hormones play in your mental agility and emotional stability because you've dealt with menstrual cycles and, in some cases, pregnancy. When estrogen levels drop and progesterone levels rise before your period, you might get those annoying PMS symptoms such as fuzzy thinking, mood swings, fatigue, and restless sleep.

As hormone levels jump around during perimenopause, these bothersome symptoms may become more commonplace. Estrogen plays a role in managing a number of brain operations, and when estrogen levels take a dive during perimenopause, it's like guiding a boat that periodically loses its rudder. Here are some of the mental functions that estrogen helps manage (and some of the symptoms you may experience when estrogen takes a dive):

- ✔ Serotonin production. (*Serotonin* regulates sleep, pain, libido, mood, and other mental functions. Less estrogen can mean problems in all these areas.)

- ✔ Body-temperature control. (You experience hot flashes and night sweats.)

- ✔ Pain threshold. (You're more sensitive or intolerant to pain.)

- ✔ Attention, mental focus, and concentration abilities. (You have mental lapses.)

- ✔ Communication between nerve cells related to memory. (You become forgetful.)

Your perimenopause may be longer or shorter than those of your friends. The average length of perimenopause — from the start of symptoms until the one-year anniversary of your last period — is about four years. But it's not abnormal for perimenopause to last only a couple of years, or for as many as ten or more years.

## Meeting menopause

The onset of menopause, by definition, takes place a year after your last period. Very few medical conditions use an anniversary date as a basis for diagnosis, but lucky us, menopause is one. That's why figuring out who's in the club and who's not is so hard. After menopause, you're technically *postmenopausal* (for the rest of your life). The term *postmenopausal* hasn't really caught on in common usage (maybe because it's such a mouthful). So we generally use the term *menopause* to refer both to menopause and the postmenopausal years.

As far as your body is concerned, reaching menopause is almost a nonevent. Your ovaries have been slowing down for several years, producing lower and lower levels of estrogen and only releasing eggs sporadically. Stopping your periods is a logical outcome of all these changes.

Most of the symptoms ascribed to menopause generally begin during peri-menopause. But back-to-back (to back) years of lower estrogen-production levels can result in health issues that you don't notice until menopause proper has set in. Over time, lower levels of estrogen (estradiol in particular) contribute to osteoporosis, cardiovascular problems, and other diseases. Due to these possible complications later in life, gynecologists and internists begin measuring your height, keeping a closer eye on your cholesterol levels and blood pressure readings, and monitoring your lifestyle habits (such as exercise and diet) as you approach midlife.

Menopause is the time to review your diet, exercise routine, and unhealthy habits (smoking or excessive consumption of alcohol, for example). In your earlier life, your body was very forgiving. During menopause, it won't let you get away with unhealthy habits — you'll pay. During menopause, gaining weight is easier, and losing it is harder. And getting a good night's sleep and waking up feeling refreshed and ready to take on the day isn't as easy as it used to be. Make some healthy resolutions and stick with them so you don't wind up saying, like composer Eubie Blake said when he turned 100, "If I'd known I was going to live this long, I'd have taken better care of myself." We'll talk more about the benefits of a healthy lifestyle during and after menopause in Chapter 20.

# Seeking Out Support

One thing's for sure as you look down that menopausal rocky road — and we don't just mean the kind in your freezer, though that might come in handy from time to time. No, we mean it's time to do what women do best: gather your reinforcements and find some support.

Repeat after us: Menopause is a normal stage in a woman's life. When symptoms make you uncomfortable and seem to last for years, going through menopause can almost make us feel as if we're ill. This is when it's helpful to have friends and family members make you repeat over and over "Menopause is not a disease. Menopause is not a disease. Menopause is not a disease."

In the case of perimenopause, menopause, postmenopause — whatever you want to call it — this means three things:

- ✔ **Girlfriend power:** Find some friends to rely on, women who have already been there, done that, and bought the perspiration-wicking t-shirt. Your mom, your aunt, your sister, your best friend, or 600 strangers on an Internet message board — they're all there for you. Just remember — everyone's menopause experience is different. Take all the comfort and information your fellow gals can offer, but also take everything you hear with a tiny (or not so tiny) grain of salt. If someone tells you they're fatigued, it's appropriate to sympathize and wonder whether that's what you've been feeling. If you hear that someone is so tired they spend most of their days in bed, feel free to suspect there might be something else going on in their life. In which case it's time to turn to.

- ✔ **A supportive partner:** You know the old saying, "If Mama ain't happy, ain't *nobody* happy!" It's the same with menopause. Just because your true love isn't sweating bullets in the middle of the night, or changing moods as quickly as the local weather guy changes the forecast, doesn't mean that your sweet baboo isn't affected by what you're going through. Family dynamics are like that: What one person experiences affects everyone. If you're single, you probably still have someone who plays this role for you — someone who's got your back when you're facing a deadline at work, your last good blouse is at the cleaners, and your hormones are raging. It's true what they say: We all need someone to lean on.

- ✔ **Medical expertise:** By this point in your adult life you probably know how you feel about your healthcare provider — general practitioner, internist, gynecologist, nurse-midwife, or alternative medicine practitioner. You might love one of these and look forward to seeing the others with the joy normally reserved for a root canal appointment. Or you may have established a great relationship with one or two medical practitioners whom you trust and respect. This is a good time to take stock: Do you trust the person who takes care of you? Do you see eye to eye on the approach you want to take when the time comes to consider whether to use hormone replacement therapy or alternative (sometimes called complementary) treatments or a balance of the two? Or is it time to find someone new you can turn to for information and support (and to tell you at 11 o'clock at night that you're probably not having a heart attack, but you can come in anyway if you'd feel better)?

The point is clear. You don't live in a vacuum, and neither should you go through menopause in one. There are people and resources out there to help you. And we're here to be one of those.

# Chapter 3

# Fooling Mother Nature:
# Early Menopause

*T*hough it's not something you think about a lot, you probably expected all along to go through menopause sooner or later. Mostly later. But if you're one of the roughly 25 percent of women who experience early menopause because of surgery or some other health factors, you're now facing a whole new game plan. You may be one of a significant number who find themselves experiencing menopause way too early, often without much warning. You find that the bookstore shelves aren't exactly sagging under the weight of books on early menopause, and that your own physician may not even recognize the symptoms for what they truly are.

Early menopause isn't just regular menopause with bad timing. If you're already in early menopause, we don't have to tell you that it's far more complicated than menopause arrived at the old fashioned way — by aging. And if you're facing this possibility now, the best thing you can do to protect your health and your lifestyle is to educate yourself (and your friends, and your family, and your doctor).

Which (blush) is why we're here for you. We're here so you can figure out what's going on. And why. And what to do about it. In this chapter, we discuss some different ways in which menopause can sneak up on you and shout "Boo!" before you are even remotely ready for it. While your girlfriends are still stocking up on tampons and asking, "Is it hot in here, or was that my first hot flash?" you're looking menopause in the face. We'll help you here with an introduction to menopause — the early edition.

# Understanding the Lingo

As if one kind of menopause isn't enough to go around, there are actually several kinds, each with its own designation. And even though each one leads to more or less the same outcome (the end of menstruation and fertility), there are differences among them that will color your experience.

Here's the obligatory "your mileage may vary" notice. Every case is different. One woman might breeze through chemotherapy and still be fertile, while a woman with a similar diagnosis experiences ovarian failure after such treatments. Keep in mind that no two people or sets of circumstances are exactly alike, so no two outcomes will be the same. So many variables are involved: your personal health history, your genes and your family's health history, your age, body type, general level of health and fitness, environmental circumstances, lifestyle, and, of course, the nature, history, and extent of your medical problem.

## Induced menopause

Induced menopause occurs when your periods end because of some kind of intervention that removes or damages your ovaries. In many cases this is the result of surgery (surgical menopause), but radiation therapy, chemotherapy, and some medications can also cause your ovaries to quit functioning (medical menopause).

### Surgical menopause

Most cases of surgically induced menopause result from either the removal of both ovaries (oophorectomy) or from a hysterectomy (surgical removal of the uterus) that includes removal of the ovaries or results in the cutting off of the blood supply to the ovaries. After your ovaries are removed, you are immediately in menopause.

If you have just one healthy ovary, you can continue to produce estrogen and stave off menopause, at least for a while. Women who have had a hysterectomy but whose ovaries remain intact tend to go through natural menopause a few years earlier than they might have otherwise.

You can enter surgical menopause in a number of ways. Hysterectomy is the most typical cause of surgical menopause. Oophorectomy (ovary removal) may also be performed along with an elective hysterectomy in the case of conditions that are not necessarily life-threatening but that have not responded to any other medical treatments.

Fewer hysterectomies are performed these days for non-life threatening conditions than was the case in even the recent past. Certainly this surgery is an appropriate option under some circumstances. It is, however, an irreversible option with long-term consequences. Don't assume that the first suggestion that you have a hysterectomy is the right decision for you. Get a second (and a third and a fourth) opinion. Be sure to weigh in the potential for early menopause when weighing up the costs and benefits of this procedure when it is genuinely an elective choice.

Don't be afraid of offending your doctor by asking for a second opinion. If your doctor is truly looking out for your best interests, he or she should applaud you for investigating all your options before having major surgery.

Some surgeries intended to treat non-reproductive health conditions may also result in surgical menopause. Surgical treatment of colon cancer, for example, may involve removal of the uterus and ovaries. The ovaries may also be removed to treat disorders driven by or made worse in the presence of plentiful estrogen. These might include breast cancer or endometriosis.

### Medical menopause

Medical procedures and treatments beyond those requiring surgery can also put you into menopause. These can include radiation therapy, chemotherapy, and certain medications.

The fact that radiation and chemotherapy have been associated with medical menopause in many cases doesn't *necessarily* mean this will be true in your case. Understand the risks and possible outcomes, but don't give up hope too soon. Every case is different.

Surgical removal of ovaries results in an immediate end to fertility. In cases in which ovarian functioning has been damaged by medications or radiation, fertility may decline more slowly and unpredictably. Be sure to talk with your healthcare provider about the best way to protect against unplanned pregnancy during this transitional time.

# Premature ovarian failure

Premature ovarian failure (POF) can occur at almost any age prior to the time at which menopause would be considered natural. Finding out that you are in menopause in your 30s, even in your 20s, can be devastating, particularly because it means the end of your fertility.

POF not caused by one of the diseases or conditions described below affects about one out of 100 women. Sometimes the cause of premature menopause is never found, but it can be linked to a variety of conditions, among them:

✔ Immune system disorders

✔ Severe anorexia

✔ Genetic disorders

✔ Polycystic ovarian syndrome (PCOS)

✔ Chronic, severe physical stress, such as that sometimes experienced by professional athletes or those with exercise anorexia

✔ Nutritional deficits

✔ Pituitary tumors

Because POF can occur so much earlier than you would expect to start identifying perimenopausal symptoms, those first hot flashes and skipped periods might not make you jump up and say, "Aha! This could be menopause!" Trouble is, it might not make your doctor say this, either. Although POF is rarely reversible, there are cases in which an early diagnosis and treatment of the underlying problem could mean the salvation of your ovaries — derailing that menopause train that's pulled out of the station way ahead of schedule. If you even suspect that what you're experiencing sounds similar to menopause, bring this concern to the attention of your healthcare provider, and do whatever gentle prodding (or jumping up and down) it takes to get the blood tests that could point you to a correct — and well-timed — diagnosis.

# Coping with Sudden Change

After you pull the plug on estrogen production — either in one big whoosh or one prolonged trickle — unless you begin taking HT, your body is going to be subject to the same changes (see Chapter 4) and risks (see Chapters 11 through 14) that you'd experience in natural menopause. The biggest difference is in the timing: when it occurs, and how fast it happens. The younger you are when you experience early menopause, the greater the number of years you will have to cope with the consequences. Making decisions about your health and whether to take replacement HT early on, as well as continued monitoring of your hormone levels (see the next section "Knowing when you hit menopause"), are crucial.

## Knowing when you hit menopause

We define menopause as reaching the one-year anniversary of your last period. But if your uterus is gone, you can't have a period. How do you know when you clear that hurdle? The only way to know is by keeping an eye on your other symptoms — restless sleep, hot flashes, heart palpitations —

the whole nine yards. If you experience the classic perimenopausal symptoms, you're probably entering perimenopause and your hormones are dipping and cresting like waves in a storm. You're probably menopausal when your symptoms settle down and the seas are calmer. If you're not sure, ask your physician for a hormone test that can tell you what your menopause status is.

Women who have had hysterectomies but who still have one or both ovaries often go through menopause one to three years earlier than women who haven't.

## Getting the help you need for your body and mind

Estradiol (or E2), which your ovaries produce, is like a magic serum for your body. In addition to promoting breast development, bringing on your menstrual cycles, and helping you get (and stay) pregnant, estradiol has lots of other roles to play in promoting and protecting your health. It keeps your tissues (inside and out) moist and supple, helps you to grow strong bones (and you thought it was just the Wonder Bread), promotes normal sexual development, and plays many other roles throughout your body.

If the source (that is, your ovaries) of this wonderful stuff dries up — regardless of whether the cause is surgical, pharmaceutical, genetic, or something altogether different — then you may not even have achieved your peak health and strength by the time your hormones disappear. Not having had the full benefit of your hormones to start with can make it doubly hard to keep your whole body in its best working order when menopause begins to make demands on your bones, your sexual health, and your overall well-being.

Women in induced or premature menopause who are not taking hormone therapy are faced almost immediately with increased risk of a number of health problems. All these are associated with loss of estrogen, so hormone therapy does alleviate these risks. (We say more about these risks in Chapters 11 through 14.) Your caregiver can help you to cope with these sudden changes by working with you to find a medical regimen that minimizes menopausal symptoms while maximizing your overall health outlook.

Even if children (or more children) weren't officially in your plans, losing your ability to conceive can be a shaker (for you and the people who care about you). Losing your *options* can be difficult, too. Seeing your periods come and go every month can also be a marker, a healthy part of your functioning. It's okay to grieve this loss (and to get help in doing so), even if you are still figuring out what it means for you. Recognize your feelings and talk with a counselor or therapist about what's happening to you.

# Prepping for Surgical Menopause

If your physician anticipates that your ovaries will both be removed or damaged during your surgery, she knows that you'll wake up in an uncomfortable state of hormone depletion. To help you make a slightly smoother transition to this new state of affairs, she may start you on hormone supplements prior to your surgery (if she's not sure about what she'll find during surgery, she may want to wait and start HT after your operation). Although every situation is different and most are more complex than this, the type of hormone therapy you are given depends largely — to put it bluntly — on what had to be removed during your surgery. If you still have a uterus, you will most likely be given combination hormone therapy (HT) with estrogen and progesterone balanced just for you to prevent cancer. If you've had a hysterectomy, then you will be given estrogen therapy (ET) because it can replace your missing estrogen with no increased risk of uterine cancer (the uterus now being gone, remember).

A hysterectomy with your ovaries left in place technically shouldn't slow down the ovaries' production of hormones. You should go through natural menopause (though perhaps a little sooner) if your ovaries are still intact and producing hormones.

While you are preparing for the hysterectomy you will have lots of questions for your surgeon and your general practitioner, internist, or gynecologist. Before surgery is a good time to talk about what to expect in the way of hormone-related effects, both immediately after surgery and in the long run. Because this is a very stressful time, especially if you only found out recently that you have a condition that requires surgery, you may find yourself a little rattled. Right near the list of the top 10 things that make you forgetful is having your doctor look up and say brightly, "Do you have any questions?" This is the universal signal for forgetting everything you wanted to ask, which is why it's a good idea to keep a running list. No question is too small — or too large — to tackle. Questions to ask about menopause-related outcomes of your surgery might include:

- ✔ How likely is it that my ovaries will still be functional after my uterus is removed? How great a risk is there that the ovaries will have to be removed, too?

- ✔ If my ovaries are removed or damaged, how will that change how I feel after the surgery? What sorts of symptoms might I experience? How soon will these begin?

- ✔ What kinds of decisions will I need to make about hormone therapy following the surgery?

✔ Do you recommend that I begin any hormone therapy *before* my surgery?

✔ I have concerns about some of the risks I've heard about from women taking hormone therapy. How do these apply in my case?

If your surgery is to treat a severe or life-threatening illness, don't let anyone make you feel that you're being petty or trivial worrying about menopause when all you "should" be worrying about is beating your breast cancer or curing that chronic infection. Certainly you will have questions about both the reasons for the surgery and the possible outcomes — that's entirely normal. But if your doctor says, "We can talk about all that after your surgery," be persistent. She may not be able to give you all the answers you need yet, but it's entirely justifiable to want — and get — some sense of what you may be facing after the surgery.

# Taking Advantage of Assisted Living

No, no, we don't mean the kind your Great Aunt Natalie lives in, with the hot meals and the Bingo games on Saturdays. But under your new circumstances your doctor will most likely suggest very strongly that you go — and soon — on some form of hormone therapy. Hormones got you into this strange new place, by leaving you — literally — in the lurch. And hormones —administered with care and patience — can get you out again, or at least play an important role as you try to get a grip on the changes in your body and your mind that accompany induced or premature menopause.

As with natural menopause, whether you decide to take hormone replacement therapy is entirely your call. The difference that you need to factor in as you make this decision is all about the timing. Many women experiencing natural menopause take hormones for just a few years, until they are over the most bothersome of their menopausal symptoms. You will need to rely on hormone therapy indefinitely to ward off the effects of menopause until you reach the time at which you and your doctor feel you'd be postmenopausal even by natural menopause standards. At that point, you can work together to decide whether remaining on hormones is in your best interest, or whether it's time to wean you off of them.

## Estrogen alone

If you have had your uterus removed, you no longer need to fear that taking estrogen will contribute to uterine cancer. This means you can control your menopausal symptoms and reap the benefits of replacement estrogen as it wards off the health risks described above.

The especially good news for you (you knew there had to be some good news *somewhere*, right?) is that new findings coming out of the 15-year-long Women's Health Initiative Study says that for women *who have had a hysterectomy and who are between the ages of 50 and 59,* and *only* for this group, estrogen therapy not only doesn't damage the heart, but it can actually protect you from heart disease.

## Combination therapy

With progesterone (and perhaps testosterone) added to the recipe to help balance the risks of uterine cancer, women who have had their ovaries removed but who still have an intact uterus can minimize their risk of other menopausal health problems.

It's important to note that, especially with combination therapy, one size definitely does not fit all. What worked for your mother may not work for you. The balance of hormones that puts your best friend in the pink may leave you feeling bluer than blue. Be patient as your physician works with you to find the right balance — and the right dosage — of therapeutic hormones.

You may also hear a lot about the synthetic hormone DHEA if you surf the Internet or cruise the shelves of your local natural foods store. To listen to the manufacturer's claims, you'd think that DHEA is the ultimate wonder drug, replacing or supplementing your body's natural hormones to cure what ails you. Be very careful, though. Although there have been many claims about its symptom-relieving, vitality-giving qualities, no long-term studies have proven DHEA to be either effective or safe. Some of its known side effects (deepening of the voice, thickening of the skin, facial hair growth, and headaches) are as troublesome as the symptoms you're trying to free yourself from. If you're interested in learning more about this steroid hormone, ask your physician before you try it on your own.

If you *do* decide to use DHEA by itself or in combination with other forms of HT, do not use or suddenly discontinue its use without the supervision of a physician.

Got a uterus? Your hormone therapy will probably be a balanced mix of the hormones normally produced by the ovaries: estrogen and progesterone, or even estrogen, progesterone, and a bit of testosterone. If you've had a hysterectomy (no uterus), you can take estrogen-alone therapy (ET).

## And your grandmother on your mother's side?

If you experience induced or premature menopause at very nearly the age at which you would have expected to start natural menopause, you may have more leeway when it comes to deciding whether to take hormones. Here are some things you need to consider when making this decision:

✔ Your age and general health

✔ Any family history of DVT (deep vein thrombosis), pulmonary embolism (blood clots that have traveled to your lungs), or other blood clots; any family history of stroke

(hormone therapy can increase the risk of these)

✔ Any family history of breast cancer (estrogen therapy can promote the growth of breast cancer cells)

✔ Whether you smoke (hormones and smoking are a time bomb combination, greatly increasing the risk of other dangers, such as that of stroke or blood clots)

✔ Any family history of osteoporosis, which hormone therapy would help to prevent

## *Alternatives to HT*

Certainly if you are still wary of hormone therapy, there are practical, situational remedies you can try. Some women find relief in simple approaches to symptom control:

✔ **Find fixes for your hot flashes.** Sleep in a cool room with a window partly open, even in cold weather. Keep a pitcher of cool water on your nightstand, and sleep on 100 percent cotton sheets. If you find that alcohol or spicy foods contribute to your hot flashes, avoid them.

✔ **Get a good night's sleep.** Make your bedroom a calming place and don't use it for work or exercise. Get plenty of exercise every day, but not within an hour or two of bedtime. A warm, caffeine-free drink before bed — warm milk, herbal tea, or hot lemonade — can help you relax. If you wake up for long periods during the night, get up and read quietly, or engage in a simple activity such as knitting or reading so that you don't come to associate your bed with sleeplessness.

✔ **Calm your moods.** Practice meditation or yoga and breathing exercises every day.

✔ **Take good care of yourself.** Get plenty of rest, maintain a healthy weight, and don't smoke.

✔ **Protect your bones.** Do some weight-bearing exercise at least five days a week. Smoking also compromises bone health — if you smoke, stop.

Ask your physician for recommendations for herbal remedies to fight hot flashes and insomnia if you want to. Bear in mind, though, that few herbal preparations are regulated in the United States, so you may be getting more or less than the label indicates, and the product may not be as clean or free from additives as you'd like to think. Remember, too, that herbs aren't necessarily any safer, or any more effective, than pharmaceutical hormones. Keep an open mind, but make sure your health and safety are your first concern, whether you rely on traditional medicines, alternative products, or a combination that balances the best of both.

# Finding Support: Birds of a Feather

Taking care of yourself and getting support from people who understand your situation is especially important for women experiencing early menopause. Your issues, in many cases, are different from those of women who go through natural menopause at the expected time in their lives and you may need to go a little further out of your way than to the next cubicle at the office or your best friends to find women who know what you're going through.

People who don't "get" premature menopause are usually people who just haven't been educated yet. Try to keep this in mind when people ask you questions about your situation or assume they know what you're going through (when they don't). Even people who care a great deal about you may say things to you that cause you pain or distress.

Ask your healthcare provider whether she knows of a support group in your area for women with early menopause. Or find a supportive message board online (feel free to lurk a while, or read the boards without becoming a member) until you find one that seems to offer genuine help and accurate information.

And don't forget that the answers to your questions may be found in the upcoming chapters in this book. Although your situation may be different from that of most women, in many ways you are all going through the same things, even if you're on different timetables.

As you're making decisions about hormone therapy and your continuing care, try to find at least one woman to speak with who went into early menopause years ago. Get the benefit of her hindsight by asking whether she is happy with the decisions she made, and whether — given ongoing advances in our understanding of hormone therapy — she thinks she would make the same decisions today. Are there things she wishes she had done differently? What things were relatively easy to handle, and what were some that were the most difficult? What surprised her the most? Did she find any unexpected silver linings in this cloud?

# Chapter 4

# Getting In Sync with the Symptoms

. . . . . . . . . . . . . . . . . . . . . . . . . . . . . . . . . . . . . . . . . . . . . . . . . . . . . . . . . . .

*In This Chapter*

▶ Getting in touch with the changes before the change

▶ Discovering the physical and emotional effects of menopause

▶ Talking to your doctor

. . . . . . . . . . . . . . . . . . . . . . . . . . . . . . . . . . . . . . . . . . . . . . . . . . . . . . . . . . .

**Y**ou're irritable for no reason, you have trouble sleeping, you experience heart palpitations, and you're sure somebody keeps sneaking the thermostat up when you're not looking. Sound familiar? If so, you're almost certainly starting down the road to menopause.

Every human body is unique — that's no surprise. But the path to menopause reveals just how different we really are. Some women breeze through the change, experiencing very few physical discomforts or emotional upsets. Other women experience a whole menu of disturbing symptoms for a number of years. Fortunately, for most women the symptoms often pass as you move into menopause and beyond.

In this chapter, we provide an introduction to the perimenopausal and menopausal symptoms you may experience. We go into much greater detail concerning the biology of menopause and how to alleviate these symptoms in other chapters of this book (especially in Chapters 5 through 10).

The symptoms we discuss in this chapter are all symptoms of perimenopause or menopause, but they're not unique to just perimenopause or menopause. Other medical conditions — or even normal variations — cause these symptoms as well. If you experience any symptoms that worry you, though, don't just assume that they're a result of perimenopause or menopause. Your doctor will help you rule out any more serious causes.

# Kicking Things Off with Perimenopausal Symptoms

In this section we give you the laundry list of symptoms that have been attributed to the sudden drops of estrogen during perimenopause. Individual women experience none, a few, or quite a few of these symptoms. If you think we sound a little vague about what perimenopausal symptoms are like, we're guilty as charged, but we have to hedge our bets because everyone's experience with menopause is unique.

In fact, many women in the United States report experiencing no perimenopausal symptoms at all. For women who do experience symptoms, the symptoms can range in severity from being somewhat annoying to interfering with their ability to enjoy life.

## Getting physical

If you do have physical symptoms as you enter and go through perimenopause and menopause, though, you may find them hard to ignore. They're just, well, different. People often compare reaching menopause with hitting puberty, but approaching adolescence didn't bring on hot flashes, hair loss, insomnia, or heart palpitations.

Many of the physical symptoms are the result of a string of events that are set in motion when *estradiol* (the active form of estrogen — the "good" stuff) levels suddenly drop — a typical occurrence during perimenopause. The drop causes a chain reaction within your body, which we describe in the "Revealing the biology behind the symptoms" sidebar later in this chapter.

The relationship between estrogen and serotonin plays a role in many of the mental symptoms, but it also has a hand in some of the physical symptoms — such as interrupted sleep. *Serotonin* is a compound that helps the body regulate sleep and moods. Though all the details aren't in, estrogen plays some kind of role in the production and maintenance of serotonin. It's amazing how all this stuff gets connected, huh?

### Turning up the heat

*Hot flashes* (also called hot flushes) are the traditional, highly recognized symptom of menopause — 85 percent of women have them at least a time or two as they enter perimenopause, and 10 to 15 percent of women report having them often enough or severely enough to seek medical treatment. When you have a hot flash, you suddenly feel intensely warm and very flushed — especially in your face and upper body. Increased perspiration — anything from a moist upper lip to enough sweat to leave your clothes or bedsheets uncomfortably wet — usually accompanies this feeling of warmth. And sometimes, dizziness, heart palpitations, and a suffocating feeling can precede or accompany hot flashes. As many comediennes have said, it feels as though your inner child is playing with matches.

A sudden drop in estrogen levels triggers a hot flash. This drop in estrogen sends a message to your brain that something is terribly wrong, so your brain sends out a power burst of adrenaline (norepinephrine). *Norepinephrine* is the hormone that triggers the fight-or-flight response in humans, so your body moves into ready mode, which gets your blood pressure up and your heart pounding and also causes the blood vessels in your head, neck, and chest to dilate. All this commotion brings on that sweltering feeling.

Until 1970, doctors didn't acknowledge hot flashes as a real physical phenomenon; they attributed the sensation to a woman's imagination or to a psychological problem. In fact, though, the effect of hot flashes is real and measurable — ask anyone who's ever slept next to a woman when her internal thermostat goes haywire. The temperature of your skin may go up as much as six degrees, as if you had a fever. The symptom is only temporary, though, typically lasting no more than 10 minutes or so. Hot flashes aren't dangerous, but the first time or two that you have one, it can be mighty scary unless you've been warned to expect them.

### Sweating your lack of sleep

*Night sweats* are essentially hot flashes that occur at night. The same estrogen drop that triggers hot flashes during the day triggers night sweats.

Night sweats can also be caused by infection, thyroid problems, or other types of illness, so if this is the only seemingly perimenopausal symptom you experience, check with your doctor.

### Losing your snoozing time

With all the weird symptoms going on during the day, getting a good night's sleep so you can wake up feeling rested doesn't seem like a lot to ask for, but lack of sleep during this period can be a real problem. Hot flashes in the middle of the night often result in interrupted sleep. You wake up, often perspiring (and sometimes cursing), with damp bedsheets and skin that may end up being itchy as you cool off and all that sweat dries, and have a hard time going back to sleep. If your sleep is often interrupted this way, you can build up quite a sleep deficit, which in turn leads to irritability, anxiety, and mood swings.

Serotonin is a neurotransmitter that's found throughout your body, especially in your brain. A neurotransmitter is a chemical that sends messages from one nerve cell to another. There's still a lot we don't know about serotonin and its functions, but it's clear that it can act to affect our muscles, nerves, and moods.

A rapid drop in estrogen also affects your serotonin levels. Serotonin helps regulate mood and sleep patterns. (Drugs such as Prozac and Zoloft work on the principle that serotonin regulation is key to relieving mood swings, irritability, and so on.) Estrogen makes serotonin more available by prolonging its action. When estrogen drops, it affects your serotonin levels, which contributes to interrupted sleep.

### Getting to the heart of the palpitation issue

Butterflies in your stomach often accompany rapid heartbeats, or *palpitations*. The sudden drops in estrogen that are so common during perimenopause cause reactions all over your body (see the "Revealing the biology behind the symptoms" sidebar later in this chapter), including heart flutters. The drop in estrogen causes your body's natural painkillers and mood regulators (*endorphins*) to drop. Your body interprets this state of affairs as trouble, so a command is issued to send out a burst of adrenaline (norepinephrine, the fight-or-flight hormone). Your body is responding as though you had just encountered a big grizzly bear. The only trouble is you don't see the grizzly bear, and you're left wondering why your body suddenly decided to get ready to flee from it just when you sat down to a nice candle-lit dinner.

### Expecting menstrual irregularities

The approach to menopause can be blamed for a number of menstrual changes. But remember that you can't blame all irregularities on perimenopause. Consult your healthcare provider about the following irregularities and all other symptoms before simply writing them off to perimenopause:

- **Irregular periods** are quite common in perimenopausal women because fluctuating hormone levels can interrupt the ovulation cycle. Some months you ovulate; some months you don't. If you don't ovulate, you don't produce enough progesterone to have a period, so the lining of your uterus builds up.

- **Heavy bleeding** during perimenopause is usually caused by an "eggless" cycle. You make estrogen during the first part of your cycle, but for some reason (often unknown), you just don't ovulate. Therefore, you don't produce progesterone, and you develop an unusually thick uterine lining, which you shed during your period. This process translates into abnormally heavy bleeding.

- **Bad timing** has probably struck every woman at one point or another. We just don't want you to think that perimenopause is going to make dealing with your periods easier. As long as you still have periods, they're liable to show up at inconvenient times (which can help make getting rid of them not sound like a bad thing at all).

# Revealing the biology behind the symptoms

As you may have suspected, the symptoms of menopause are all tied to plunging hormone levels. You may feel these symptoms more frequently during perimenopause than menopause itself because your hormone levels fluctuate more during perimenopause. Sometimes they rise to fairly normal levels, and then they come crashing down. The *fluctuation* is the trigger for a lot of the symptoms. In menopause, hormone levels are consistently lower than they are during your reproductive years, so they don't pop up and drop down so frequently, though symptoms can still occur.

Here's a step-by-step guide of what happens to your body when your estradiol (the active form of estrogen) levels drop:

1. Your ovaries produce lower levels of estradiol, which causes a drop in the amount of estradiol reaching the brain.

2. Less estradiol in the brain causes a decrease in your endorphin levels. *Endorphins* are your body's natural painkillers and mood regulators. (If you're a runner, you're probably familiar with the effects of endorphins — they cause the "runner's high.")

3. Lower levels of endorphins in your brain cause it to think that something is terribly wrong, so it sends out a burst of adrenaline, namely *norepinephrine* (the hormone that triggers the fight-or-flight response).

4. The burst of norepinephrine causes your body to kick into ready-for-anything mode by increasing your heart rate (which causes those palpitations and flutters), raising your blood pressure, and dilating your blood vessels. Dilating blood vessels cause the hot flashes and sweating. If you're asleep, you may wake up suddenly. You may also experience diarrhea or get a feeling of anxiety and butterflies in your stomach.

**WARNING!**

If you have unusual bleeding in-between your cycles though, you should consult your doctor. This may be a sign of abnormal cells developing in the lining of your uterus that should not be ignored.

## Handling the headaches

For women who experience migraine headaches immediately before or during the first few days of their periods, we have some bad news — you may have more headaches during perimenopause. Headaches during the first few days of your period mean that you're sensitive to low estrogen levels, which are typical at that time. When estrogen levels drop quickly, which happens during perimenopause, the drop may trigger another one of those headaches. Just as your estrogen level has become unpredictable, so might your headaches. Just as you're congratulating yourself for being headache-free in June, July might bring on a doozy.

### Facing the fibroid factoids

*Fibroids* are simply balls of uterine muscle tissue. Nearly one-third of women have fibroids by the time they're 50. Fibroids tend to get bigger as you approach menopause, but they usually don't continue to grow in size after menopause.

You really don't need to do anything about fibroids unless they cause symptoms such as pain, pressure, or increased bleeding. As with other symptoms, talk with your doctor if you're having any problems you feel may be related to fibroids.

## Playing head games

The mental/emotional symptoms associated with perimenopause can be very frustrating given that many women don't associate their recent irritability or depression with perimenopause.

The symptoms we list generally pass when your hormones settle into their new, lower levels after menopause. However, these symptoms severely inconvenience or otherwise bother many women during perimenopause. If this description mirrors your situation, there's no need to sit there suffering in silence.

Be sure to inform your medical professional about these mental and emotional symptoms. They may be more closely related to hormonal imbalances than to psychological issues. But, either way, your healthcare professional can ensure that you get the proper treatment to alleviate your symptoms. (For more detailed information on the mental and emotional issues associated with perimenopause, check out Chapter 10.)

### Sitting on the mood swings

Mood swings are common among perimenopausal women. But remember that mood swings are also common before your period (part of premenstrual syndrome) and after pregnancy. Although medical researchers don't know all the details, low levels of estrogen are associated with lower levels of serotonin, which can lead to mood swings, in addition to irritability, anxiety, pain sensitivity, and insomnia.

### Worrying about anxiety

Anxiety is another common symptom perimenopausal women face. As with mood swings, anxiety seems to be tied to low levels of estrogen. The lower levels of endorphins and serotonin associated with low estrogen levels may trigger anxiety. Another theory is that low levels of estrogen, serotonin, and endorphins leave you more vulnerable to the emotional stressors in your world. According to this theory, lower estrogen, serotonin, and endorphin levels don't trigger anxiety; they simply limit your ability to deal successfully with stressful situations.

### Touching on irritability

The same hormonal shifts that cause mood swings and anxiety (see the previous "Sitting on the mood swings" and "Worrying about anxiety" sections) cause irritability. As with these other symptoms, marked irritability is a temporary condition that seems to blow over after you're officially menopausal (if you can put up with yourself for that long).

### Recalling memory malfunctions

Memory problems during perimenopause sneak up on you. You forget your friend's name one day; you leave your keys somewhere in the grocery store another day. Pretty soon you start remembering how many times you couldn't remember something. We're not talking about dementia or Alzheimer's disease here; we're talking about forgetfulness and a lack of focus. This category covers relatively minor memory glitches: You forget where you're going with a thought in mid-sentence, or you get to the store and forget what you need to buy. Thank goodness for sticky notes and grocery lists.

Estrogen seems to facilitate communication among *neurons* (nerve cells) in the brain. Much of memory is a matter of the brain sending information from one memory storage center to another. Because estrogen helps maintain connections and grow new ones, shifting estrogen levels can stymie communication between memory storage areas. Memory problems seem to be a short-term issue; some women seem to lose the memory lapses after menopause.

Indications from later stages of the Women's Health Initiative seem to be that *for women 65 and older only,* hormone therapy is associated with an *increase* in the risk for dementia and overall cognitive functioning. Because this is the opposite of what researchers in this large, 15-year study predicted they'd find, follow-up studies of the relationship between hormone therapy and a decline in cognitive functioning are continuing. There's no official word yet on the effects of hormone therapy in younger women on dementia, cognitive functioning, or memory.

Even though the Women's Health Initiative Study reported a statistically significant increase in the risk of dementia among women between 65 and 79 who were using either combination (estrogen plus progestin) hormone therapy, the overall risk of Alzheimer's in the United States is still extremely low.

### Thinking through a haze

Fuzzy thinking is common when you're deprived of sleep or your hormones are in flux. When we say *fuzzy thinking,* we mean the feeling that you're just not with it today — as though you're walking through a fog or you just can't concentrate on what you're doing. Fuzzy thinking can be the result of interrupted sleep (which is extremely common during perimenopause).

Fluctuating hormone levels also cause fuzzy thinking (as you may have experienced during pregnancy or at certain points in your menstrual cycle). Fuzzy thinking is a temporary thing. It generally clears up when your hormones settle down and your sleep patterns chill out during menopause. Experiencing little brain farts now and then doesn't mean that you're on the slippery slope to premature senility — this will pass.

# Visiting the Menopausal Symptoms

All the symptoms we describe as *perimenopausal* have long been attributed to menopause. But after you're menopausal (without a menstrual period for a year), things begin to settle down a bit. Hot flashes subside and your moods stabilize. Your body and psyche seem to get used to some aspects of lower estrogen production. A small percentage of women may continue to experience menopausal symptoms for years after their periods end.

The symptoms experienced after menopause may even be a bit more uncomfortable physically. If this describes you, don't just suffer — work with your physician to help you find a hormonal or non-hormonal treatment to keep you comfortable.

Long periods of low levels of estrogen encourage conditions such as osteoporosis, cardiovascular disease, heart attack, stroke, colon cancer, and other diseases discussed in Chapters 5 and 6 of this book.

To avoid wordiness, we use the term *menopause* in this chapter (and most others) to refer to the time period that incorporates both menopause and postmenopause.

## Figuring out the physical facts

After you officially reach menopause (after 12 full months without a menstrual period), you produce lower levels of estrogen without the sudden spikes and drops typical of perimenopause. Your hormones calm down — way down. As time goes by, these long periods of low estrogen levels result in some physical changes.

In this section, we discuss what these conditions feel like. We go into greater detail about the biology behind these conditions and how to alleviate the symptoms in other chapters of this book. (Chapter 7 deals with vaginal and urinary issues; Chapter 8 covers your skin and hair during menopause.)

Some of the symptoms are the result of lower levels of estrogen, pure and simple. We call these primary symptoms. Some of these primary symptoms can actually cause further unpleasantness, which we call secondary symptoms.

### *Looking first at the primary symptoms*

The primary symptoms include

- ✔ **Vaginal dryness:** The medical establishment refers to this condition as *vaginal atrophy.* Because estrogen keeps vaginal tissues moisturized and pliant, continuous periods of low estrogen can result in the drying out and shrinking of vaginal tissue. Between 20 and 45 percent of women in the United States experience vaginal dryness. They often notice it when intercourse becomes painful due to a lack of lubrication.

- ✔ **Vulvar discomfort:** Itching, burning, and dryness of the vulva isn't uncommon among menopausal women. But remember that many conditions and diseases that affect the vulva have nothing to do with estrogen, so have your doctor check out any vulvar changes.

- ✔ **Urinary incontinence:** This condition is much more prevalent in women during perimenopause and menopause than it is during their earlier reproductive years. The tissues of your urinary tract become drier and thinner, and the muscles lose their tone as estrogen levels diminish. You know you're experiencing urinary incontinence if you have a hard time holding it when you laugh, exercise, or sneeze. Your urinary tract, especially your urethra, depends on estrogen to maintain its form and muscle tone. The urethra has a hard time sealing off the flow of urine after years of diminished estrogen levels.

- ✔ **Urinary frequency:** Similar to incontinence, urinary frequency results from sustained, low levels of estrogen that define menopause. Urinary frequency simply means that you have to urinate frequently. You may leave the bathroom and quickly feel as though you have to go again. This condition can be very frustrating during the day — and even more frustrating at night. Urinary frequency can also cause interrupted sleep, which understandably, turns into irritability.

- ✔ **Headaches:** Women who experience their first migraine during perimenopause often find that the migraines go away after menopause.

- ✔ **Skin changes:** Lower estrogen levels cause your skin to lose firmness and elasticity. Estrogen doesn't literally prevent sagging or wrinkles. But estrogen does keep your skin supple and help your skin retain fluid, so it remains "filled out" rather than becoming loose and droopy.

✔ **Hair changes:** Your hair becomes thinner and more brittle with menopause, though some women report that their hair feels as soft and fluffy as cotton several years into menopause. Estrogen seems to promote your body's natural moisturizers, so with lower levels of the stuff flowing through your body, your hair takes a hit and becomes more brittle and wiry. You also have a tougher time keeping a perm permanent. Some women, though, also note that their hair has more body than it used to, and find that they no longer need to shampoo every day to keep their now somewhat drier hair looking good.

✔ **Weight changes:** Your weight shifts to the center of your body — around your waist. Instead of the lovely hourglass shape you once had, you take on more of an apple-shaped appearance due to shifting hormone levels. Although you may gain a bit of weight, you probably can't directly blame that on hormonal changes. Your body simply becomes less forgiving about nutritional imbalances and poor eating, drinking, and exercise habits.

### Leading to the secondary conditions

It's not over yet. One or more of the primary symptoms can trigger even more unpleasantness. Here you go:

✔ **Painful intercourse:** Vaginal dryness and changes in the shape of the vagina can lead to discomfort or pain during intercourse. As low levels of estrogen cause your *urovaginal tissues* (tissues of the vagina and urinary tract) to become thinner and the supporting muscle to lose its tone, your organs naturally shift position a bit.

✔ **Interrupted sleep:** Hot flashes, urinary frequency, anxiety, and a variety of other menopausal symptoms can cause interrupted sleep during the night. You wake up tired and feel fatigued throughout the day because your body isn't able to enter the deep stages of sleep at night that make you feel resilient and energetic.

✔ **Fatigue:** If you consistently don't get a good restful night's sleep or you experience insomnia, you may become fatigued. But fatigue can also be the result of low testosterone levels.

## Discovering that it's more than skin deep

The mental/emotional aspects of menopause are more of a mixed bag. Some symptoms experienced during menopause usually decrease or go away completely; others are a bit more difficult to deal with.

✔ **Anxiety:** The anxiety common during perimenopause is often caused by the rapid drop in estrogen, which initiates a chain reaction (see the "Revealing the biology behind the symptoms" sidebar earlier in this chapter). After menopause, unexplained anxiety often dies down, and you return to your normal self.

✔ **Depression:** Women who have had hysterectomies are more likely to experience menopause-related depression than are women who go through a natural menopause. Researchers don't yet understand why this is the case, but it's likely that physical, mental, and cultural factors all play a part.

Also, women who have been on estrogen and suddenly quit taking it, rather than going through a weaning process, also have more problems with depression. Estrogen assists in the production of serotonin (a substance which helps regulate moods), so lower levels of estrogen can mean lower levels of serotonin.

✔ **Lower libido:** Decreased sex drive is a problem for many menopausal women, but the good news is that 70 percent of women remain sexually active during their perimenopausal and menopausal years. Lower libido can be traced to hormonal imbalances and may be the result of testosterone levels being too low. (For more information on menopause and your libido, take a look at Chapter 9.)

✔ **Memory lapses and fuzzy thinking:** Though memory lapses and fuzzy thinking are common during perimenopause, most women notice their concentration and memory return to normal after menopause. Aging can cause mental impairment later in life, but you can't blame everything on menopause! Remember, though, that recent research has found an association between continued use of hormone therapy after age 65 and a heightened (but still small) risk of dementia. If you are still using hormone therapy at this point, talk with your doctor about whether the reasons you continued hormone use to this point are still valid.

# Understanding That It's Not Your Imagination

Many people associate the word *symptom* with disease, but the definition we use throughout this book is much closer to the dictionary definition — a condition or event that accompanies something. If you're like many women, you may feel that weird things keep happening to your body or your emotions.

Maybe you feel a flutter in your chest, and you become convinced that you're on the verge of a heart attack. If you go to a cardiologist to check out heart palpitations, she probably won't even think to check your hormones because she's looking for something in your heart to answer the riddle.

Or maybe the "weird things" going on with you aren't physical at all. Maybe they're emotional — such as becoming easily frustrated at work or chewing your kids out 50 times a day for the last two weeks. Many women may think twice about these symptoms, but they don't bring them up with their doctor. If you do mention them to your doctor, she may say something such as, "It's nothing." Nothing? We know what you're thinking, "Try telling that to my co-workers and my kids."

Even gynecologists sometimes overlook a hormonal imbalance as the source of symptoms. Women may suspect that their problem is "chemical" or hor-monal only to have doctors say that they're too young for menopause or that they're still having periods, so they aren't menopausal.

Some gynecologists go so far as to give a blood test to check your FSH (follicle-stimulating hormone) level to rule out menopause. High levels of FSH are indicative of *menopause.* But during perimenopause, your hormone levels go up and down. One month your FSH may be perfectly normal; another month it may be high. Without getting tested month after month, determining whether you're *perimenopausal* is difficult.

But women's estrogen and testosterone levels can (and usually do) get out of whack even before they officially become menopausal, and the imbalance trig-gers the annoying symptoms often associated with menopause. Sometimes you can become even more frustrated after seeking medical advice because the experts tell you, "It's nothing," or they alarm you with the number and types of tests they want you to take.

The reality is that the symptoms you experience are often more intense before menopause, during perimenopause, than they are after you make the change. After you get a hot flash or two, you may figure out that these "weird things" aren't part of your imagination and that you're getting close to menopause. If you figure out the connection, consider yourself lucky. Few women realize that the heart palpitations and the irritability can be part of the same condition — perimenopause. Having read this book, you can be the local expert — it's up to you to coach other women through this!

# Part II
# The Effects of Menopause on Your Body and Mind

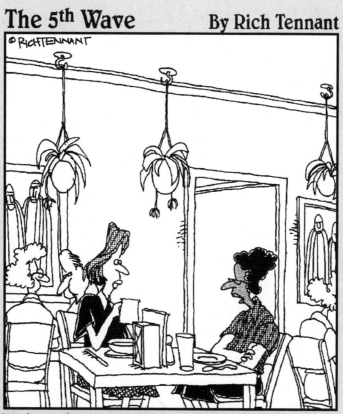

The 5th Wave     By Rich Tennant

"I think they're typical symptoms of menopause — gaining weight, feeling tired, locking your husband in the basement because he finished the double-chunk peanut butter."

## In this part . . .

Are you convinced that the goldfish is deliberately trying to aggravate you? Has your family recently taken to wearing gloves and parkas in the house in August because you insist on keeping the air-conditioning cranked all the way up? We jest because we've been there. But the years before and after menopause can bring a whole host of symptoms and conditions with them — from the simply annoying to the potentially dangerous. Don't worry: Knowledge is power! In this part, we cover the physical, mental, and emotional symptoms and conditions that women run into. We deal with your bones, cardiovascular system, female organs, skin, hair, sex life, and mental and emotional outlook. Pretty thorough, huh?

# Chapter 5

# The Business of Your Bones

. . . . . . . . . . . . . . . . . . . . . . . . . . . . . . . . . . . . . . . . . . . . . . . . . . . . . . .

## In This Chapter

▶ Understanding how bone stays healthy

▶ Recognizing estrogen's role in bone loss

▶ Understanding the medical tests that help identify osteoporosis

▶ Taking steps to protect your bones during and after menopause

▶ Discovering whether you have osteoporosis

▶ Finding out the best ways to treat osteoporosis

. . . . . . . . . . . . . . . . . . . . . . . . . . . . . . . . . . . . . . . . . . . . . . . . . . . . . . .

*M*ost of us don't want to just live through menopause, we want to dance through it and keep dancing for another 40 or 50 years. Healthy bones keep your get-up-and-go from turning into sit-down-and-wait — or worse — fall-down-and-call-for-help.

*Osteoporosis* literally means "porous bone." It's a disease in which your bones become thin and fragile and more likely to break. In fact, bones can become so fragile that they're crushed by their own weight. When the grocery clerk throws apples on top of the soft bread in your grocery bag, the bread becomes smashed and deformed from the weight of the apples. A similar thing happens when your bones in your back press on each other — you lose height.

If you've seen women, maybe your own mother and grandmothers, shrinking, developing a stoop, or being treated for fractures, you begin to understand the toll that losing bone can take on your health, your longevity, and your ability to remain independent as you age. In this chapter we'll tell you how to lower your risk of developing osteoporosis by building healthy bones before menopause and making some healthy choices in your lifestyle after menopause. Knowledge and prevention can keep you dancing.

# Homing In on Bone Health

Knowing how your body makes bones and what it takes to keep them healthy is a good place to start when outlining the relationship between the change and the health of your bones. Your bones don't quit growing after you become an adult. They're alive and changing throughout your life.

## Growing big bones and strong bones

When you're a kid, it's obvious that your bones are growing. As your bones get longer, you get taller. But your bones don't just grow longer; they also get thicker — denser. The denser the bone, the harder it is to break. Think of your dinnerware. Those thick earthenware plates are much more difficult to break than the fragile, translucent, fine china found in expensive restaurants. People with strong bones have dense bones. Your bones continue to increase in density until you're about 30 years old, at which age you reach *peak bone density*. If you start building strong, dense bones when you're young, the effects of bone loss in midlife are less problematic. The higher your peak bone density, the better chance you have of keeping your bones healthy.

If illness, surgery, or some other factor causes you to go through menopause prematurely, your bones are at extra risk. Not only are you subject to bone loss at an earlier age and for a longer period of time than women who enter menopause in their 40s or 50s, but — depending on the age at which you go through menopause — your bones may never reach peak bone density before you begin to lose bone mass. It will be especially important for you to follow the advice in this chapter and work with your doctor to monitor your bone density and stay up to date on advances in bone care.

In general, human males tend to be bigger than females; men also tend to have denser bones than women. On average, African-American women have denser bones than Caucasian and Asian women. This is why men and African-American women generally have less trouble with osteoporosis than Caucasian and Asian women.

## Understanding peak bone density

*Peak bone density* is the maximum amount of bone that you'll ever have. Most people reach their peak by about age 30. Maximizing your peak bone density is important because, after 35, you lose more bone than you build.

## Remodeling your house of bones

To better understand osteoporosis, it helps to look at how bone is "built." Each bone contains cells that build bone (*osteoblasts*) and cells that clear away bone (*osteoclasts*). Just as in home remodeling, one crew comes in to knock down walls, after which another crew comes in to build the new room. Even medical professionals refer to the bone-growing process as "remodeling" because this life-long process fixes wear and tear caused by everyday living.

At some point, a section of bone is selected as a remodeling site. Scientists don't fully understand how this happens, but at least some of this takes place as daily wear and tear — and, yes, exercise — bring on minute microfractures. This kind of wear actually gives your body a chance to make itself stronger through rebuilding. Osteoclasts remove bone by dissolving it with acid, which creates a cavity. This process of breaking down bone is referred to as

bone *resorption.* What happens to the dissolved bone? The body is an efficient recycler — the calcium and other minerals that made up the bone pass into the bloodstream and are used by other parts of the body. In fact, whenever your body needs extra calcium, the osteoclasts get busy dissolving more bone. That's why it's important to keep the body well supplied with calcium so your osteoclasts don't cannibalize your bones for calcium.

After the osteoclasts have done their thing, the osteoblasts get to work building new bone by spreading a gel-like substance in the cavity. Over the course of a month, this gel hardens into bone. The bone-remodeling project takes about two to three months. That's probably quicker than your last home-remodeling project, but it's a slower healing process than those associated with other tissues such as muscle or skin.

Your peak bone density depends on a number of factors such as genetics, diet, and exercise. You can't control the genes that control the size of your frame and your ability to produce bone. But you can control your diet, get plenty of calcium, vitamin D, and magnesium, and exercise early in life so that you maximize your peak bone density. Using alcohol only in moderation and not smoking also helps you reach a high peak bone density.

# Keeping Pace with Bone Reconstruction

Even after you grow to your full height, your bones keep gaining and losing bone material. Your body's maintenance process, called *remodeling,* keeps your bones strong and healthy day in and day out. Hormones help regulate the maintenance process. So you can imagine that as your hormones change, it messes up the bone maintenance process. (Check out the "Remodeling your house of bones" sidebar earlier in this chapter for the ins and outs of bone remodeling.) During your first 30 years on this planet, bone building exceeds bone destruction in the remodeling process, and your bones stay nice and healthy. After the big 3-0 or thereabouts, the teardown crew stays active, but the builders have a harder time keeping up.

## *Making the calcium connection*

Calcium is the central figure in the bone story. Your body needs calcium to build bones and to keep every cell in your body in shape. Calcium helps muscles contract, nerves respond, and blood clot. Bones store the calcium your body uses until they release the calcium to a part of the body that requests it.

Findings from the Women's Health Initiative study give calcium a thumbs up. Calcium and vitamin D supplements were found to help preserve bone mass. Calcium and vitamin D also serve to protect against hip fractures, especially in older women. These supplements *weren't* shown to be significantly effective at preventing other types of fractures. Still, taking these supplements is easy and inexpensive, so there's no reason not to add them to your regimen. A slight increase in the risk of kidney stones is the only risk detected. Table 5-1 lists calcium requirements by age. As your bones grow larger, your body needs more calcium. Your calcium requirements level off during your reproductive years but increase after menopause. The reason — estrogen helps your body absorb the calcium in your food. What happens to the calcium that's not absorbed? It goes out with the trash (other waste products). So to get the same amount of calcium into your bones, you have to take in more calcium.

| Table 5-1 | Calcium Requirements by Age |
| --- | --- |
| *Age* | *Calcium Recommendation (in Milligrams)* |
| 1–3 | 500 |
| 4–8 | 800 |
| 9–18 | 1,300 |
| 19–50 | 1,000 |
| 51 and older | 1,200 |

You may think that keeping your bones building and rebuilding is simply a matter of getting enough calcium, and you'd be partly right, but a number of vitamins and hormones help your body digest and absorb calcium. These vitamins and hormones have to be working right for the calcium in your diet to get incorporated into your bones (see the "Nutrition" section later in this chapter). The calcium must be digested and absorbed by your body to help your bones and other tissues that need it.

MEDICALESE

## Losing ground inside and outside your bones

*Osteopenia* is a condition in which bone density shows some decline, but not enough to cause fractures. Left untreated, osteopenia can lead to *osteoporosis*, a disease characterized by weak, porous, and brittle bones.

Doctors actually group osteoporosis into three types. Type 1, called "postmenopausal osteoporosis," describes bone loss, linked to the failure of estrogen production. The loss occurs mostly on the *inside* of your bones (you might hear your doctor call it *trabecular* bone). Fractures of the vertebrae and hip are typical of Type I osteoporosis.

Type II osteoporosis affects people over 65 — men as well as women. Time is the big culprit here: It's just been a lot of years since your 30s, when your bones were in their prime. In Type II osteoporosis there's excess *cortical* bone loss — from the outside of the bone. These folks can also have hip and spine fractures, but pelvic, shin, wrist, and arm fractures are also common, as is the "dowager's hump."

Type III ospteoporosis is sometimes called *secondary* osteoporosis because it's secondary to (caused by) some other factor, such as hyperthyroidism (excess thyroid hormone), alcoholism, a bone tumor, surgical menopause, and some medications taken on a long-term basis, including the anticoagulant drug heparin and anticonvulsant meds.

If the calcium in your blood drops below a certain level, your *parathyroid glands,* which monitor the amount of calcium in your blood, send the parathyroid hormone out into the bloodstream to deliver the following messages to your kidneys and to your osteoclasts:

- ✔ Your kidneys get a message: "Save the calcium, don't put it in the urine!" In response, your helpful kidneys start activating the vitamin D they've been storing so you can better absorb the calcium you eat.

- ✔ Your *osteoclasts* (the destruction crew) get a message, too: "Start mining calcium from the bones to beef up supplies in the bloodstream."

Your body cannibalizes its own bone to supply calcium to other cells if it doesn't get enough calcium or vitamin D. As a result, you suffer bone loss. This can happen, for instance, when you're pregnant or nursing. If your body decides there's not enough calcium in your blood for two, it will place a takeout order for more calcium to be pulled from your bones so the baby's needs can be met.

There are two ways to resolve this problem: Either get more calcium in your diet or slow down the remodeling process so that the builders can keep up with the destruction crew. You can get more calcium into your system by taking supplements, and exercising promotes remodeling. To slow down the destruction crew, you need medication (see the "Treating Osteoporosis" section later on).

## Recognizing the role of sex hormones

Sex hormones also play a big role in helping your body absorb the calcium you eat and manage the remodeling process. Hormone imbalance caused by estrogen deficits affects your bones.

Estrogen helps absorb the calcium and magnesium you eat and deposits it properly into your skeleton to give you strong bones. Estrogen also has a calming effect on bone destruction and lets the bone builders stay more or less caught up with the bone destroyers. As your estrogen supply dwindles during menopause, the bone destroyers get more active. What's more, you aren't able to digest as much of the calcium and magnesium you get from your food as your estrogen supply declines. If your eating habits don't change, the old amount of calcium and magnesium won't go nearly as far in helping to build bone. That's why most women add calcium and magnesium supplements to their diet after menopause.

Some of the other sex hormones that help in the bone building process include progesterone and testosterone, both of which your ovaries produce:

✔ Testosterone is actually a better bone builder than progesterone. It not only triggers the osteoblasts to build bone, but it also helps them build stronger bones.

✔ Progesterone helps the bone builders repair bone, but only if estrogen is also present.

The slowdown of estrogen and testosterone production is another one of the reasons the bone builders have a hard time keeping up with the destruction crew after menopause.

So, sex hormones are an important player in the osteoporosis game because they regulate bone remodeling. If you let the bone destroyers get too rowdy and don't force the bone builders to keep up with them, bone deteriorates and becomes less dense.

# Boning Up on Osteoporosis

The real danger of osteoporosis is that it sets the stage for literally breaking a leg (or a hip, or a wrist, or another bone). As you age, breaking a bone becomes more than an inconvenience — it can be deadly. A hip fracture carries the same mortality rate as breast cancer in the elderly! And half of hip-fracture victims become dependent on caregivers for the rest of their lives.

# Linking osteoporosis and women

First, the bad news about osteoporosis and women: About 25 million Americans have osteoporosis, and most of them are women. The good news is that the disease is preventable and treatable, even after menopause.

Women lose bone at very different rates, so the following generalizations reflect averages for the *perimenopausal* (premenopausal), menopausal, and postmenopausal years and don't necessarily apply to every woman:

- **Perimenopause:** Most women begin losing bone from their spine before or during perimenopause at a rate of 1 percent per year.

- **Menopause:** After a woman becomes menopausal, the rate of bone loss increases to about 3 percent per year if she doesn't receive hormone therapy.

- **Postmenopause:** Sometime during the ten years following menopause, bone loss slows back down to a rate of about 1 percent per year.

In the first five to seven years following menopause, a woman can lose as much as 20 percent of the total bone she's expected to lose during her lifetime. By the time a woman is in her 80s, she may have lost as much as 47 percent of her total bone density. If you think skeletons are scary, imagine losing almost half of yours!

There is some good news, though: Only 25 to 33 percent of women develop osteoporosis. However, it's like a thunderstorm. You may only have a 33 percent chance of rain, but if it's your picnic that gets rained on, you're gonna get wet.

# Defining and diagnosing osteoporosis

Osteoporosis literally means porous bone — bone that is weak and brittle. Too little calcium in the bone is the cause of this disease. Both men and women can develop osteoporosis, but it's more common in women than men for a couple of reasons:

- Women's bones are less dense than men's bones.

- Testosterone stimulates bone growth and helps build stronger bones. Men have more testosterone than women.

- More women live further into their senior years than men.

In your grandmother's day, doctors only diagnosed patients as having osteoporosis if they actually broke a bone because of the disease. Today, technology exists that can help identify osteoporosis before it results in painful and often debilitating fractures. We baby boomers are definitely into prevention.

How does a healthy bone differ from a fragile bone? Imagine cutting the bone in half so you can see it in cross section (as we illustrate in Figure 5-1).

✔ A healthy bone looks like Swiss cheese — lots of cheese separated by small holes.

✔ A fragile bone looks like lace — lots of holes separated by thin, string-like structures.

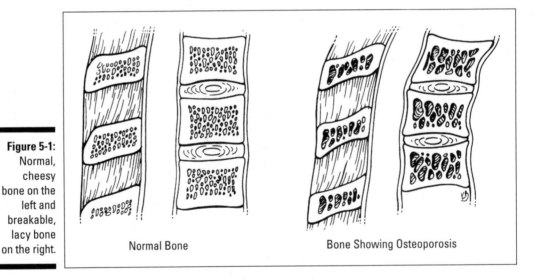

**Figure 5-1:**
Normal, cheesy bone on the left and breakable, lacy bone on the right.

Normal Bone                    Bone Showing Osteoporosis

Osteoporosis today is defined in terms of how your bone density compares with the peak bone density of a healthy, 35-year-old woman, (which serves as the basis for the Young Adult category in Table 5-2):

✔ If your bones are just slightly less dense than the bones of an average 35-year-old, the diagnosis is *osteopenia* — low bone density.

✔ If they're significantly less dense than the bones of an average 35-year-old, the diagnosis is *osteoporosis* — brittle bones. Table 5-2 shows the National Osteoporosis Foundation's criteria used to diagnose osteoporosis as of 1998.

| Table 5-2 | Criteria for Diagnosing Osteoporosis |
|---|---|
| *Category* | *Bone Density T-Score* |
| Normal | Less than 1.0 standard deviation below Young Adult |
| Osteopenia | 1.0–2.5 standard deviations below Young Adult |
| Osteoporosis | 2.5 or more standard deviations below Young Adult |
| Severe osteoporosis | 2.0 or more standard deviations below Young Adult and evidence of fractures |

The threshold that separates osteopenia from full-blown osteoporosis comes from research that shows how much bone you can lose before significantly increasing your risk of fracture. Folks with osteoporosis have low bone density, but they also have a higher risk of fracturing a bone.

## Looking at causes

Sixty years ago, doctors noticed that osteoporosis occurred primarily in menopausal women. They suspected that osteoporosis was related to sex hormones — specifically to estrogen deficiency. Hundreds of research grants later, medical professionals and ordinary folks know that estrogen levels affect bone density.

Does menopause *cause* osteoporosis? The short answer is no. Osteoporosis is caused by calcium deficiency in the bones, and estrogen plays a role in getting calcium to your bones and keeping bones healthy. (Check out the "Making the calcium connection" section earlier in this chapter for more on calcium's role.)

Deficiencies of other vitamins, minerals, and hormones can influence the amount of calcium that gets absorbed by your bone, thereby contributing to the development of osteoporosis. Lack of exercise can promote osteoporosis as well. Finally, lifestyle choices, such as the use of tobacco and excess alcohol, can also play a role in the onset of osteoporosis.

## Avoiding the effects

Osteoporosis weakens every bone in your body, leaving them prone to breaking. The bones most likely to break include the spine, hip, and wrist bones. Breaking your wrist may inconvenience you for a few weeks or months. Hip fractures are much more debilitating. Crushed vertebrae, so often associated with osteoporosis, can cause you to become shorter. Crushed vertebrae can leave you with a stooped appearance, too.

Here's how fractures of different bones occur and how they might affect your functioning:

- **Spinal fractures:** Osteoporotic fractures of the spine are called compressions. The weight of your body crushes, or compresses, the round body of the vertebra, which provides these fractures with their name, *compression fractures.* Compression fractures in your spine can leave you stooped with what appears to be a hump in your back (called a *dowager's hump*).

Between 5 and 15 percent of 50-year-old women get compression fractures in their spine (as in osteoporosis in general, Caucasian and Asian women are at greater risk than Hispanic or African-American women). By age 70, that number grows to between 40 and 55 percent. (It depends on whose research you're looking at.) Often, these crushed or wedged vertebrae cause little or no pain. You simply begin to notice poor posture that you can't correct by standing up as straight as you can.

You may notice the first sign of crushed vertebrae during your annual medical exam. After age 40 or 45 your doctor starts measuring your height. Women with crushed or wedged vertebrae are often shorter than they were before. If you find yourself getting shorter, the measurement may not be a mistake — it could be a sign of osteoporosis. Figure 5-2 shows the possible changes in your spine that accompany osteoporosis.

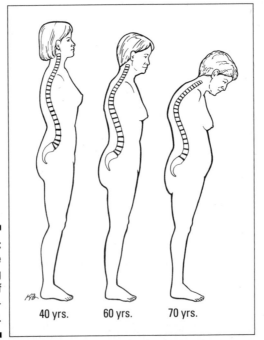

**Figure 5-2:**
The shrinking effects of osteoporosis.

40 yrs.     60 yrs.     70 yrs.

# Your hip bone's connected to . . . your molars?

Menopausal bone loss can have a devastating impact on your dental health as well as on your spine and hips. The loss of bone mass in the jaw is common in older women (and men), and can lead to tooth loss when the bone that holds your teeth in place is weakened. As with so many health problems, dental bone loss is lowest in people who have never been smokers, and highest in long-time smokers who haven't quit.

---

Most women experience little or no pain when the vertebrae collapse, which is both the good news and the bad. Nobody wants to be in pain, but the lack of a clear signal that your spine is in trouble means it could be months or years before the damage is detected and addressed. Some compression fractures do cause pain, but it's usually mild and can be controlled by using an over-the-counter painkiller such as ibuprofen or aspirin. The pain rarely lasts more than a few months. If you suspect compression fractures, though, don't try to take them on by yourself. Work with your doctor to determine the extent of the problem and the best course of action.

✔ **Hip fractures:** This problem is generally the result of a fall that breaks the *femur,* the long bone of the thigh that connects your knee to your hip. This break often occurs at the head of the femur where it connects to the hip socket. In some cases, however, it's the other way around: The fragile bone simply breaks, causing a fall.

More than 90 percent of hip fractures occur in people over 70. So even though osteoporosis can begin during perimenopause, it can be corrected or held at bay so that you don't experience the debilitating aspects of the disease — the fractures. But don't underestimate the trauma of experiencing a broken hip at age 70. Only one-third of all women who have hip fractures regain the functionality they had prior to the fracture. Another third wind up in nursing homes. And unfortunately, about 20 percent die of complications within a year of the fracture.

✔ **Wrist fractures:** Wrist fractures are common. When you fall, your first reaction is to catch yourself by sticking your hands out in front of you. You don't have to guess why wrist fractures are common in women with osteoporosis.

# Preventing Osteoporosis by Managing Your Risk Factors

Your risk of developing osteoporosis is higher than your risk of getting breast, ovarian, or uterine cancer combined. After your 50th birthday, your risk of developing osteoporosis grows. Forty percent of women over 50 will sustain a fracture due to osteoporosis in her lifetime. Again, the risk for Caucasian women is nearly twice as high as the fracture rate for African-American women. So, the next time you're sitting in a Mother's Club meeting, look to one side. Depending on your ethnicity, it's likely that either you or the friend next to you will break a bone because of osteoporosis.

Some women develop osteoporosis as they age, and others don't. It's important to understand why this happens and how to be one of the women who doesn't fall victim to this disease.

If you're a young woman, you can start preventing osteoporosis today. If you're over 35, finding out how healthy your bones are right now is a good place to start. In either case, prevention and treatment are easier if you understand how your bones stay healthy, how osteoporosis develops, and why your risk of developing brittle bones increases after menopause. (Check out the preceding "Keeping Pace with Bone Reconstruction" section.) Risk factors vary by age. From childhood through your 20s, you can lower your risk of osteoporosis by getting enough calcium, vitamins, and minerals; by exercising; and by avoiding unhealthy activities such as smoking and drinking too much alcohol. (We discuss exercise in Chapters 19 and 23.)

If you have children (whether they're toddlers or young adults), they can begin taking measures right away to prevent this disease. The stronger your bones are early in life, the more you have to work with as you grow older. Having really dense bones when your bone density peaks (when you're about 30) gives you more bone to work with during and after menopause. Young people can develop strong bones by eating properly and staying fit (see Chapters 18 and 19).

After your 30s are in your rearview mirror and you begin to go through perimenopause and menopause, menopausal-related shifts in sex hormones and other factors increase your risk of osteoporosis. (Check out the "Recognizing the role of sex hormones" section earlier in this chapter for more on the connection between osteoporosis and these hormones.) Risk factors boil down to three basic categories:

✔ Genetic factors and family background

✔ Personal health history

✔ Your lifestyle

We devote a subsection to each of these topics.

# Blaming your genes: Genetic factors and family background

Your genes establish a lot of the rules concerning how your body develops and how it ages. So it's no surprise that genetics plays a role in increasing or reducing your risk of osteoporosis.

Caucasian and Asian women have higher risks of osteoporosis than women of African ancestry, particularly during perimenopause and the early years of menopause. African Americans have a 6 percent lifetime risk of osteoporosis, but Caucasian and Asian women each have a lifetime risk of about 14 percent. The lower incidence of osteoporosis in African-American women is probably due to the fact that African-American women have higher peak bone densities than Caucasian and Asian women. Even though everyone loses bone with age, African-American women have the advantage of having stronger bones from the start.

### Body build

Large-boned people generally build more bone than small-framed people, and they often start out with more bone mass when they hit their bone-building peak. As they age, large-boned people draw from a larger supply of calcium, so bone deterioration takes longer. But large-boned people aren't completely safe; they get osteoporosis too. Small-boned, or petite, women have lower peak bone densities, so they have less bone to lose.

### Family history of osteoporosis

Medical folks have found that daughters of osteoporosis sufferers tend to have lower peak bone density than normal for their age. Genes help determine our ability to make bone, and some women just don't make as much bone even with a proper diet and exercise.

# Reviewing your personal health history

A number of aspects of your personal history influence your risk of osteoporosis, including menstrual and menopause-related issues and the medications that you take.

### Menstruation

Because estrogen prevents bone loss, the more estrogen you produce during your lifetime, the less your risk of osteoporosis. Not surprisingly, many factors relating to your periods affect how much estrogen you produce and, therefore, your risk for osteoporosis. Check out the following:

- ✔ **Age at your first period:** After you begin menstruation, your body produces more estrogen. Most girls begin to menstruate sometime between the ages of 11½ and 13. If you get your period early, you may produce more estrogen in your lifetime than the average woman. With the additional estrogen, your bones may have a higher peak bone density than the average woman. Of course, this assumes that you followed a proper diet and got appropriate amounts of exercise. If you start out with higher bone density, you can lower your risk for osteoporosis.

- ✔ **Age at the onset of menopause:** Most women go through menopause between the ages of 45 and 55. Women who go through menopause earlier begin losing bone earlier than women who start the change later in life. This is particularly true if you go through premature menopause in your 20s or 30s because of ovarian loss or failure linked to surgery, medications, illness, or other variables. Women who have their ovaries removed before age 35 often develop osteoporosis even with hormone therapy. Women who have their uterus removed (*hysterectomy*) can go through menopause two years earlier than other women. The earlier onset probably results from cutting off some of the bloodflow to the ovaries. The earlier onset of menopause increases your risk of osteoporosis a bit because you have fewer years of estrogen production.

Your body produces much less estrogen after menopause than it did during your reproductive years, and the more estrogen you produce in your lifetime, the lower your risk of osteoporosis.

### Eating disorders

Anorexia and bulimia (along with over-exercising) can lead to low estrogen levels, which can cause you to skip periods and your body to begin losing more bone than it builds. Losing more bone than your body builds leads to osteoporosis. These conditions also rob you of bone-friendly nutrients.

### Medications

Some medications affect peak bone density, raising your risk of osteoporosis. Ask your physician or read the literature that accompanies the medications to determine if you're at risk of bone loss from using a specific medication. Some of the medications that can affect your bones include

- ✔ Corticosteriods used to treat chronic conditions such as asthma, rheumatoid arthritis, psoriasis, and chronic obstructive pulmonary disease (COPD) can cause bone loss. These drugs increase bone loss by inhibiting calcium absorption. Women who take corticosteroid dosages greater than 5 milligrams for more than two months increase their risk of bone loss. Sometimes, physicians prescribe Fosamax, a drug that slows down bone destruction and encourages bone building, along with certain steroids if long-term steroid use is necessary.

✔ Excessively high dosages of thyroid-replacement medication or an over-active thyroid (as with Grave's disease) can decrease bone strength. Excess thyroid hormone causes bone loss.

✔ Some of the medications used to treat endometriosis and breast cancer contribute to rapid bone loss.

✔ Certain types of diuretics used to treat heart disease or high blood pressure cause the body to excrete more calcium. When used for prolonged periods of time, they can raise your risk of bone loss. Thiazide diuretics, on the other hand, actually reduce the amount of calcium excreted in the urine. They also seem to inhibit bone breakdown.

### Surgeries

Certain surgeries can increase your risk of osteoporosis because they impact your body's ability to absorb or digest calcium or the vitamins and minerals needed to get calcium from your diet into the bone. These surgeries include

✔ **Gastrectomy:** Removal of all or part of the stomach. This surgery impacts your ability to digest calcium and other nutrients needed to build bone.

✔ **Intestinal bypass:** Surgery to remove a portion of your intestine. This surgery impacts your ability to absorb calcium and other nutrients needed to build bone. Gastric bypass weight-loss procedures can have the same effect for the same reason.

✔ **Thyroidectomy:** Surgery to remove part or all of the thyroid gland. If your thyroid is removed, you must take thyroid-hormone medication. Too much thyroid-replacement medication triggers excessive bone loss and a decrease in bone strength.

# Looking to your lifestyle

Now we come to the section about lifestyle issues, most of which you have some control over. You can't do much about your age (even if you claim to be 39 years old for the rest of your life, your body knows the truth). But you can take steps to lower your risk of osteoporosis by picking up some new healthy habits and eliminating the unhealthy habits.

## Age

From the time you're born until you're about 30, your main job is to build the strongest skeleton you can by following a healthful diet, exercising regularly, and avoiding tobacco and alcohol. After you reach your 30s, your body loses bone faster than it makes it.

By the time you're 70, you've probably lost about as much bone as you're going to, but other aspects of aging increase your risk of falling and breaking a bone. By 70 or 80, your body has lost much of its flexibility, you may have less balance, your eyesight and depth perception may be poor, and you may be taking medications that affect bone loss or physical conditioning.

### Smoking

Smoking is clearly associated with compromised bone health. It accelerates bone loss, contributes to the development of osteoporosis, and — in the event that you do break a bone — impairs healing. Smokers have a 41 percent higher incidence of hip fractures than non-smokers do. The dangers are greatest for long-time smokers, but even if you haven't smoked for very long, you will take longer to heal if you break a bone. The good news is that it's never too late to quit and see improvement. If you don't smoke, don't start. If you do, this gives you another good reason to quit.

### Alcohol use

More than three drinks a day is considered excessive as far as raising your risk of osteoporosis. Excessive alcohol consumption decreases bone density. Moderate drinking, however, actually appears to have a protective effect. If you don't drink, don't start just to give your bones a buzz. If you have an evening glass of wine, though, it looks like you may be helping your bones.

### Exercise

Exercise is the kindest gift you can give your bones after you give them calcium. It's critical to building strong bones. Exercise puts stress on your bones, which is a good thing as far as bone density is concerned. Stress forces the bone tissue to absorb calcium and promotes remodeling; therefore, it gets stronger. Exercise also stimulates the muscles around the bone so that the muscles get stronger and provide more support for your bones. Exercise also can help decrease your chances of falling and having a fracture by training your muscles to respond quickly to a trip or accident.

Exercise during childhood and early adulthood is important in preventing osteoporosis because it helps your bones achieve their full potential strength. Later in life, exercise helps your bones continue to absorb calcium so that they stay strong.

Add 30 to 40 minutes of weight-bearing exercise to your routine most days of the week. Exercises that emphasize core strength (focusing on your core — back and abdominal — muscles) and balance are especially helpful and can help prevent falls. Try tai chi, yoga, Pilates, or working out with a balance ball. Swimming, although one of the best exercises for your overall muscle strength, heart and lungs, and stamina, doesn't do much for your bones (because the water does all the work holding you up).

Although physical activity helps protect your body against osteoporosis, too much strenuous activity can lead to low levels of estrogen. Unless you're training for the Olympics, you probably aren't exercising too strenuously. Skipping periods can be a sign that you're over-exercising.

## Nutrition

Calcium helps your body build bone. But calcium does much more than the TV advertisements proclaim. Calcium is also fundamental to regulating your sleep and moods and to proper muscle function.

Dairy products are the best source of calcium as far as food goes. A variety of vegetables also contain calcium, but vegetables contain less calcium per serving than dairy products. The fiber in vegetables makes it harder for your body to extract and use the calcium in them — strange, but true.

Are soft drinks getting the best of you? Drinking carbonated soft drinks every day can zap the calcium out of your foods and supplements before it ever gets into your system. The phosphates in the soda bind with the calcium and magnesium, making them unusable. If you drink sodas regularly, try to stop or cut back on them, or increase your consumption of calcium. Doctors recommend menopausal women get 1,200 milligrams of calcium every day after age 50 (check with Table 5-1).

Many women find it easier to use calcium supplements than to get all the calcium they need from dairy products. With supplements, you know exactly how much calcium you're getting each day and most have the appropriate amounts of two other nutrients critical to bone building — vitamin D and magnesium. When choosing a supplement, avoid those made from oyster shell and dolomite. These supplements can be contaminated with toxic heavy metals. Calcium-carbonate antacids are one of the cheapest and easiest calcium supplements to find. As long as the calcium-carbonate antacid has no aluminum, it's safe to take every day. We personally prefer a calcium supplement that also contains vitamin D and magnesium, two other nutrients critical to healthy bone maintenance.

Women should get 400 to 600 milligrams of vitamin D and magnesium every day to maintain healthy bones. In other words, you should have about half as much vitamin D and magnesium every day as calcium. Magnesium prevents bone loss by playing an active role in bone growth. It also supports nerve cell communication (preventing wild mood swings), helps regulate blood pressure, and aids in muscle contraction. The last two functions help prevent heart attacks. The heart is essentially one big muscle so magnesium helps keep the contractions regular. Also, magnesium seems to prevent spasms of the blood vessels, particularly in the arteries around the heart.

Calcium supplements with magnesium help prevent the constipation that some women experience when they take calcium supplements. Magnesium is a natural laxative and one of the main ingredients in milk of magnesia. Dividing your daily dose of calcium into two parts (say, 500 mg with breakfast and another 500 mg with dinner) also seems to help.

Vitamin K helps keep the body from cannibalizing bone for calcium by maintaining proper levels of calcium in the blood. Vitamin K also produces a protein used to build bone called *osteocalcin.* You can get vitamin K in green, leafy vegetables such as spinach and broccoli. You should get at least 100 micrograms of vitamin K a day. (Half a cup of broccoli has about 150 micrograms of vitamin K.)

Take your calcium faithfully every day. Findings from the Women's Health Initiative show that women who did so had 29 percent fewer hip fractures. Women who were more haphazard about their calcium supplements had only marginally fewer hip fractures than women who didn't take them at all.

### Caffeine

Women who drink four or more cups of coffee a day increase their risk of fractures due to osteoporosis. Caffeine promotes bone loss by increasing the amount of calcium in your urine. Because coffee has more caffeine than most teas or colas, curbing your coffee habit is one of the best ways to reduce your caffeine intake in the quest for healthier bones. If you just can't get that coffee monkey off your back, at least drink a cup of milk for each cup of coffee you drink. You can also switch to decaffeinated beverages.

### Foods to watch

You know about the vast array of diets and dieting products available today to help you lose weight. Be aware that high-protein foods and diets may not be good for your bones. Acids are sent into the bloodstream to help digest the protein, and your body hits the bone up for calcium to neutralize these acids. This leads to bone loss.

Women who eat a lot of red meat each week (5 servings or more) increase their risk of fractures by 20 percent. Proteins from vegetables, grains, and fish don't seem to cause the same responses as proteins from meats.

Lactose intolerant? Good sources of dietary calcium that won't give you the collywobbles include yogurt; some hard cheeses; leafy, green vegetables such as broccoli, spinach, and kale; and fish canned with the bones left in, such as sardines and salmon. The many foods now available that have been enriched with calcium are helpful if you're no longer friends with milk: look for juices, breads, and cereals with added calcium.

### Sunshine

Soaking up some rays can actually help your bones soak up the calcium. Vitamin D is crucial to your body's ability to absorb calcium, and sunshine helps your body make vitamin D. Don't overdo it, though — this advice isn't a free pass to spend hours at the beach courting wrinkles and melanoma. As little as 15 minutes of sunlight a day can help without turning you into a crispy critter. Work in your garden, take a walk, or read the paper on your sunny porch.

# Finding Out Whether You Have Osteoporosis

Unfortunately, most women find out they have low bone density only after they've had a fracture. Other women first notice it in the mirror — their posture seems poor, even when they stand up as straight as they can. Still other women have a chest x-ray for some unrelated reason and the doctor notices crushed vertebrae, indicating brittle bones.

Among women 45 to 75, 75 percent have never asked their healthcare provider about osteoporosis. And many doctors don't think to bring it up unless you're being treated for a fracture. Start the ball rolling by asking your doctor about whether you need a *bone mineral density (BMD)* test. Having a test sometime around your 40th birthday gives you a baseline — that is, a sort of "before" picture your doctor can use in coming years to compare with new tests to help determine whether you're losing bone. These baseline tests often measure bone in your spin and your hip, but may also include one or both of your wrists.

Because "official" recommendations, such as those from the U.S. Preventative Services Task Force, recommend that all women have their first bone density test after they turn 65, you may have a tough time convincing your insurance company to cover the cost of this test if you haven't yet reached this age. If you have one or more risk factors for osteoporosis, though, it may be possible to persuade the insurance company to pony up. Bone-density tests can help your doctor answer three important questions:

1. How much bone, if any, have you lost?

2. How quickly are you losing bone?

3. What's the best therapy to get your bones healthier and keep you from losing more bone?

## Reading a DEXA report

The first thing you'll notice on the DEXA bone-density report is the colorful graphic image of your hip or spine. The report you receive looks almost like an x-ray except it displays colors that correspond to different bone densities. Typically, a legend shows the color gradient going from low-density bone to high-density bone. This allows you to see exactly where the low-density areas are.

Statistics that compare your *bone mineral density* (BMD) measurements to the average density derived from BMD readings of a large number of 35-year-olds are displayed next to the image. When they compare your bone density to this "standard," the difference is represented as a percentage. In other words, if your bones were half as dense as the average 35-year-old's, your statistics would read 50 percent; if your bones were the same, it would read 100 percent.

Suppose your comparison shows that your bones are within 85 percent of those of a 35-year-old. Is this terrible, or is it terrific? To determine if this percentage is statistically significant

(something worth treating), the report also includes a *T-score* and a *z-score*. For those of you who weaseled your way out of taking statistics, T-scores show how much your score differs from "normal." In this case, *normal*, or +1, is the score of a healthy 35-year-old woman of your ethnic background. Negative T-scores aren't so good. A T-score of –1, (1 standard deviation below normal) isn't too bad (unless you have already experienced unexplained fractures). Your doctor will probably diagnose you with *osteopenia*, which means you have low bone density (see Table 5-2 for the criteria used in diagnosing osteoporosis). If your T-score is 2.5 standard deviations below normal, or lower, your doctor will probably diagnose you as having osteoporosis and recommend a course of treatment or some kind of dietary/fitness intervention.

Your test will also give you a z-score. This is similar to your T-score except this test compares your bone density to that of other women of your age, weight, and ethnicity.

The bone-density test produces a graphic image of your bone as well as statistics that compare your bones to healthy bones. You can find out how quickly you're losing bone by having these tests repeated every two or three years. The results of your bone-density test will guide your physician in choosing an appropriate therapy for bone loss, if one is needed.

## Doing the DEXA

To measure bone density, most physicians use a test called a *dual energy x-ray absorptiometry*, or DEXA for short, which uses a fraction of the radiation a chest x-ray uses.

Preparing an image of your hip only takes a few minutes, and preparing an image of your spine only takes a few minutes more. The technician can see the results immediately, although you often receive your report a few days later. (They don't want the insurance company to think that the procedure isn't worth the money.)

The report shows colored images of your spine and hip reflecting different bone densities. The statistics that accompany the images compare your bone density to that of the average 35-year-old woman and to women your own age. (See the "Reading a DEXA report" sidebar nearby.)

If you're at high risk for osteoporosis due to genetics or life events (such as premature menopause), have your initial bone-density test during your early 30s, and have subsequent tests every two years after that.

## Opting for another type of test

The DEXA bone-density measurement is probably the most commonly used procedure, but you or your doctor may opt for another procedure. Several devices work on the same principle as the DEXA bone scanner, including:

- **Dual photon absorptiometry (DPA):** Introduced in the early 1980s, DPA was one of the first devices that could measure bone density in areas covered by heavy muscle, such as the spine and hip — the best bones to use as predictors of total body bone density. This machine is a bit slower and less precise than DEXA and can't measure small changes, so using it for comparisons is more difficult.

- **Quantitative computed tomography (QTC):** Also known as *CAT scans* or *CT scans,* QTCs can measure bone density anywhere in the body. The advantage of this procedure over the others is that it can accurately measure the center of each vertebra in the spine. DEXA measurement can only measure a certain type of vertebrae because other bones are in the way.

  CAT scans aren't typically used to measure a patient's bone density on a yearly basis because it exposes the patient to more radiation than the other techniques — and they're pretty expensive.

- **Ultrasound:** This test is sometimes used to measure bone density in the heel or kneecap. These machines are portable, so theoretically, more people can be screened using this quick, inexpensive bone-screening procedure. On the down side, this machine is limited to measuring bone density in *peripheral* sites — places other than the preferred spine and hip sites. If an ultrasound detects low bone density, you should have a follow-up DEXA test.

✔ **Urine tests:** As bone dissolves, some of the byproducts show up in urine. When performed every few months, urine tests can tell whether bone loss is increasing or decreasing. This test isn't an accurate diagnostic instrument for osteoporosis because you can have low bone density but be losing bone slowly. The test is generally used with patients on a treatment program for osteoporosis to monitor progress.

X-rays are *not* used to test for bone density because changes in the "whiteness" of the bone on the x-ray can't be detected until you've lost 30 percent of your normal bone mass. Clearly you want to take some action before you lose 30 percent of your bone mass.

# Treating Osteoporosis

The first step in reducing bone loss is eliminating unhealthy habits (smoking and excessive alcohol use, for example) and picking up healthy habits (such as a healthful diet and an exercise program). Even simple treatment measures, such as calcium supplements and increased exercise, can slow bone loss and improve bone density.

More aggressive treatment programs include medications and/or hormone therapies. These programs can slow and even reverse bone loss. Many physicians recommend that women at high risk of osteoporosis begin hormone therapy during menopause. Estrogen levels need to be at least half of the level that they are during a normal menstrual cycle to prevent bone loss. Some women who have lost a significant amount of bone may have testosterone added to their hormone regimen. Hormone therapy should be started early in menopause in addition to the other treatment programs. We'll talk more about hormone therapy and bone loss management in Chapter 16.

## Battling bone loss with medication

There are several classes of prescription medications that help prevent or repair the damage done by osteoporosis. Because they may have side effects and risks of their own, you will need to work closely with your doctor to decide whether medication — and which one — is right for you. Even if you take medication to keep your bones healthy, you will still need to supplement your diet with calcium and vitamin D, exercise, and follow other bone-protecting health guidelines.

# Examining the link between bone density and diabetes

Type I diabetes has long been associated with low bone density, though the reasons are still poorly understood. Because Type 1 diabetes tends to be diagnosed relatively early in life, however, one factor seems to be that diabetes develops before bone density has had an opportunity to peak.

People with Type II diabetes often actually have better-than average bone density, but recent research shows that a surprising number are prone to osteoporotic fractures. It may be that, because this type of diabetes is associated with obesity and a more sedentary lifestyle, as well

as with nerve damage that impairs sensitivity in the feet, falls may simply occur more often, leading to osteoporotic fractures.

The incidence of both diabetes and osteoporosis are increasing as longevity increases, and the complex factors at work here need more study. In the meantime, follow medical advice consistent with managing both conditions: exercise and eat right. Make sure you talk with your doctor about how these conditions might be related, and how treatment for either disease might have an impact on your experience with the other.

# Using hormones

In 1991, the U.S. Department of Health and Human Services, Department of Health, and the National Heart, Lung, and Blood Institute launched the Women's Health Initiative (WHI), a group of long-term studies of health issues in the lives of more than 160,000 postmenopausal women.

## Estrogen-alone therapy and bone health

One of these researchers looked at the effect of estrogen-alone (without progestin) hormone replacement on bone health.

For such a long study, the findings that relate to the estrogen-alone study are short — and not particularly sweet. This type of therapy *was* associated with decreases in the risk of hip fracture in post-menopausal women. This protection came at a steep price, though: women taking the estrogen also suffered a significant rise in the risk of stroke. In fact, the risk was so great that the WHI voluntarily suspended the estrogen-only trials before the eight-year follow-up period was over. The FDA currently advises that estrogen-alone therapy should be used for as brief a time as possible, and in the smallest effective dose, to control menopausal symptoms, and should not be prescribed just for the prevention of disease, including osteoporosis.

### Estrogen plus progestin therapy and bone health

Women taking estrogen and progestin together also got a good news/bad news message from the WHI about HT and osteoporosis. Postmenopausal women taking this combination therapy had 24 percent fewer fractures of any kind, and a one-third reduction in hip fractures compared with women taking a placebo (a fake pill with no active medical ingredients). Not only that, but hip bone density actually *increased* in this group by a small percentage: about 3.7 percent after three years. But this study, too, was stopped early. In the case of the combination HT study, the increased risk of breast cancer was the main concern. Again, the FDA recommends against the use of HT just to prevent osteoporosis because of this increased breast cancer risk.

Does this mean that HT is universally bad for all women? No, of course not. Every woman's case is different, and you'll need to take your own experiences, feelings, and history into account when working with your doctor to decide what's right for you. But the findings from the WHI studies at least give us a good place to start.

# Chapter 6

# Getting a Handle on Heart Health

· · · · · · · · · · · · · · · · · · · · · · · · · · · · · · · · · · · · · · · · · · · · · · · ·

## In This Chapter

▶ Uncovering estrogen's connection to cardiovascular disease

▶ Getting the goods on "good" and "bad" cholesterol

▶ Understanding cardiovascular diseases

▶ Laying out the risk factors for cardiovascular disease

▶ Preventing cardiovascular conditions

· · · · · · · · · · · · · · · · · · · · · · · · · · · · · · · · · · · · · · · · · · · · · · · ·

**W**omen usually don't have heart trouble until after they reach menopause, at an average age of 51, and your risk for cardiovascular disease increases after menopause because you lose the protective benefits of estrogen. Plus, if a woman has a heart attack during mid-life, she's more likely than a man to die from it. Why? One reason is that women have different symptoms than men. The crushing chest pains that warn men of a heart attack aren't as common in women when they experience a heart attack.

Uncertainty about whether your symptoms signal a potentially serious heart problem can lead to delays in seeking treatment. So be sure to check out the section, "Holding off heart attacks," later in this chapter to review the warning signs of a heart attack for women, one of the many heart-healthy tips you can find in this chapter.

In this chapter, we discuss heart attacks and many other types of cardiovascular disease that can affect your health during and after menopause. But you can keep your heart healthy even after menopause. And what would this chapter be if we just covered the bad news? We also discuss ways to keep your heart happy after the change — adopting a heart-healthy diet, getting a bit of exercise, and eliminating some bad habits.

# Keeping Up with All Things Cardio

Okay, we're not discussing the latest craze in cardio workouts (although Chapter 19 gives you some great ideas on fitness!); instead, in this section, we bring to light how your heart and blood vessels work so you can better understand both the role estrogen plays in your cardiovascular system as well as the connection between menopause and your cardiovascular health.

In its simplest form, your cardiovascular system consists of your blood vessels and that big pumping muscle you know as your heart. As seen in Figure 6-1, blood carries oxygen to the heart and picks up garbage on the way back.

## Revealing estradiol's role in heart health

Estrogen (in particular, the active form, estradiol) does a lot to keep your blood vessels and heart healthy and free from disease. The following list of ways estradiol protects you from getting an achy-breaky heart pulls together all the studies that have been done on estradiol and the cardiovascular system:

✔ Estradiol lowers your blood pressure by dilating blood vessels.

✔ Estradiol increases the good cholesterol and lowers the bad.

✔ Estradiol keeps platelets (part of your blood) from clotting too quickly.

✔ Estradiol acts as an antioxidant to keep fat deposits from forming on the walls of your arteries.

✔ Estradiol facilitates the release of a chemical that relaxes blood vessels, which helps reduce vessel spasms and increase blood flow.

## Linking cardiovascular disease and the menopausal woman

Estrogen, the female hormone produced in the ovaries, is good for your heart. *Estradiol,* the active form of estrogen, is the most beneficial form of estrogen, but (you guessed it) it's also the type of estrogen that decreases as you become menopausal. (Chapter 2 is full of information about what your hormones do — check it out.)

Basically, estradiol is our secret weapon against all kinds of cardiovascular diseases. It's what every man wishes he had so that he could avoid the early onset of heart problems. (See the section, "Revealing estradiol's role in heart health," earlier in this chapter.)

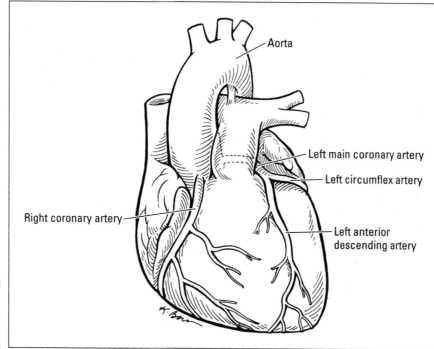

**Figure 6-1:**
The healthy
heart.

You may have heard that before age 50, women are about half as likely as men their age to have heart disease. This statement has led many people to perceive heart disease as largely a male problem. It isn't. Men do tend to develop heart problems about ten years earlier than women — so on average, a woman has the heart of a man ten years her junior. But just because men develop heart disease at an earlier age doesn't mean that heart disease isn't deadly for women. Just as many women as men die of heart disease each year.

Cardiovascular disease (disease of the heart and blood vessels) increases in women as estradiol levels decrease. After menopause, your risk of cardiovascular disease shoots way up. Between 45 and 65 years of age, men experience three times more heart attacks than women. But after age 65, watch out — women have more heart attacks than men.

We want to give you the total picture here, and unfortunately, that includes some info you may not want to hear. Of all the ways a menopausal woman can pass into the hereafter, cardiovascular disease is the most likely culprit. In fact, after menopause, you're ten times more likely to die from cardiovascular disease than from breast cancer.

For some reason, the word hasn't gotten out to women or their doctors. Heart disease kills more women each year than lung, breast, and colorectal cancers combined. Also, diagnoses of heart disease and heart attacks are often delayed in women because the symptoms aren't recognized and taken seriously. See the section, "Holding off heart attacks," later in this chapter for more information on symptoms.

The term *cardiovascular disease (CVD)* encompasses conditions that affect your heart and blood vessels such as heart disease, heart attack, high blood pressure, coronary-artery disease, and stroke. All these diseases restrict the flow of blood to the heart or brain.

# Considering Cholesterol

You probably hear a lot about cholesterol — from your doctor, and from commercials for cholesterol medications. And you're not getting forgetful when you begin to think the cholesterol goals your doctor sets for you get lower and lower. The more doctors learn about the dangers cholesterol plays in our health, the more they encourage you to avoid it.

Lowering your cholesterol isn't the only important factor in keeping your heart healthy, but it definitely plays a strong supporting role.

At its basic level, *cholesterol* is fat — waxy, yellowish, oily fat. However, this fat (also known as a *lipid* in med speak) is critical to keeping your well-oiled body running. Your body uses cholesterol to build and repair cells and to produce hormones, such as estrogen and testosterone, vitamin D, bile (used to absorb fat), and myelin (coats the nerves). If your blood contains too much cholesterol, the cholesterol gets deposited with other crud on the inside of your blood vessels. Cholesterol travels through your bloodstream on the back of proteins, so the particles are named *lipoproteins* (get it? — lipid plus protein equals lipoprotein). Lipoproteins with more protein than fat are called high-density lipids (HDL), and those with more fat than protein are called low-density lipids (LDL). By the time you're menopausal, your LDL levels have risen and often exceed those of men your age.

## Breaking down the types of cholesterol

Not too long ago doctors thought that the most important cholesterol number to look at was the ratio of your total cholesterol to your HDL, or good cholesterol. Now groups such as the American Heart Association and others recommend looking instead at your *individual* cholesterol numbers. Lucky you, you have *four* of these, one for each aspect of your cholesterol:

- ✔ **High-density lipids (HDLs):** These lipids are called the "good" cholesterol because they help prevent the buildup of plaque. Because HDLs are mostly protein with just a little bit of fat, they can carry the extra bad cholesterol back to the liver so that the body can (literally) flush it away.

- ✔ **Low-density lipids (LDLs):** Also known as the "bad" cholesterol, LDLs are mostly fat and only a small amount of protein. At normal levels, they carry cholesterol from the liver to other parts of the body where it's needed for cell repair. When LDL cholesterol is too high, it adheres to the walls of the arteries and attracts other substances. The combined glob is called *plaque.*

- ✔ **Triglycerides:** In addition to the fat known as cholesterol, your blood contains this other type of fat in small quantities. Triglycerides have very little protein. They're almost pure fat, and the body uses them to store energy.

- ✔ **Total cholesterol:** This isn't literally another type of cholesterol. The term refers to a measure of the total amount of cholesterol in your blood.

To help separate the good cholesterol from the bad stuff in your mind, just remember **Lousy DeaL:** Low-density lipids (LDLs) are the "bad" cholesterol behind plaque formation.

You really don't need to eat *any* cholesterol after the age of one because your liver produces enough cholesterol on its own. Animal products such as meat, eggs, and dairy foods are especially high in cholesterol. Even though people don't need to eat these types of food to get enough cholesterol, most folks enjoy meat, cheese, birthday cake (which is full of butter and eggs), and other good stuff packed with cholesterol.

To find out the shape your blood is in, your doctor checks your cholesterol and triglyceride levels by taking a blood sample. The results, a *cholesterol profile* or *a lipoprotein analysis,* include your LDL, HDL, total cholesterol, and triglyceride levels. Using this information, your doctor can identify problems with your lipids and evaluate your risk of atherosclerosis.

## Decoding your numbers

The more we know about cholesterol, the more complex our cholesterol reports get. Once upon a time we just got numbers that told us whether our good and bad cholesterol were good, borderline, or bad. It's not so simple any more. Each of those four cholesterol numbers we mentioned before presents a whole range of possibilities. In the case of some of them (total cholesterol, for instance) lower is better. In others (HDL — remember, that's your *good* cholesterol), a higher number is more favorable. Here's how to decipher your report:

- ✔ **Total cholesterol,** roughly speaking, is considered to be good if it's under 200, bad if it's over 240, and marginal or borderline if it's somewhere in between. Your doctor may help you set a more specific individual goal, though, if you're at high risk for heart disease based on weight, lifestyle, or family history. In such a case you may be advised to get far less than 100.

- ✔ **HDL** (good cholesterol) tends to be higher in women than in men, though it often drops after menopause. Recent recommendations put *good* HDL ranges at 60 or more, marginal HDL between 41 and 59, and worrisome HDL levels at about 40 or below.

- ✔ **LDL**, or bad cholesterol, has even more specific ranges. Optimal is less than 100, but anything between 100 and 129 is probably fine. Numbers between 130 and 159 are considered borderline high, 160 to 189 is high, and anything over that means you need to work with your doctor, pronto, to get your bad cholesterol down to a safer level.

- ✔ **Triglycerides** have their own numbers, too: less than 150 is normal; 151 to 199 is borderline; high is 200 to 499; and any triglyceride level charted at 500 or above is considered very high.

## Looking at the factors

We all know that you are what you eat, but diet isn't the only thing that controls your blood cholesterol. Exercise, insulin, obesity, and age also influence cholesterol levels.

Your genes probably have the biggest influence on your cholesterol profile. Your mother, for example, might nibble on salads, avoid desserts, and banish butter from her plate. Despite her low-fat eating habits, your mother's cholesterol profile could actually be worse than your dad's — even if he loves to eat cholesterol-intensive grilled cheese sandwiches and enjoys milk shakes with his grandchildren (when he's not snacking on a cream-of-something soup). It may not seem fair, but it happens. Genes are powerful things. (Want to read more on the respective roles of genes and diets in controlling your cholesterol? Check out *Controlling Cholesterol for Dummies* by Carol Ann Rinzler and Martin W. Graf., M.D. [Wiley])

## Regulating estrogen's role

*Estradiol* (the active type of estrogen) plays a major role in the way lipids are produced, managed, broken down, and eliminated from the body. Estradiol also seems to help dilate the blood vessels and keep them from having spasms. This may be part of the reason that women are prone to cardiovascular problems after menopause.

Natural estradiol is one thing, but hormone therapy is another when it comes to protecting your cardiovascular system. Take a look at Chapter 11 for more details on this subject, but here's the most recent word on hormones and your heart. Fair warning — it's a little bit surprising.

First, we know that estrogen increases the level of good cholesterol (HDL) in the blood, and lowers the level of bad (LDL) cholesterol. We also know that lowering bad cholesterol and raising good cholesterol is generally associated with better heart health.

But new findings on the effects of hormone therapy on heart disease and women seem to contradict this. In fact, the study found two surprising things. First, women in the study taking estrogen and progestin were 29 percent more likely to have a heart attack, and *twice* as likely to have a stroke than women taking a placebo, or mock drug. Furthermore, women taking estrogen alone received no significant heart benefits from taking estrogen therapy.

The bottom line on heart health and hormones hasn't been written yet. Women from both groups — estrogen alone and estrogen plus progestin — will continue to be followed up for a number of years. During this time, researchers will try to figure out this apparent contradiction. We'll talk more in Chapter 11 and in Chapter 16 about how to figure out what this means for you as you make your own decisions about hormone therapy.

## Connecting the dots between cholesterol and cardiovascular disease

If your artery walls are injured (as a result of smoking, cocaine-use, diabetes, or other factors), your body may react too aggressively in repairing the walls. White blood cells come to the rescue and bring cholesterol with them to patch over the damaged area. After a while, other stuff adheres to the spot and this patch becomes harder, similar to a callus. This harder stuff is called *plaque*. This is how bad habits or disease can lead to hardening of the arteries — what your doctor refers to as *atherosclerosis*.

Sometimes people have way too much LDL cholesterol and not enough HDL to carry it out of their bloodstream. When this happens, LDL cholesterol gets deposited on the artery walls and rots. (Antioxidants can prevent the rotting, which is one reason that nutritionists tell folks to get plenty of antioxidants if they want to be good to their hearts.) Other substances then collect with the rotting cholesterol to form plaque. This is how high cholesterol can lead to hardening of the arteries.

Antioxidants are substances, such as vitamins A, C, E, or beta-carotene, that protect cells from damaging oxidation, which appears to encourage aging and certain diseases.

The latter process is a lot like the buildup that causes the drains in your kitchen sink to clog. Garbage goes down your sink every day, and every day, a little bit of gunk gets stuck on your pipes. Pretty soon the gunk buildup slows down the water as it moves through the pipes.

With time, calcium begins to form on the plaque, hardening the arteries. Now your arteries are narrowed and hardened, and blood has a hard time flowing to the heart. Just as the water backs up in your sink because of the clog, the blood backs up in your arteries when they become stopped up. Narrowing arteries can force your heart to pump harder to get the blood around your body. When your blood needs more pressure than normal, you have *hypertension* (high blood pressure).

Sometimes the plaque in your artery breaks off and gets lodged in a blood vessel, as shown in Figure 6-2. Imagine pouring clog-busting chemicals down your drain; except instead of dissolving the clog, the chemicals just loosen the gunk. Then the chunk o' gunk gets stuck in the curve of the pipe. When a piece of plaque gets stuck in a blood vessel, the area of heart muscle that gets fed by that vessel dies, and you have a heart attack.

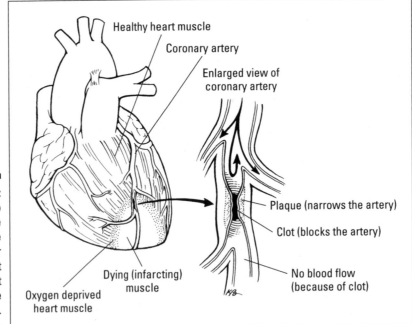

**Figure 6-2:** The thing to look at is the clog on the right. Your heart shouldn't look like this.

Healthy heart muscle

Coronary artery

Enlarged view of coronary artery

Plaque (narrows the artery)

Clot (blocks the artery)

No blood flow (because of clot)

Dying (infarcting) muscle

Oxygen deprived heart muscle

# Understanding Cardiovascular Diseases

A whole family of diseases affects your cardiovascular system, and a lot of inbreeding goes on in this family. For example, high cholesterol can lead to hardening of the arteries. Hardening of the arteries can lead to heart attack or stroke as well as angina. Hypertension can lead to heart attack or stroke. It goes round and round and your risk of all these conditions increases as your natural estrogen levels decline after menopause.

In this section, we introduce you to the members of the cardiovascular-disease family. Don't worry, we talk about preventing and treating unexpected visits from these conditions, too.

## Containing coronary artery disease

*Coronary artery disease (CAD)* affects the blood vessels (the *coronary arteries*) that supply blood to your heart muscle. If these vessels are damaged, or if you have too much cholesterol in your blood, coronary arteries become narrowed or blocked by plaque as cholesterol and calcium build up inside them. This process is called hardening of the arteries, or *atherosclerosis.* When the heart doesn't get enough oxygenated blood because of partially or totally blocked arteries, your heart muscle pays the price. The result is *coronary heart disease.* Coronary heart disease may cause angina (chest pain that we talk about in the "Avoiding angina" section later in this chapter) or a heart attack (check out the "Holding off heart attacks" section also found later in this chapter). Here's a depressing factoid: Nearly a million women in the United States develop coronary heart disease during the course of a year.

 Women often underestimate the severity of their chest pains or don't realize that the chest pains are related to heart problems; therefore, they play down the symptoms to their physician. A couple of the reasons women give for not seeking help immediately are that they didn't want to inconvenience anyone and that they thought that heart disease was a guy thing.

## Avoiding angina

To function properly, the heart muscle needs a constant supply of oxygen and nutrients delivered by the blood. If your veins or arteries become narrowed by fatty buildup in the artery walls (atherosclerosis), you may experience severe chest pain called *angina.* You feel pain because insufficient amounts of blood are getting through your veins into your heart muscle, and your heart is straining to pump enough blood to keep your body going strong.

Angina can also be caused by spasms in the blood vessels that block blood flow to the heart. Spasms can occur even if no blockages are present. Women are much more likely than men to suffer angina with no evidence of blockages.

Symptoms sometimes begin during physical activity or emotional stress. They typically last about ten minutes and go away after several minutes of rest. But many women experience chest pain while they're resting. This is typically triggered by spasms or an *arrhythmia* (irregular heartbeat).

Pay attention to warning signs. As a woman, you may not feel the typical crushing, squeezing, heaviness, or burning chest pain that many men feel prior to a heart attack. Instead you may experience one or more of the following symptoms:

- Back pain
- Bloating
- Chest pain while resting
- Fatigue
- Heartburn or abdominal pain
- Jaw pain
- Joint pain
- Lightheadedness/fainting
- Shortness of breath
- Sweating

Attention all women! Angina is a very common early warning sign of coronary artery disease (CAD). Because CAD is so lethal in women, heart specialists typically schedule further tests right away for women with severe chest pains. (For more on coronary artery disease, check out the "Containing coronary artery disease" section earlier in this chapter.)

Unfortunately, a survey studying how emergency-room doctors treated patients with severe chest pain showed that men received much more aggressive and quicker treatment than women did. Also, men were twice as likely as women to be sent for *coronary arteriography* (a special test that looks at the coronary arteries) and bypass surgery after complaining of chest pain. If you go to the emergency room with chest pain or anything else that could be symptoms of a heart attack, insist — or make sure whoever accompanies you insists — that a heart attack be taken into serious consideration as a possible cause.

# Holding off heart attacks

Menopausal and postmenopausal women are at an increased risk of heart attack (*myocardial infarction* in medicalese). Most women experience heart attacks after age 60, but heart disease may begin as early as the preteen years. Cholesterol accumulations have been found in girls as young as ten years old. These accumulations in young children, called *fatty streaks,* sometimes turn into more significant buildup later in life.

Blocked arteries often cause heart attacks. Either plaque breaks loose or a *blood clot* (a mass of solidified blood) blocks an artery cutting off blood supply to the heart. If the blockage remains in place for 5 to 10 minutes or more, the piece of the heart muscle fed by that artery begins to die.

Vessel spasms and arrhythmia are two additional causes of heart attacks, and evidence suggests that they're more common triggers of heart attack in women than in men. *Spasms* constrict your coronary arteries so blood can't get to the heart. Spasms can also cause plaque to break away from the vessel and get lodged in an artery, cutting off blood supply that way. *Arrhythmia,* or an irregular heartbeat, can mess up the pumping action of the heart and cut off blood supply as well.

Women often have different symptoms before a heart attack than men do. The symptoms are easy to overlook because they're often subtle and typical of many other, less serious problems. Often, women look back and say, "Oh yeah, now that you mention it, I felt that way yesterday," after the heart attack has already occurred.

An unfortunate byproduct of a heart attack is a condition called ventricular fibrillation. *Ventricular fibrillation* refers to an irregular heartbeat that happens when the main pumping chambers of the heart, the *ventricles,* can't get coordinated; therefore, the blood can't get to the far reaches of the body.

African-American women are at one-third greater risk of heart attack than are Caucasian women, probably because of their increased level of risk for two prominent risk factors for heart attack: diabetes and hypertension. If you're African-American, be especially vigilant about living a heart-healthy lifestyle and monitoring your cholesterol and blood sugar.

# Fending off hypertension

High blood pressure is another one of those health issues that's more likely to pop up as you get older. Until age 55, women usually have lower blood pressure than men. Between 55 and 65 years of age, women and men are about equal in the incidence of high blood pressure. After 65, more women than men have high blood pressure. So, just when you're dealing with all the symptoms connected with menopause, you may develop high blood pressure (your doctor may call it *hypertension*).

About half of all Caucasian women and three-quarters of African-American women over 50 have hypertension. For some reason, African-American women are more prone to hypertension than Caucasian women. Mexican-American women have about as high a chance of having hypertension as Caucasians, but Cuban-American and Puerto Rican women have lower incidence of hypertension.

No one knows why people develop high blood pressure. About 5 percent of the time, high blood pressure is caused by a condition such as diabetes or pregnancy, and it often goes away with treatment or resolution of the precipitating condition.

To visualize high blood pressure, think of blowing up a balloon. As you hold the balloon opening to your mouth and blow, the air in your mouth is under a great deal of pressure because you're trying to pass it through the small opening in the balloon. Now, think of your heart as your cheeks and your arteries as the balloon opening — the smaller the balloon opening, the more pressure in your cheeks as you try to blow. So, if your blood vessels get smaller due to cholesterol buildup, or whatever, your heart has to pump harder to pass the blood through these narrower openings. The result: Your blood pressure rises.

High blood pressure can lead to heart attack, kidney damage, bleeding in the retina behind your eyes, and stroke. For these reasons, having your blood pressure checked routinely after you reach 40 (or at any age) is critical.

Many women develop high blood pressure because of obesity. Fortunately, these women often can reduce their blood pressure dramatically by switching to a heart-healthy diet (see Chapter 18) and losing weight.

If you're not overweight, you may need to try some other types of intervention. Some women are able to regulate their blood pressure by reducing anxiety through meditation or other relaxation techniques. If these techniques don't work, medication may be the answer to getting your blood pressure under control. You may have to work with your doctor to find just the right type of drug and dosage. One drug may work for others but not for you. And, for some reason, drugs used to control blood pressure are more effective in men than women.

## Staving off stroke

A stroke can occur for one of two reasons: either a blood clot blocks the flow of blood to your brain or a blood vessel in your brain ruptures. In either case, oxygen-rich blood can't get to the brain to nourish it. The problems a stroke causes depend on the location and severity of the stroke, but speech problems, physical weakness, paralysis, and permanent brain damage are all possible stroke complications. Many stroke victims go through rehabilitation programs that restore full or partial function to the affected areas of the body.

Here are the symptoms associated with strokes:

✔ Difficulty talking or understanding speech

✔ Dizziness

✔ Loss of vision, particularly in just one eye

✔ Unexplained numbness or weakness in the face, an arm, a leg, or one side of your body

A *transient ischemic attack (TIA)* is like a mini-stroke. During a TIA, blood flow to the brain is interrupted (usually by a blood clot). The symptoms of a TIA usually last only 10 to 20 minutes and end when blood flow returns to normal. At worst, the symptoms of a TIA last 24 hours; symptoms of a stroke can last a lifetime. Pay attention to TIAs because they can be early warning signs of an impending stroke. Half the people who have a TIA suffer a stroke within a year.

If you have any of the symptoms listed in conjunction with the stroke discussion, call your doctor or 9-1-1 immediately. Seeking *immediate* treatment for stroke is critical to your best chances of a full recovery.

# Checking Out Your Risk Factors for Cardiovascular Disease

Many of the risk factors for complications related to cardiovascular disease are more risky for women (particularly menopausal women) than men, but many are risk factors for both men and women — even men and women who seem to be in good health:

✔ **Alcohol:** Women don't produce as much of a specific enzyme used to break down alcohol (*alcohol dehydrogenase*) as men do. So women tend to feel the buzz from alcohol earlier than men, and alcohol stays in their systems longer. Three or four drinks a day will cause a noticeable rise in blood pressure. (We outline the dangers of high blood pressure in the earlier "Fending off hypertension" section.) In large doses, alcohol acts as a poison and kills heart tissue.

✔ **Cholesterol:** Low HDL levels and a high LDL-to-HDL ratio increase a woman's risk for cardiovascular disease. After menopause, most women's HDL levels drop a little bit. A bigger change takes place in your LDL level. As women age, LDL levels keep rising — especially between the ages of 40 and 60. So your HDL and LDL levels and your LDL-to-HDL ratio are usually worse as you age.

✔ **Cocaine use:** Cocaine and its relative — crack — are seriously danger-ous drugs. Cocaine, whether snorted, smoked, or injected, can cause serious damage to women's arteries and heart. Cocaine and crack use can cause spasms in the coronary arteries, restrict oxygen flow to the heart, and cause arrhythmia. If a woman has a previous coronary-related condition such as a *mitral valve prolapse* (heart murmur), cocaine can cause sudden death.

✔ **Diabetes:** High blood pressure, excessive weight, and inactivity can lead to adult-onset diabetes in women. Although adult-onset diabetes isn't real common, it's very serious for menopausal women. Diabetes can cause a host of other problems, one of which is an increased risk of heart disease. Here's the scoop on women, diabetes, and cardiovascular disease:

  • Women over 45 (menopausal women) are twice as likely as men their age to develop diabetes.

  • Women with diabetes are more than five times as likely to have some type of coronary "event" (we're not talking about a gala here; we're talking about a heart attack, angina, and so on) than women without diabetes.

  • Women with diabetes are four times more likely to die of a heart attack. In fact, 80 percent of all people who suffer from diabetes die of heart attacks

Fortunately, adult onset diabetes can often be prevented or controlled through weight loss, exercise, and a healthy diet.

✔ **Excessive weight:** If you weigh 20 percent or more than your target weight, you're overweight. (Chapter 18 has a chart you can use to deter-mine where you are in relation to your target weight.) For example, if your *target weight* (how much people your height and build should weigh) is 125, you're overweight if you weigh 150 pounds or more. Excessive weight increases your risk of high blood pressure, heart dis-ease, stroke, and even diabetes. Because excessive weight leads to many diseases and complications, it only makes sense that losing the exces-sive weight can lower your risk for many diseases and complications. Excessive weight is a huge and growing problem (no pun intended) — more than one-third of all Caucasian women and half of all African-American women in the United States are overweight.

✔ **High blood pressure:** High blood pressure can lead to heart attacks and stroke because it stresses out the blood vessels. Stress on your blood vessels can constrict the arteries and cause plaque to separate from the vessel wall and clog your arteries.

**Inactivity:** For women, inactivity is the most common risk factor for cardiovascular disease. Most women never had the time or chance to incorporate a "workout" into their busy schedules. Chauffeuring chil-dren and performing household chores, intermingled with a 40- to 50-hour workweek, often leaves women with no time or desire to take a walk or regularly attend an exercise class. Husbands and children (aren't they precious?) may question how you can waste an hour on an activity that doesn't directly benefit them or the household. Well, the fact is that you must make the time (just as your husband or kids do) for physical activity. Physical activity is not a waste of time — it lowers a woman's risk of heart problems by a whopping 50 percent. And keep in mind that half of all women die of cardiovascular disease. Take a look at Chapter 19 for some ideas on increasing your activity level.

✔ **Personality:** Many people believe that too much stress results in high blood pressure and heart attacks. Whether you're talking monkeys or people, the research indicates that it's a control thing, not a just a stress thing. Women (and monkeys) who feel in control of their lives are much less likely to have heart disease. Cholesterol profiles are also much better for women who feel in control of their jobs, lives, or homes. When you feel out of control, you're more likely to feel cynical or hostile, or you may feel sorry for yourself. Researchers have also linked these personality traits to a higher incidence of heart disease.

✔ **Smoking:** Cigarette smoking triples your risk of heart attack and angina. Even women who smoke fewer than five cigarettes a day double their risk of heart disease. When you inhale smoke, your heart beats faster, your blood vessels constrict, and your circulation slows down. The nicotine in cigarettes promotes blood clots (which can lodge in your arteries to cause heart attacks or stroke). Smokers also have a greater risk of high blood pressure and emphysema.

# Being Smart about Your Heart

Eating a healthy diet, watching your weight, exercising routinely, avoiding unhealthy habits, and getting annual medical examinations are the best ways to prevent cardiovascular problems.

## Weighing an ounce of prevention

Keeping your blood clean and lean really helps prevent hardening of the arteries, which is the source of many serious problems. Controlling your cholesterol boils down to eliminating unhealthy habits (smoking, drinking too much alcohol, using recreational drugs, and so on), sticking to a healthy diet (check out Chapter 18), and exercising five days a week for a half-hour (turn to Chapter 19).

If you're not able to control your cholesterol through lifestyle changes, you and your doctor can consider alternatives. A variety of medications are available today that can lower your cholesterol.

But many people develop hypertension even though their cholesterol levels are terrific. Doctors always seem to check your blood pressure as soon as you step in the door. So keep those doctor appointments and, if your blood pressure is high, seek help. Your doctor will work with you to find the right medication for you, but you're the one who has to take it every day if it's going to work.

Routine checkups (that means at least once a year) with your internist and gynecologist should prevent cardiovascular problems from sneaking up on you.

## Treating what ails you

If you maintain regular appointments and seek help when you feel any weird happenings in your heart (such as palpitations or pain), you should be pretty safe. Of course, you have to follow the advice given to you by professionals when problems are detected. If you have high blood pressure, you need to take your medication. Even though you usually have no symptoms with hypertension, not taking your medication can cause trouble — same goes for cholesterol. Many people have no symptoms when their cholesterol is high, but if they go untreated, faulty cholesterol levels can cause a world of problems.

Today, a variety of medications are available to treat these conditions. Sometimes you and your doctor will have to experiment a bit to find out which medicines work for you, but the effort is worth it because the reward is a prolonged life.

# Chapter 7

# Dealing with Vaginal and Urinary Changes

....................................................................

*In This Chapter*

▶ Getting the scoop on vaginal and urinary changes

▶ Starting a dialogue with your doc

▶ Treating vaginal dryness

▶ Understanding the shape urine

....................................................................

*I*f you think it's difficult talking to your mom about menopause, envision talking to her about the vaginal and urinary problems associated with the change. Probably not going to happen? Join the club. Many women live with discomfort because they're too embarrassed to discuss these problems with anyone — not even their doctors.

In this chapter, we open the discussion so you can not only understand the potential vaginal and urinary issues you may encounter, but also so you can feel free to discuss these problems openly with your doctor and get the treatment you need.

## Understanding the Normalcy of Vaginal and Urinary Changes

Someday, you may notice that your vagina doesn't seem to be performing its lubricating duties like it used to when you're about to engage in sex. Or maybe sex is becoming a bit uncomfortable. Your private parts may be dry, and you may experience itching around your vulva or in your vagina, a watery vaginal discharge, or a burning sensation when you pee. The medical term for this is *atrophic vaginitis,* or *vaginal atrophy* in more common terms.

Vaginal and urinary issues are not unique to menopausal women — some women experience vaginal dryness during sex long before they're menopausal, and other women who have been menopausal for several years have no problems with vaginal dryness. Some women experience vaginal irritation only temporarily; others find it gets worse with age. It's a very individual thing.

If you live long enough, without hormone therapy or some type of treatment, your vaginal lining is going to thin and become drier, but you may never experience any of the symptoms, pain, or discomfort. You may never even know that it's happening. Some women notice dryness during sex or itching that lasts a few months while their bodies adjust to the lower estrogen levels. Other women may experience discomfort during sex at first and then more intense symptoms as time goes on. If you do experience discomfort, you don't have to simply put up with it — many treatments are available.

Your urinary tract and your female organs are located next to each other, and both systems rely on estrogen to function properly. These two facts explain why problems can arise in both systems during the change and why changes in your vagina may affect your urinary tract.

# Talking Shop with Your Doc

Before you can do anything about urinary-tract or vaginal problems, you must have a doctor diagnose your condition. Many vaginal symptoms have nothing to do with menopause, so seeing a medical expert is critical.

You may think that talking to your doctor about painful sex or problems with your plumbing is embarrassing, but get over it. Your doctor has heard it all before. Doctors are supposed to ask you about them, but if they don't, you should bring the issues up.

Here are some tips for talking to your doctor about your symptoms:

- **Keep track:** You need to plan ahead for your visit to the doctor. If you experience vaginal or urinary-tract pain, keep track of when it hurts, where it hurts, the presence or absence of discharge, the color of the discharge, and any other details. If you experience urine leakage, write down what time you urinated, how much urine was involved (use any measure you're comfortable with — cups, ounces, teaspoons, whatever — and let the doctor do the conversion), and what triggered the accident. Also note any type of discomfort and the level of pain.

- **Be specific:** When you discuss matters with your doctor, don't just say that you're uncomfortable "down there" and then lift your eyebrows to make your point. Tell the doc specifically what symptoms you're experiencing.

> ✔ **Be persistent:** If the doctor's response isn't helpful — "That's normal for women your age" — press him on the issue to get the advice and help you need to deal with the problem. Just because "it's normal" doesn't mean that it can't be helped.

# Overcoming Vaginal Changes

Many women fear that the natural result of menopause is that their vagina dries out, shrivels up, and becomes a sexual wasteland. Well, that doesn't have to happen. In fact, *fewer than half* of all postmenopausal women complain of vaginal dryness or other symptoms of vaginal atrophy.

Who came up with the term *vaginal atrophy?* The term *atrophy* makes you think of stagnant, dead things, doesn't it? When we hear *atrophy,* we think of those plump little worms that get stranded on a sidewalk after a rainstorm and end up dried out and dead. Look up the word *atrophy* in the dictionary — it means "wasting away" and "failure to grow because of lack of nutrition." But don't worry — you have way more options than that poor little worm does.

## Understanding what vaginal atrophy is and what it isn't

We're going to start by describing what vaginal atrophy is not. It's not a condition that occurs only in women after menopause, and it doesn't mean your vagina is going to shrivel up and blow away.

So what is *vaginal atrophy?* Glad you asked. Because estrogen keeps your vagina moist and elastic, loss of estrogen can cause it to become drier, thinner, and less elastic. The downturn in estrogen production can also cause your vagina to shrink slightly in terms of width and length.

An atrophic vagina has lost some of its plumpness and firmness because the lining has thinned, and it doesn't have the furrows and folds typical of a fertile vagina. (Yes, this is one case in which wrinkles are a sign of youth.) The vagina appears red instead of pink. Also, with less mucous, the vagina becomes less acidic, so it's easier for bacteria to grow, which causes the watery discharge some women experience.

Talk to your doctor about vaginal changes if you experience discomfort. Dryness and other vaginal-atrophy-related symptoms may prompt you to avoid sex just when you have more time for it. Don't be embarrassed to bring it up — your doctor knows of plenty of ways to fix this one.

# Looking at what less estrogen means for your vagina

Estrogen bathes the vagina (and your urinary tract), keeping the tissue lubricated and flexible. Estrogen is the secret behind keeping the female organs working like a well-oiled machine.

Here's what the relative lack of estrogen that menopause brings about can mean to you:

- ✔ Your vagina becomes more susceptible to tears or damage from friction.

    Sexually transmitted diseases have an easier time invading your body through tears than through an intact lining. So, step up your protection after menopause. Also, because tearing your vagina is easier after menopause, watch the rough stuff.

- ✔ As vaginal tissues lose their elasticity, your vagina may become less pliant and sometimes smaller. Sex may be less enjoyable if you don't intervene with some type of therapy to improve pliability and lubrication.

- ✔ Your vagina may not get as lubricated during sexual arousal as it did before menopause, so intercourse may be painful if you don't use a lubricant.

- ✔ Vaginal mucous keeps your vagina an acidic kind of place. This acidic environment destroys much of the bacteria introduced into the area (through sex or wiping after you go to the bathroom). When your production of vaginal mucous declines, infections find it easier to grow in your vagina. After menopause, you become more susceptible to vaginal bacteria, so you can develop *bacterial vaginosis* (inflammation of the vagina caused by bacterial infection).

# Doing something about vaginal atrophy

For some women, the easiest way to prevent or slow down the progress of vaginal atrophy (and probably the most enjoyable one) is to practice regular sexual activity. Sexual activity increases blood circulation and lubrication and promotes vaginal elasticity. If you don't have a sexual partner, masturbation provides the same benefits.

If dryness inhibits your sexual desire, or makes you anxious or nervous about sex, try one of the many lubricants available over the counter. Some of the lubricants are for use during sexual activity; others act as moisturizers and cause your vagina to absorb water. Some women also find that vitamin E relieves dryness. Break open a capsule and apply the oil directly to your vagina. Even if you use an over the counter product, though, you should still mention the problem to your doctor, who may have better options to recommend.

Avoid any lubricants that contain mineral oil or ingredients that begin with "petro." These can promote bacterial infections, and can also damage diaphragms and condoms.

Applying estrogen cream to the vagina also provides relief from the pain and itching associated with vaginal dryness. Your best bet is to use these medications as prescribed by your physician. If you have a history of any condition that prevents you from taking hormone therapy, be sure to discuss the use of hormone-based vaginal creams with your doctor to make sure they're safe for you.

Vaginal estrogen creams seem more effective for relieving discomfort due to dryness than oral hormone treatments. Although most of the estrogen stays in your vagina, some is absorbed into your bloodstream. However, doctors usually prescribe such a low dosage for this problem that using a vaginal estrogen cream shouldn't substantially increase your risk of endometrial cancer or breast cancer as oral estrogen does. In fact, vaginal creams are often prescribed for women who don't want to take hormones orally because they're at higher risk of endometrial or breast cancer. Still, there have been some reports of increased breast development in *men* whose sexual partners use estrogen creams, so we know they can get into your bloodstream (or his).

As with hormone therapy (HT) and estrogen pills, you need a prescription from your doctor for these creams.

By the way, you can use a lubricant during sex in addition to the estrogen cream to keep things slippery.

Before we change subjects, here's one last tip: Drinking plenty of water keeps your entire body hydrated, including your vagina. Think of yourself as an athlete in training and follow an athlete's regimen: Drink more water. Drink less alcohol and coffee.

# Talking about Urinary Problems

A healthy urinary tract depends on healthy tissue and toned muscle around the plumbing. About 40 percent of women between the ages of 45 and 64 have urinary-tract problems, which mainly take the form of *incontinence* (inability to hold back urine). You may never have a urinary-tract problem, but if you do, you'll know the basics because in this section, we arm you with the information you need to know.

## Getting a grip on types of urinary problems

Urinary-tract problems are no longer kept in the closet as they once were. Everyday, it seems another famous actor appears on a TV commercial confessing his or her problem. Many products are available to help control or eliminate urinary disorders so that you can enjoy all the activities you've always participated in. Ask you doctor about appropriate courses of treatment.

Your *urinary tract* moves liquid waste from your kidneys, through your bladder, and out to the toilet. For the most part, it consists of your kidneys, bladder, *ureter* (the duct that carries urine from the kidney to the bladder), and urethra. But never mind the technicalities, the relevant fact is that urinary-tract conditions are more common in women after menopause.

Bet you didn't know this: The end of the *urethra* (the little tube that your urine flows from) is more dependent on estrogen than any other part of your urinary tract. After menopause, when estrogen has been low for a period of time, that tube can become inflexible. Simultaneously, the collagen and connective tissue (the fleshy stuff) around your urethra that supports your plumbing gets thinner. So three problems can occur:

- ✔ With less flexibility and thinner tissue in and around your urethra, you're more likely to get some microscopic tearing that makes it easier for bacteria to enter the urethra. Therefore, urinary-tract infections (UTIs) can get started more easily.

- ✔ An overall decrease in your level of estrogen occurs at about the same time that some women develop a painful and little-understood bladder disease called interstitial cystitis.

- ✔ The urethra has a harder time sealing itself using pressure, so you may leak or dribble urine when you least expect it and have instances of incontinence.

Nearly one of every six women over 45 develops one of these urinary-tract problems. So don't feel embarrassed when you talk to your doctor. These problems are quite common and very treatable. But infections only become worse with time, so go to the doctor right away if you think you've got problems with your plumbing.

Take a look at the "Talking Shop with Your Doc" section earlier in this chapter for recommendations on recording your symptoms in preparation for your visit to the doctor. For urinary-tract problems, you can talk to either your gynecologist or primary-care physician. Your doctor will refer you to a specialist if needed, but most of the time, a gynecologist or primary-care physician can handle these issues. We're not here to diagnose your problems, but in the following sections, we tell you a bit about each of these conditions and what your doctor might do about them.

# Tracking urinary-tract infections

A whole slew of urinary-tract infections (UTIs) are out there, and they can affect areas of your bladder, kidneys, and so on. One thing all UTIs have in common is that they're mainly caused by bacteria entering your plumbing from your urethra.

The most common UTI, *cystitis,* affects your bladder. Women are more prone to bladder infections than men because we wipe after we use the toilet. That's right — just tidying up leads to problems. Wiping can sweep germs from your feces (bowel movements) into your urethra. These bacteria (especially E. coli) can travel all the way to your bladder (or further into your kidneys) and create an infection. (That's why you should always follow your mother's advice — wipe from front to back.) Your urethra is also shorter than a man's, making the trip to the bladder shorter and easier for bacteria.

Frequent or vigorous sex can harm the delicate tissue of the vulva and outer urethra, which in turn allows bacteria into the body causing urinary-tract infections. Peeing immediately after sex helps you avoid UTIs by flushing out unfriendly bacteria.

## Getting to a diagnosis

If you have a urinary-tract infection, it usually starts with a burning sensation or pain when urinating accompanied by urgency, frequency, or both. (*Urgency* refers to feeling as though your bladder is so full it's about to burst and you can't make it to the bathroom. *Frequency* is that feeling that you have to go to the bathroom constantly.)

If you have a UTI, you may find yourself rushing to the bathroom, releasing just a trickle of urine, and then a short time later, feeling as if you have to go again. This pattern is especially irritating at night. Repeatedly waking up to shuffle off to the bathroom can leave you exhausted.

You may also notice that your urine is cloudy, has blood in it, or smells badly. If the infection is in your kidneys, you may have a fever, chills, back pain, nausea, or vomiting.

Urgency, frequency, and pain related to peeing are also symptoms of other conditions. If you experience any or all of these symptoms, make an appointment with your medical advisor. You'll have to do the pee-in-a-cup routine so that the professionals can examine your urine to determine whether you have a UTI or some other condition. The tests your doctor may run include

✔ **Urinalysis:** The doc examines the urine under a microscope for white blood cells (which indicate an infection), bacteria, and so on.

✔ **Urine culture:** Your doctor sends your urine sample to a laboratory to find out exactly what type of bacteria are present.

### Trying some treatments

Treatment usually includes a short course of antibiotics and instructions to drink plenty of fluids.

Drinking several glasses of unsweetened cranberry juice every day also helps your recovery from a bladder infection. Cranberry juice makes urine more acidic, thereby making it more difficult for bacteria to grow.

Don't use cranberry juice as an alternative to visiting your doctor if you think you may have a urinary-tract infection. Some dangerous conditions can develop if a urinary tract is left untreated.

## Covering interstitial cystitis

Interstitial cystitis (IC) is often overlooked or misdiagnosed as a urinary-tract infection because the symptoms are so similar, but it's actually a bladder disease. Interstitial cystitis is often called *painful bladder syndrome (PBS)* because its symptoms include general pelvic pain or pressure.

IC is rare, yet nearly a million people suffer from it each year in the United States, and 90 percent of these are women. It can occur in women who have reached menopause, but some women also develop IC in their 20s or 30s.

Some medical professionals wonder aloud whether there's a link between hormones and IC. We've mentioned that tissues in the bladder and throughout the urinary tract rely on estrogen. Well, the nerve-endings do too. When estrogen bathes these nerve endings during your reproductive years, you don't notice any sensation in your bladder until it's quite full because estrogen keeps your sensory threshold high. But, when your estrogen levels are reduced during perimenopause and menopause, your pain threshold is lowered and you become more sensitive in your bladder area. Here are more clues that suggest a possible role for hormones in connection with IC:

✔ The average age of an IC sufferer is 42.

✔ Premenopausal women who have IC seem to have recurrences during the part of the menstrual cycle when estrogen levels are falling.

### Getting to a diagnosis

If you have IC, your doctor won't find any bacteria when he analyzes your urine sample, even though the symptoms of IC are similar to those of a bacterial bladder infection (frequent urination — especially at night — a sudden urge to urinate, and pain that becomes worse as the bladder fills up). Sometimes the pain, which can get very intense during urination, subsides after urination. The symptoms may go away from time to time. It's all quite mysterious.

Sometimes the pain is pretty generalized and occupies your entire pelvic area. You may feel pressure, tenderness, or pain in your bladder and the area around your bladder. If you're still menstruating, the pain may get worse just before your periods. You may also have pain during intercourse.

Diagnosing IC isn't easy. In their search for a cause of your symptoms, doctors initially go through a process of elimination, testing for UTIs and other conditions. After they eliminate these other possible causes, docs may take a peak at your bladder by inserting a scope up through your urethra into your bladder (this is called a *cystoscopy*, and though it's about as much fun as it sounds, you are given an anesthetic to help you through it) to look for scarring or microscopic tears on the walls inside your bladder.

### Trying some treatments

The treatment options range from the least invasive — modifying your diet — to the most invasive — bladder surgery to repair the walls or remove the entire bladder.

Some women find that eliminating certain foods from their diet helps relieve bladder irritation. These foods include alcohol, coffee, tobacco, sharp cheeses, artificial sweeteners, preservatives, and acidic foods. Dyes used in food and medicines have also been found to irritate the bladder or cause bladder spasms.

Between modifying your diet and having surgery, you may find success with some medications: There are several medications in use for the treatment of IC, including antidepressants, antihistamines, and mild analgesic narcotics can manage the pain. Only one, Elmiron, has been approved just for IC; it has been found to repair some of the damage on the bladder wall.

Antibiotics are ineffective in treating an IC. Women misdiagnosed with a urinary-tract infection find that the antibiotics prescribed for that condition do little to help relieve the symptoms of IC.

## Encountering incontinence

Three-year-olds have a hard time "holding it" when they don't recognize the signal telling them that they have to pee until it's too late. Later in life (after babies, surgery, and menopause) some women again have trouble "holding it," but for different reasons. Sometimes, your body doesn't follow the orders your brain calls out.

When you can't hold back urine, or urine leaks out when you don't want it to, you may be *incontinent*. Lower levels of estrogen contribute to reduced muscle tone in the urethra, so you can lose bladder control. Wear and tear on muscles from bearing children or surgery can make the problem even worse.

The urethra (the tube through which urine flows from the bladder out of your body) is controlled by having more pressure around the urethral tube than in the bladder, keeping it closed. Estrogen helps increase muscle tone that leads to increased pressure, which prevents leakage. With lower estrogen levels, the muscle fibers lose their flexibility. The urethra has a hard time making a nice tight seal where it connects to the bladder.

### Getting to a diagnosis

Incontinence comes in a couple of varieties:

- **Stress incontinence:** Urine leaks when you laugh, sneeze, or cough, or when you jump vigorously during exercise (jogging and jumping jacks can be problematic). Many women whose pelvic muscle tone is shot because of bearing children or having surgery suffer stress incontinence.

  The *stress* in *stress incontinence* has nothing to do with psychological pain you may or may not be feeling; it refers to the stress in your abdomen. When you cough or laugh, you create pressure in your abdomen, which puts pressure on the bladder, causing the bladder pressure to become greater than urethral pressure. So laughing and coughing set off a chain reaction that ends in leakage.

  About a third of the women who suffer from stress incontinence are pre-menopausal. After menopause, it can get worse.

- **Urge incontinence:** A less common type of incontinence. With urge incontinence, you feel a tremendous urge to urinate, but before you can get to the bathroom, you begin leaking. You get "caught short" because you just can't make it to the bathroom fast enough.

  Spasms in your bladder cause this type of incontinence. Urge incontinence is usually caused by a more serious medical problem such as a herniated disk in your back, *fibroids* (little, noncancerous wads of tissue), nerve damage, or even bladder cancer. Contact your doctor right away so he or she can check out this condition.

### Trying some treatments

See your doctor if you experience any type of incontinence. Incontinence may be a symptom of another medical condition, and treating the symptom may not be the best way to treat the whole disease.

Incontinence due to weakened muscles in the pelvic floor can be treated with *Kegel exercises,* which strengthen the muscles around your urethra. If you went to childbirth classes, you may have heard of these exercises. Well, Kegels are as useful in menopause as they were after childbirth.

Strengthening the muscles supporting the urethra keeps you from leaking urine when you laugh, cough, or exercise. Kegel exercises also can help you improve the muscle tone in your *pubococcygeous (PC)* muscle — the muscle you use to stop urine from flowing.

The biggest problem with Kegels is that most women aren't taught the right way to do them, so they don't get the full benefit. The nearby "Strengthening with Kegels in three easy steps" sidebar starts your Kegel program off on the right foot. Kegels can be especially effective when combined with biofeedback techniques.

Kegels can improve muscle tone, but they don't strengthen thinned tissue. If thinning tissue is the cause of incontinence, surgery may be the appropriate treatment.

Some other methods you can use to handle incontinence caused by weakened muscles include

- ✔ **Pads:** These pads are similar to the pads you wear during your menstrual period, and they function the same way — the pad absorbs leaked urine, and you change a used pad when you go to the bathroom. Gel-affixed, foam pads are also available. These little devices are either inserted like a tampon or worn over the opening of the urethra. You have to change them after urinating. This type of pad is most useful for women whose incontinence problem is primarily limited to certain activities such as exercise.

- ✔ **Watching your weight:** Maintaining a normal weight helps to relieve stress on your pelvic floor.

- ✔ **Silicone caps:** Silicone-rubber caps inserted into the urethra are now available and seem to reduce leakage by about 50 percent.

- ✔ **Teflon or collagen injections:** Some doctors are currently performing these procedures. The injected Teflon or collagen strengthens the tissues around the urethra or bladder neck by making them thicker. You normally need multiple injections.

✔ **Vaginal cones:** This approach uses little weights (vaginal cones) to strengthen muscles related to controlling urine flow. You insert a tampon-like cone into your vagina and hold it there. The goal is to gradually increase the weight and the amount of time you hold the cone in place.

Talk to your doctor about these solutions and others (such as electrical stimulation and vaginal urethral rings). Medications are available that inhibit bladder contractions, increase the fortitude of the bladder lining, or relax smooth muscle in both the urethra and bladder — all of which can help curb symptoms of incontinence. These medications include probanthine, flavoxate, oxybutynin, and imipramine — all of which control bladder spasms. As always, medications have side effects.

If your sleep is interrupted by incontinence, you restrict the amount of fluids you drink after dinner. Be sure to drink enough fluid during the day to make up for the curfew.

---

## Strengthening with Kegels in three easy steps

Every time you go to the bathroom, end the outing with a series of Kegel exercises. Although medical professionals usually say you only need do these exercises three times each day, you won't have to tax your memory if you just do them every time you urinate. If you follow this advice, you'll ensure that you're exercising routinely and frequently — two requirements for successfully strengthening the pubococcygeous (PC) muscle, which helps you stop urine from flowing. Here are the three steps to a stronger PC:

1. While you're urinating, squeeze the muscle you use to stop the flow of urine. Now that you've found your PC muscle, you're ready for the workout.

2. Squeeze the PC muscle for 3 seconds (one one-thousand, two one-thousand, three one-thousand) and then relax for 5 seconds.

Try to squeeze only your PC muscle, keeping your thigh, abdomen, and buttocks muscles relaxed. Squeezing the other muscles actually works against the exercise because it creates pressure above the urethra, which makes it difficult to squeeze the PC muscle. Do this exercise five times every time you go to the bathroom.

3. Work up to holding each squeeze for 10 seconds and relaxing for 5 seconds in between squeezes. Continue doing five of these each time you go to the bathroom.

After 6 to 8 weeks, you should notice an improvement in your ability to control the flow of your urine. Practice while you're actually urinating to see if you can completely stop the flow.

# Chapter 8

# Examining Your Skin and Hair on Menopause

### In This Chapter

▶ Ironing out the hormone-induced wrinkles and other skin changes

▶ Putting a cap on thinning hair

▶ Telling substance from snake oil

*N*o, you're not going crazy or losing your mind if you think that your skin has gotten drier over the years. Face it — dry skin happens. And it's likely to be related — at least in part — to menopause. Depending on which scientists you believe, the sags and wrinkles in your face may or may not be due to lower levels of estrogen. Don't worry — we give you both sides of the story in this chapter.

Dealing with your hair can get a little, well, hairy, too. If you're like us, as a child, you watched an aunt or grandma in total amazement, wondering how that one hair on her chin got so long. Does grandma have to shave? Read on to find out why the hair on your head seems to get thinner even as it pops up in unwelcome places like your face.

We'll be the first ones to admit that no one is going to win a Nobel Prize for discovering a pill to relieve the conditions described in this chapter. In the grand scheme of things, these conditions may be mosquito bites in relation to the other issues that women face during and after menopause. But they're really annoying, and they vex our vanity! So it's nice to know why they happen and what you can do about them. We're also here to help you figure out what you can't do (and thus avoid those sounds-too-good-to-be-true products you see on the late-night infomercials or the shelves of your local drugstore). That's what this chapter is for.

# Getting the Skinny on Skin

Usually, during perimenopause (the years leading up to menopause) and menopause, you're on a heightened state of alert, looking for the changes you know are happening. You expect your periods to change, and you're probably not all that surprised by vaginal and urinary changes. But one day you look down and realize the texture on the skin on the back of your hands has become less like satin and more like crepe. Suddenly you have a few extra laugh lines or crow's feet around your eyes. You may also notice dry skin or dry scalp that you never had before. But wait — menopause can't affect the *outside* of you, too, can it?

## Making the skin and hormone connection

Menopause (more specifically the associated decline of estrogen levels) probably accelerates many of the little annoying changes that accompany aging. But separating the skin changes due to low estrogen from those that come as a result of being on this planet for a long time can be difficult. Think about it. Forty plus years of gravity is going to contribute to sagginess. No matter whether you're a woman or a man, your skin has been fighting gravity's weight ever since you could sit upright. By the time you approach your 70s, you're left with jowls instead of cheeks and a turkey wattle instead of a nice, tight neck, and you've learned never to look down into a mirror.

### Placing blame for skin woes

Besides gravity, a lot of other things contribute to the aging of your skin. The first one is age itself — simple wear and tear. We just can't expect to go on looking like dewy skinned children forever. Muscle movement, sun damage, inflammation, medications, and other medical treatments can all take the bloom off the roses in our cheeks.

But estrogen (and its loss during menopause) does play a role in the great skin caper. The collagen and elastin fibers that keep your skin supple, pliant, and nicely molded to your frame slowly deteriorate as the active form of estrogen declines. The degeneration of collagen and elastin fibers leaves room for wrinkles. Wrinkles (creases in your skin) show up where muscles contract. For example, when you smile, several facial muscles pull tight, forming one or more lines in the skin adjacent to your mouth. With age, these lines stay behind even when you're not smiling. Other wrinkles resemble straight or branched lines finely etched all over the weakened skin. These wrinkles are also the result of the double dip of low estrogen levels and aging.

The fatty layer under your skin disappears over time as well, and your skin loses its flexibility — which leads not only to facial wrinkles, but to a loss of firmness and smoothness to your whole birthday suit. If your skin were clothes, you'd probably go to the tailor to have it taken in. (In fact, some women do go to the tailor, also known as the plastic surgeon, to have the sags tucked.)

Medical folks are divided on how much blame to apportion to gravity and how much to assign to declining levels of estrogen. Some scientists claim that skin changes are just part of aging, but others feel that low levels of estrogen during the years leading up to and after menopause hasten a lot of these changes in your skin.

The hormone-imbalance crowd points out that estrogen helps bring moisture to body tissue. Menopause causes lower levels of *estradiol* (the active kind of estrogen), which causes tissues and mucus membranes all over your body to act strangely. How strangely? Some women develop pimples and dry skin *at the same time*.

But the bottom line here is that during perimenopause and menopause your skin loses its elasticity and tightness — it becomes thinner and saggier. As the fatty layer under your skin thins out over time, it will be easier to see your blood vessels, and you'll bruise more easily. Because your skin is less pliant, it tears more easily than it used to — so you may encounter more minor cuts and scrapes.

Also, the skin-maintenance process slows down as part of the normal aging process in both men and women, so your body doesn't regenerate skin as quickly as it used to — another reason you may bruise and cut more easily and heal more slowly.

### Slowing the process down

Whether estrogen treatments are effective in slowing the skin-aging process in menopausal women is still debatable. (Especially because some experts don't believe that shifting hormones has anything to do with skin changes in the first place.) Experts sit on both sides of the fence.

If you want to try an estrogen treatment, skin creams (you can call them *transdermal estradiol therapies* if you're feeling pretentious) seem to be more effective than oral estrogen in preserving skin collagen. But don't get overly optimistic about the results. When you see those smiling, wrinkle-free faces on the estrogen-cream advertisements, you can be sure that it's not the estrogen skin cream that gives those women their smooth skin, big breasts, and girlish figures.

# Shining a light on the sun's dangers

The sun is public enemy number one for the skin. Sun exposure can cause wrinkles when you're in your 20s or early 30s, and it can cause your skin to become leathery and unevenly colored years before perimenopause.

### Reining in UV rays

The sun's *ultraviolet rays (UV)* inflict the greatest harm on your skin. UV rays from the sun destroy collagen fibers. Remember, the collagen fibers hold the skin tight and keep it from sagging and wrinkling. The skin has a normal maintenance process in which old skin is sloughed off and new skin is rebuilt. UV radiation messes up this process so that the collagen fibers become disorganized and form "solar scars." Just 5 to 15 minutes of sunbathing for fair- to moderate-skinned people can trash the skin-maintenance process for a week. UV radiation from the sun also causes a buildup of a substance that causes the skin to stretch (*abnormal elastin*).

If you use skin creams containing AHA (alpha-hydroxy acids) in an effort to combat wrinkles, you can create another reason to be careful in the sun. These substances increase your skin's sensitivity to the sun, and thus heighten your risk of sun damage. If you're using products containing AHA, shield your skin from the sun and wear a sunblock with an SPF of at least 15 or higher.

SPF, or sun protection factor, is described as a number that tells you how long you can remain in the sun, while wearing the product, without beginning to burn. Other factors (such as sweating, swimming, or friction from playing sports) can shorten sunblock's period of effectiveness.

---

# Working on wrinkles

Nothing prevents wrinkles like staying out of the sun. But if the damage has already been done, you can check out products that claim to retard the wrinkling process:

✔ **Retinoid creams:** These products often make use of the terms *retinoic acid, tretinoin,* and the trademark *Retin-A.* Retinoids are vitamin-A acids. To the extent that they work, they do so by smoothing out skin pigmentation (color), reducing brown spots and wrinkles, and giving skin a rosy appearance. Usually, several months of use are necessary before you notice any improvement.

✔ **Alpha-hydroxy creams:** Alpha-hydroxy acids work like a skin peel. They help remove surface skin cells, making your skin look rosier and smoother. Some advertisers claim that alpha hydroxy helps your skin *produce* new collagen and elastin. If this were true, alpha hydroxy would actually improve the layers under the skin, filling the wrinkles in from the inside out and reversing the aging process. Yeah, we wish. Some of the side effects of alpha hydroxy include burning, itching, and general skin pain. Newer products that contain beta-hydroxy acids incorporate a mild aspirin-like substance into the product, which is supposed to eliminate skin irritation.

✔ **Botox:** Wrinkles are caused by contraction of facial muscles (as we discuss in the "Making the skin and hormone connection" section earlier in this chapter). Botox, a purified form of the botulism toxin, is injected into the facial muscles. It temporarily removes the wrinkle because the toxin temporarily paralyzes or weakens the affected muscles. When the muscles relax, the wrinkle disappears. After several months, the paralysis wears off and the wrinkle returns.

# Being a skin-savvy consumer

If snake oil were an effective moisturizer, thousands of women who've spent hundreds of thousands of dollars on questionable anti-aging skin care products would have absolutely radiant skin. Aging and menopause aren't for sissies, but feeling good about our appearance is important. That's why it's so upsetting that a number of companies prey on our fears about aging and losing our youthful good looks.

Many of the creams and lotions and potions we hear about every day do give at least the *temporary* appearance and feel of smoother, younger looking skin. Some of them just make us feel good. And if you think all the claims you hear and read are legitimate, that would be understandable. After all, doesn't the government regulate stuff like this for our protection?

Well, yes and no. The U.S. Food and Drug Administration doesn't have the authority to regulate what goes into cosmetics. They can only get involved if they've received reports that a product has caused harm, or if the sellers of a particular skin product makes claims that it works like a medicine or actually changes the structure of a part of your body — such as curing wrinkles. When in doubt about a particular product, ask your doctor or a dermatologist about how realistic its claims are.

Be wary of products that claim to use "scientific" or "high-tech" breakthroughs to make your body produce more collagen (creams and lotions can't get inside your skin to make this happen), turn back time, restore aging skin, or permanently cure wrinkles. You may get plumper (and thus less visible) wrinkles, but you could also end up with a much thinner wallet.

Taking extra-large doses of vitamin A in an effort to improve your skin won't work. Mega-doses of vitamin A are toxic — don't try it!

## Caring about skin cancer

Along with lesser problems, UV radiation can cause skin cancer — a serious side effect of too much sun. Skin cancer can show up years after long-term exposure to the sun.

By the time you're menopausal, your risk of skin cancer is higher because you've been exposed to UV radiation for quite a few years. *Malignant melanoma* is a rather rare but deadly form of skin cancer. It's most commonly diagnosed in folks in their early 50s.

When you're in the sun for too long, the sun's UV radiation penetrates your skin and gets down into the DNA inside the skin cells. It zaps and damages the DNA — serious stuff because cell reproduction is based on DNA. Any mistakes in the DNA can have serious ramifications down the line. Sometimes, genetic mutations produce cancerous skin tumors. UV rays also suppress the skin's immune system, leaving your skin susceptible to cancer cells.

# Preventing premature skin aging

If you worry about the appearance of your skin, you're probably wondering how you can combat the skin changes that accompany the aging process and menopause. Well, here you go. These are a few ways to keep your skin looking youthful and firm for as long as you can:

- ✔ **Don't smoke.** On average, smokers have thinner skin and more wrinkles than non-smokers. A heavy smoker is five times more likely to have a wrinkled face than a non-smoker of the same age. A 40-year-old, heavy smoker has the face of a non-smoking 60-year-old in terms of wrinkles.

- ✔ **Drink plenty of water.** Internal hydration can help your skin look plumper (which makes wrinkles look less evident) and more youthful.

- ✔ **Follow a regular and sensible skin care regimen.** Cleanse your skin daily with a mild cleanser suitable to your skin's level of oiliness, follow with a mild toner, and finish with a good, basic moisturizer (no need to break the bank). You may not turn back the clock, but you'll probably be happier with how your skin looks and feels.

- ✔ **Avoid exposure to the sun.** Exposure to ultraviolet radiation accounts for 90 percent of the symptoms of premature skin aging. It's also the most significant cause of skin cancers.

An awful lot of products that claim to reverse the aging of our hair and skin are advertised by "Dr." this and "Dr." that. Sometimes they're real medical doctors and sometimes they're not. Some legitimate doctors even market their own skin care product lines. Even some of these may cross a different line — an ethical one — when they claim to cure wrinkles or restore youth. Shame on them — be skeptical and take your questions to your own doctor.

# Handling Hairy Issues

Gray hair has nothing to do with menopause, except that both tend to occur in women over 40. But menopause does bring about changes in hair patterns in ways you may never have imagined, including losing hair on your head and growing it on your face.

The hormonal imbalances of menopause can be responsible for those few hairs on your chin or other spots on your face. Hormone therapy helps restore some of the balance between hormones in your body, thus helping to preserve your hair (on your head) and protect your chin from hair growth.

Here's why hair loss is more likely to happen after menopause: Hair follicles are receptive to hormones. Female hormone (estrogen) levels decrease faster than male hormone (androgen) levels, so where you once had very high levels of active estrogen and very low levels of androgen, you now have low levels of androgen but much lower levels of active estrogen. These lower levels of estrogen aren't enough to block the effects of the androgen, one of which is hair loss.

## Losing it — your hair, that is

We all lose a little hair every day. As hair grows, a few of the older strands jump ship every day. You see them in your hairbrush, but you might not think much about them until you wonder whether some day there will be more in your brush than on your head. As you age, hair growth slows, and the hairs that fall out aren't replaced as rapidly. About one-third of women between the ages of 40 and 80 find their hair thinning all over their scalp but more so on the crown of the head. This is called *female pattern baldness*. The amount of hair loss varies from woman to woman.

Hair loss in women tends to be hereditary. There are other causes of hair loss in gals, too. These include thyroid disorders, pituitary tumors, stress, polycystic ovarian syndrome (PCOS), lupus, stress, and chemotherapy. So if your hair begins leaving you at an alarming rate, check with your doctor before you assume that it's "just" a normal symptom of aging.

## Taking care of your hair

Some women have had success using minoxidil, the same treatment recommended for balding men. This medication is better at preserving hair than retrieving what was lost, so if you're going to try it, seek help quickly.

Let's face it — our hair is important to us. It's one of the first things people notice about us. It's a built-in accessory. There are things we can do, though, to minimize the impact of lock loss:

- ✔ **Be kind to your hair.** Use soft brushes with gentle bristles. Only brush your hair as needed and treat your hair tenderly when you do. Avoid styles that involve pulling the hair back tightly.

- ✔ **Get a great haircut that makes the most of what you have.** Soft layers maximize fullness. Shorter is better than longer — extra length can pull hair down, making it look even thinner.

- ✔ **Use a mild shampoo and don't over-condition.** Heavy conditioners can also weigh hair down and emphasize thinness.

- ✔ **After styling your hair, hang your head down and use your fingers to fluff hair up before righting yourself.** This adds height and the illusion of fullness to your hair.

- ✔ **Work with your stylist to find products that add height and texture to your hair.** Light piecing waxes or gels can work well if you take a few minutes to learn how to use them.

Unless you use a physician-prescribed medication such as minoxidil to stop falling hair, or resort to hair transplants (some women do, with varying results), restoring the lush look of your crowning glory may be a little like using anti-aging creams to fight wrinkles. Although you may not be able to reverse the effects of aging on your hair, you may succeed at keeping up appearances.

# Chapter 9

# Maintaining Your Sex Life Through Menopause

## In This Chapter

▶ Understanding how your libido can cha-cha-cha when your hormones are doing the rumba

▶ Getting the scoop on your partner's libido

▶ Warming up the sheets

▶ Facing the challenges of fertility in your 40s

*B*ravo for life's little ironies. You may discover that at about the same time your kids are moving on (and out), you finally have the leisure (and the cash) for those romantic weekends; your doctor gives you the green light to toss your contraception; your body is ready to make whoopie; but your sex organs are preparing for retirement. Or you may discover that your organs are still willing, but your hormones are not.

On the other hand, you may expect interest in and capacity for great sex to decline, only to discover that menopause is the best thing that ever happened to your sex life. Just don't just assume that the dire predictions about loss of libido and dewy freshness giving way to disinterest and dryness are the rule for everyone. Lots of women find sex after menopause to be better than ever.

There's no question, though, that sex *changes* after menopause — your hormonal shifts have repercussions for your private parts as well as your emotional parts. There's also plenty of pesky cultural silliness to deal with — an awful lot of folks still hold to the idea that women of a certain age aren't supposed to be sexy, or sexual. In this chapter we'll talk about why you shouldn't kiss your sex life goodbye just yet, why you still need to be careful about birth control (and why it may not be too late for a baby if that's where your heart lies), and suggest some ways to keep the home fires burning as you approach and enter menopause.

# Looking at Menopause and Your Libido

Menopause opens a new chapter in your life, so it's no surprise that the sexual you changes as well. In many cases, the changes are for the better. Even though there's never been a medical reason for you to abstain from sex during your period, most women and their partners refrain from sex for those days. Now that those menstrual periods have hit the road (or are at least packing for the journey), you have more opportunities for sex. And remember how you always seemed to get your period when you were on vacation, no matter how well you planned? Now you can play around until your heart's content without checking and double-checking for those red circles on your calendar. The crankiness, cramps, and headaches that characterized much of your menstrual cycle now level out into a kinder and gentler expression of you.

Libido often declines with age. Most scientific studies have found that little change in sexual activity occurs between the ages of 45 and 55. But, between 55 and 65, sexual activity slows.

And, though women in their 60s may not engage in sex as often as they did in their younger years, no change occurs in the frequency of orgasm or the level of sexual enjoyment. So, you may not do it as often, but sex is just as satisfying. (An interesting note: Research shows that activity with sexual partners often slows down long before women discontinue masturbating.) Quality doesn't have to decline just because quantity does!

The fluctuating hormones that characterize menopause and perimenopause definitely have an effect on your sex drive. Be prepared for a gradual increase — or a gradual decrease — in your libido. Of course, you may not be aware of any change at all, but most menopausal women experience at least brief periods of a higher- or lower-than-usual sex drive.

## Letting your feelings be your guide

When it comes down to it, no one knows your body better than you do, so pay attention to it. Because every woman experiences menopause a little differently, your medical advisor may not be familiar with what's normal for you — and what seems different to you. Learn to trust yourself and communicate openly with your doctor.

This advice goes double for changes in your *libido* (desire to have sex). Many doctors ignore sexual issues when treating perimenopausal and menopausal women. So it's important that *you* bring up the issue if your doctor doesn't.

Here are some helpful hints for talking to your doctor:

- ✔ Doctors have heard everything; don't feel embarrassed about your questions or concerns. If you don't feel comfortable discussing sex and sexuality with your doctor, find one who's more engaging.

- ✔ Raise your questions early in the appointment. Take a moment right after the "Hi, how are you doing today" part to raise the issue by saying something such as, " . . . and there's another problem that we need to solve before I leave today." Waiting until you're actually walking out the door to bring up a sensitive issue happens so often that doctors actually have a name for the phenomenon: "the doorknob moment."

- ✔ Keep a diary of any pain, discomfort, or discharge you experience related to sex. Track things such as how long it lasts, what activity may have caused the problem, and the level and nature of pain you felt.

- ✔ Sexual responsiveness is a natural process, not a right reserved for special people. If you're experiencing troublesome changes in your sexual desire after menopause, be direct with your doctor. The problem may be hormonal (low testosterone levels) or there may be other medical reasons for the change.

- ✔ If your doctor can rule out medical problems that might be interfering with your sexual satisfaction, but doesn't seem comfortable helping you pursue a solution, ask for a referral to a specialist — in this case, an accredited sex therapist.

## Turning up the heat

More than half of all menopausal women maintain the same level of sexual interest after menopause as before. In fact, you may feel less inhibited when the possibility of pregnancy no longer looms over the bed. After you can safely put away the contraceptive devices (after you have gone a whole year without a period), you can be freer to express yourself sexually.

The famous sex research team of Masters and Johnson proved to the world that sexual *appetite* is not tied to estrogen levels (although you may need a little lubricant to make sex comfortable after estrogen declines). It's really the *androgens* (male sex hormones such as testosterone) produced by your ovaries throughout your life that keep your sex drive running. Even after menopause (when your ovaries have gotten out of the estradiol- and progesterone-production game), your ovaries keep on producing androgens.

If you have sex with more than one partner during or after menopause, you still need to practice safe sex to avoid picking up a sexually transmitted disease or AIDS.

Even though men don't go through menopause, their testosterone levels gradually decline after 40. The physiological changes don't happen overnight. Over time, men will notice that it takes longer for them to get an erection and that they aren't aroused as easily, which may be good news for a woman who enjoys foreplay. Women whose partners suffer premature ejaculation can rejoice. That problem may go away and men gain lasting power as they age.

Even if you're having fewer periods (or perhaps you haven't had one in months), don't give up your birth control until you've been without periods for a full year. During perimenopause, your hormone levels and the chance of ovulation are wildly unpredictable. It's unlikely, but you could just have a hormonally hot month and wind up pregnant.

## Dealing with a lowered libido

A healthy self-image and adult lifestyle generally include satisfying and safe sexual activity. Yet many (but not all) women are frustrated by a declining desire for sex during and after menopause. Understanding the biology behind a declining libido can help bring about a solution.

Your sex drive can decline sooner than you'd like for several reasons. Some are mental or emotional — if your self-esteem declines because of changes in your life or in your body, you may have to address that issue before you can find your old libido. Some of the reasons are physical — painful sex is nothing to look forward to. And some are hormonal — your hormones are changing, and if you'd like to maintain your sex drive, your hormones must be balanced.

Communicating with your doctor is even more important if you've experienced early menopause. If your doctor takes your concerns about sex lightly, find another doctor. You won't be able to get pregnant after menopause, but you can still have a hot and healthy sex life.

### Adjusting your attitude

It's hard to feel amorous when you're depressed. Menopause, in itself, doesn't make you depressed, but think about the types of things happening during these years:

✔ Kids leaving home

✔ Parents aging and needing closer attention

✔ You or your spouse retiring

Add to these challenges the everyday issues of maintaining a happy relationship and just coping in a fast-paced world. Now, the one thing that used to be reliable, your body, is also changing at a faster pace than it has in quite some time. Is it any wonder that sex is the last thing on your mind?

But if the lack of physical spark bothers you, you need to get rid of the emotional stressors before you can expect your libido to kick in. It may just take allocating more time to yourself. Take some time to get an exercise program off the ground. Walking regularly by yourself or with a friend can do plenty to reduce stress. Talk with friends, a therapist, your hairdresser, or minister about your challenges. Also, remember to bring up your anxiety or depression when you talk to your internist or gynecologist.

### Making sure that sex isn't a hurtin' thing

Hormonal changes can cause the vaginal lining to become thinner, more fragile, and more susceptible to tearing *and* to produce less lubrication. You're more delicate down there — a bit more tender. Vaginal connective tissue also becomes less pliant, and nerve endings become more sensitive.

The result of this biological shuffle is that intercourse may become painful. Sexual activity that used to deliver great pleasure can now cause pain instead. The thought of the discomfort may make you want to get a headache or clean out your sock drawer when your partner makes amorous advances, but all is not lost. You can alleviate painful intercourse in a variety of ways:

✔ **Maintain an active sex life.** Regular sexual activity keeps blood circulating in your vulva and slows the drying process. So maintaining an active sex life helps postpone or altogether avoid the pain associated with dry vaginal tissues. This is definitely one of those "use it or lose it situations."

✔ **Talk to your partner about the more sensitive you.** Most men aren't aware that hormonal changes trigger changes in your vulva and vagina. Explain to your partner that the two of you need to figure out new bedroom strategies that can be mutually satisfying.

✔ **Take a firm position.** This is a great time to experiment with new positions for sex. We're not going to tell you which pages in the Kama Sutra to consult, but woman-on-top positions may give you more control over your own comfort.

> ✔ **Use a lubricant during intercourse to help keep things moving.**
> Lubricants can afford hours of interpersonal pleasure. Some women and their partners make lubricant application a part of foreplay. Water-based lubricants, such as Astroglide, are healthier for vaginal linings. Avoid petroleum-based products.

Sometimes women experience regular discomfort due to vaginal dryness — not just during sex. If you're one of them, you can use other types of lubricants on a regular basis to relieve this irritation. (See the product literature for recommended dosage, and check out Chapter 7 on tips for dealing with vaginal dryness.)

# It's not the estrogen!

Many reports and books make a huge deal about the fact that no scientific evidence links changes in estrogen levels to a declining libido. These publications then make the leap to erroneously conclude that hormones have nothing to do with libido. Although the estrogen, itself, may not play the deciding role in libido regulation, the *balance* between estrogen and testosterone likely makes a difference.

This subject is a bit controversial so we want to give you both sides of the argument. On one side are scientists who conclude that supplementing your testosterone during menopause increases your libido. On the other side are the lab coats who believe that the science doesn't exist to show that prescribing testosterone is either safe or effective for women who complain of low libido.

Testosterone is produced naturally by women's ovaries and has a very positive impact on your libido, mood, vitality, sense of well being, bone, and muscle. But, even before menopause, your body slows down its production of testosterone. After menopause, you produce about half as much testosterone as you produced during your reproductive years. So it's not unusual for your libido to decline if your testosterone levels are too low.

You don't want to have too much testosterone either — it can promote breast and liver cancer. Plus, too much testosterone relative to estrogen can unleash the effects of testosterone that estrogen had been keeping under control, such as facial hair, increased libido, redistribution of body fat (it moves to the middle of your body), and acne.

Some doctors shy away from prescribing testosterone as part of hormone therapy (HT) because they're afraid of upsetting the estrogen/testosterone balance and causing unpleasant side effects. The trick, whether you're taking HT with testosterone or not, is to keep testosterone levels high enough to avoid one set of side effects (including low libido) and in balance with the other hormones to avoid another set of side effects (facial hair or acne, for example).

Those folks in the scientific and medical communities who view testosterone as a worthy treatment for libido problems believe that the bad side effects felt by some women are caused by excessively high dosages of testosterone. Proponents of testosterone use suggest using very low dosages and maintaining a balance between the levels of testosterone and estrogen.

Don't use estrogen cream as a sexual lubricant. The estrogen cream can be absorbed by your partner and cause problems. At least one case of breast cancer has been reported in a man because his wife used vaginal estrogen cream as a lubricant. It's important to read the instructions!

# Talking Turkey about Testosterone

Don't forget that men, as well as women, experience declining libido as they age! If you're noticing changes in your sexual relationship, remember that your partner's hormones are changing too. Men produce much more testosterone than women, but when they reach 40, their testosterone levels begin declining. However, most men don't notice an appreciable change in their libido for about another 10 years. Around the age of 50 or so, the drop in testosterone causes men to stop having *psychogenic erections* (erections from just thinking about sex), and men who could have an erection at the drop of a hat find that it's a bit harder (no pun intended) to get things moving.

So, if you're worried because your partner isn't pursuing you like he used to, your menopause may not be at the heart of the matter. Your partner may be going through hormonal changes of his own, even though his change isn't as dramatic as yours. You may even find that his changes are compatible with yours. It may take him longer to reach orgasm than it used to, giving both of you more time for long, slow, comfortable lovemaking.

# Keeping Sex Sexy

If you've noticed some changes in your sexual relationship, work with your partner to make things better. Your relationship can evolve to a new level of meaning and pleasure.

First, you need to communicate with your partner and take stock of the situation. Is it a libido thing for you? Is it a libido thing for him? Is it technique? Is it timing? You need to find out what's going on.

As you and your partner get older and both your testosterone levels decline, it's time to focus on foreplay. You may both need more stimulation before intercourse — take your time! And you may need to incorporate lubricants into your foreplay if you have vaginal dryness.

Don't just focus on the anticipated orgasm (yours and your partner's). Enjoy each moment. Take time to enjoy all the feelings along the way. If actual intercourse is uncomfortable today, or just not happening, it's fine to enjoy other sensual activities together: a bath or shower, a massage, or watching a sexy movie together.

You may also have to use different techniques to provide enough stimulation for your man to get an erection — you may have to work a little magic to get his penis into position at this stage of his life. Hand stimulation or oral sex may be what it takes to get him started. You can also turn to books and counselors — two good sources of information on sexual techniques and other sexual matters for mature adults. Ask your doctor to recommend a sex therapist accredited by the American Association of Sex Educators, Counselors and Therapists (www.aasect.org). If you think your sexual issues are related to concerns about your relationship, look for a sex therapist who is also a licensed couples or marital therapist; many are both.

Although we baby boomers come from the "sex, booze, and drugs" generation, these words no longer work together. Take a look at some of the things that can douse your flame:

- **Alcohol:** One drink may make you feel relaxed and less inhibited, but several drinks can put a damper on your libido, your ability to become aroused, your performance, and your ability to reach orgasm.

- **Heavy meals:** The way to your partner's *heart* might be through a gourmet dinner, but if your intended destination is a little, um, further south, go light on the eats. You can always have dinner in bed *after*.

- **Prescription drugs:** Serotonin boosters, antidepressants, blood pressure pills, sleeping pills, and many other drugs frequently prescribed for women and men over 50 can take a toll on your libido — or your partner's. Let your gynecologist and internist know what medications you take when you discuss your libido and sexual performance. Alternative medications may be available that can alleviate some of the negative side effects.

- **Tobacco products:** The nicotine in cigarettes and other tobacco products constricts the blood vessels making it more difficult for blood to rush to your private parts. It's harder to get aroused and harder still to experience a satisfactory conclusion.

Diabetes and other medical problems also cause loss of sexual desire and performance problems. Be sure to consult with your doctor about changes in your libido because they can result from medical conditions other than menopause.

# Starting over: The good news and the bad

Here's the stereotype: you reach midlife, and your husband leaves you for a newer model. Does it happen? Sure it does. But are you ready for a little myth busting? A 2004 survey of divorced men and women aged 40 to 79, conducted by the AARP, indicates that *women* are more than twice as likely to initiate divorce in midlife than are men.

Women have a longer life expectancy than men, too, and are more likely than men to rejoin the ranks of the single when a spouse dies. About 4 percent of women between the ages of 45 and 54 have been widowed. For women between 55 and 64, though, this figure has risen to almost 12 percent.

No matter how you get there, romance doesn't have to be a thing of the past when married women become single again. Three-quarters of divorced women in their 50s, for instance, went on to have a serious sexual relationship. Many describe their sex lives at this stage as being better than ever.

Still, sex with a new partner (or partners) is not completely without its complications. It may have been years since you popped your last birth control pill or wrestled with your last diaphragm, but there are still potential risks associated with sex with a new partner:

✔ There are a lot of ugly bugs out there: neither chlamydia, human papilloma virus (HPV — some forms of which cause cervical cancer), gonorrhea, syphilis, hepatitis B, hepatitis C, nor genital herpes care how old you are. Menopausal women (and their partners) can still get STDs — sexually transmitted diseases.

✔ HIV, the virus that causes AIDS, is age-blind, too, and becoming more prevalent in older people as the population ages but stays healthy enough for sex. Ten percent of the people newly diagnosed with HIV every year are over 50.

✔ The great estrogen flight changes the environment in your vagina, making it easier to contract vaginal infections. Some of these — such as bacterial vaginosis or viral vaginitis — aren't necessarily *caused* by sex but are more common in sexually active women. Anecdotal evidence suggests that some of these may be more likely to occur when you've been with a new partner or partners. Others, such as trichomoniasis vaginosis ("trich"), can be passed among sexual partners (you and your partner must both be treated with oral antibiotics if you get trich).

Not all lubricants are friends with the latex condoms you will need to wear with new partners to prevent the spread of STDs. Vaseline and other petroleum-based lubricants weaken both male and female condoms. Petroleum-based products may also contribute to vaginal infections.

# Flirting with Fertility

For most of us, our menstruating years have been pretty much synonymous with the years when we expected to be able to get pregnant if we wanted to. We might have spent a chunk of this time wishing to conceive. Or fervently hoping *not* to conceive. Or dreaming of a little magic switch that could turn our fertility off and on according to our desires and circumstances, with none of the hassle, mess, or potential side effects accompanying our contraceptive options. If *men* were the ones who could get pregnant, we're willing to bet that medical science would have figured out a nice, neat, affordable, discreet form of birth control — years ago — but don't get us started on that one.

As it happens, the end of fertility doesn't coincide as neatly with the onset of perimenopause as we might think — or like. For many women at both ends of the wishing-and-hoping fertility continuum, this can be problematic.

## Staying fertile after all these years . . .

Maybe you just can't wait for menopause to bring freedom from the need to wonder and worry about birth control. Not all of today's available methods are right for every woman. Your own personal medical history, financial situation (some of this stuff is *expensive*), relationship circumstances, or personal beliefs can complicate the way you browse through the contraceptive menu. And, except for a few of our more dramatic choices (such as surgical sterilization or complete abstinence), few of our birth control options are completely foolproof.

The truth is, you can't tell very much about the state of your fertility from the regularity (or even the presence or absence) of your periods. Unless you've gone an entire 12 months without a menstrual period, it's entirely possible that you can still get pregnant (admit it — don't you have a friend or two with a child whose middle name is "Surprise"?). Trouble is, lots of women don't know that and quit using contraception a wee bit earlier than is medically advisable.

If you're over 40, your risk (or promise, depending on your point of view) of pregnancy is quite low. It is not, however, zero. Among women under 40, 170 women out of every 1,000 get pregnant every year. Among women *over* 40, this number drops to about 11 out of 1,000 (some of these were intended pregnancies, some were not). This means two important things for you if you *don't* want to get pregnant:

✔ You have to continue to use birth control *faithfully*.

✔ You have to use a method with a high degree of reliability in the face of decreasing predictability of ovulation. The "rhythm" method, for instance, never the most reliable of birth control methods even in earlier stages of your life, is downright risky if the number of days between your periods is becoming unpredictable.

Women over 40 rank only slightly lower than teenage girls and women in their early 20s in their rate of unintended pregnancies. Over half of all pregnancies to women over 40 are unplanned. If you don't want to get pregnant, and you haven't gone an entire year without a period, take precautions!

## Taking one more chance on the stork

Maybe, though, the signs of approaching menopause have sent you into an emotional tailspin. You aren't alone if you are still trying for a baby when you enter perimenopause. As we've said, it's certainly not impossible to get pregnant at this point, but your odds are considerably lower than they were at 30 or even 40. The hormone dance that ends in menopause actually begins years before you stop having periods. Most women don't know what time the ball begins and are shocked when they have trouble getting pregnant in their 30s.

You may have had the same experience that we had when we were teenagers: Parents, teachers, and even friends had us believing that practically all you had to do to get pregnant was to jump in a swimming pool with a boy. Okay, that's a slight exaggeration, but generally, getting pregnant is easier when you're in your teens than when you're in your 30s.

In fact, according to a recent study, a woman's fertility begins to decline in her late 20s, rather than her 30s, as previously thought. Researchers found that even women in their early- to mid-20s have only a 50-50 chance of becoming pregnant each cycle even if they have intercourse during the peak time for conception. In your late 20s to early 30s, the chance drops to 40 percent each cycle, and by the late 30s it's less than a 30 percent chance.

By the way, that study also finds that men's fertility also begins to decline sooner than expected. Men begin to lose their fertility in their 30s rather than in the 40s as was once thought. So if you're in your late 30s and your partner is five years older than you are, your chances of becoming pregnant in any given cycle could drop to 20 percent. This doesn't mean that you won't conceive if you're in your late 30s; it just means that it may take a few months longer, especially if your partner is older than you are.

### Tracing the yin and yang of conception

Many things have to happen correctly to make a baby:

- ✔ Your ovaries must produce follicles.
- ✔ The follicles have to grow big enough to release an egg.
- ✔ Your hormones have to be just right for the egg to be released and survive the journey.
- ✔ Your fallopian tubes must be unobstructed so that the egg can swim all the way through to the uterus to meet some nice sperm.
- ✔ Your hormones must create the right type of environment for the egg to get fertilized and comfortably nestled into the lining of the uterus.

All these things have to come together for you to conceive. As you begin to experience the hormonal changes of perimenopause, it becomes more likely that one or more of these essential ingredients may be missing or mis-timed.

Out-of-whack hormones (and that's the technical term — not!) are to blame for most of the infertility problems perimenopausal women face.

### Taking a dipstick to your estrogen

When you seek some assistance in your bid to get pregnant, one of the first things fertility doctors do is check to see if you're capable of ovulating. In order to ovulate, you need both the right kind of estrogen and the right amount of this particular form of estrogen in your bloodstream. This form of estrogen is called *estradiol,* and your doctor will take a blood sample to check your estradiol out.

As you approach menopause, your body produces less estradiol but continues to produce estrone. When it comes to producing follicles and ovulating, estradiol is the kind that counts: Without adequate levels of estradiol, your ovaries won't produce an egg. By measuring both types of estrogen, your doctor can see whether you're heading toward menopause or whether you have some other hormonal problems. (See Chapter 2 for more info on the different types of hormones women produce.)

Because your hormone levels fluctuate during perimenopause, you may still have periods, but you may not ovulate each month. Your estradiol levels may be sufficiently high one month and be low another month. Some months are good for getting pregnant and some months are not so good. By measuring your estradiol levels each month, your doctor will be able to see if it's a good month for producing an egg or not.

### Messing up the nest with hormones

Sometimes hormonal problems occur after the follicle releases the egg. Normally the follicle pops open to release the egg and then hangs around long enough to produce progesterone (after the follicle releases the egg, the empty sac is called a *corpus luteum*). The corpus luteum eventually disintegrates.

*Progesterone* production is necessary for thickening the uterine lining and preparing it for the egg. If the follicle doesn't produce enough progesterone, problems arise that can put an end to conception. If the lining isn't ready, the fertilized egg won't nestle into the endometrium properly.

Progesterone production slows down during perimenopause and menopause, so you may have problems making a home for a fertilized egg.

### Having periods doesn't mean you're fertile

Even for women in their prime baby-conceiving years, the planets need to be aligned to get pregnant. But as you move into your perimenopausal years, some months you ovulate, and some months you don't. As time goes by, you experience more and more cycles in which you don't ovulate.

You may have a period even if you don't ovulate.

## Taking the good with the bad

There's good news, and there's bad news when the subject at hand is conception and the older woman. Because we don't want you walking away from this chapter on a down note, we start off this section with a few gloomy stats and then turn our attention to the good stuff.

Around the time women hit the 35 to 38 mark (some experts say as early as 30), their fertility gradually declines, and it drops precipitously at 40. Unfortunately, around this time, a woman's risk of spontaneous miscarriage begins to rise. By age 45, women have a 50-50 chance of suffering a spontaneous miscarriage if they conceive. Also, by the time women reach 45, the risk of chromosomal abnormalities in the baby increases to 1 chance in 25. In other words, for every 25 babies conceived by women 45 or older, one baby has a chromosomal abnormality such as Down syndrome or spina bifida.

But there are also advantages to becoming a mom for the first time after 40.Women who have waited to have families are typically better prepared for the sacrifices they need to make to nurture children. Establishing careers, entertaining friends, travel, and other interests often preoccupy life during your 20s and 30s. Now you may be more willing to make time to raise a family, be better educated and more established in your career, and be on solid financial ground.

And, hey, the perimenopausal symptom of interrupted sleep means that you'll probably already be awake when the baby cries. You and the newborn will be on the same wavelength, and you'll have someone to talk to when you wake up.

# Chapter 10

# Mental and Emotional Issues

*M*any of us have "senior moments" even before menopause. You know — those brain hiccup moments when you're about to introduce a friend you've known for years and her name suddenly escapes you. Or maybe you find yourself spending more time thinking about the hereafter as you walk through the house — as in, "What am I here after?"

You're not alone. Many women experience these mental lapses during perimenopause or menopause. Some women even experience this type of forgetfulness long before menopause — during their menstrual cycle when estrogen levels are at their lowest. Estrogen plays a major role in memory and emotional functions.

Some perimenopausal and menopausal women also fall prey to emotional rollercoaster rides (and sometimes your friends and family are taken along for the ride). Fluctuating hormone levels prompt some emotional moments (remember being a moody adolescent?); others can come as a response to life events that — coincidentally — are more likely to occur at about the same stage of life as menopause.

Then again, you may simply not experience many mental and emotional problems at all during perimenopause or menopause. Like PMS (premenstrual syndrome), these symptoms are more severe in some women than others. Some women just seem to be more sensitive to hormonal changes. In fact, if you had memory lapses and heightened emotions in connection with your menstrual cycle in the past, they may be part of your perimenopausal and menopausal experience too.

In this chapter, we cover some of the symptoms you may be experiencing, how they're related to your hormones, and how you can tell if a symptom is hormonal or psychological.

# Understanding the Mental and Emotional Stresses of Menopause

Fortunately, with 40 or 50 years of emotional experience behind you, you're most likely quite prepared to cope with the challenges life throws your way. Midlife changes present you with plenty of new opportunities, but also with a boatload of things that may be tough to handle.

If emotional issues or serious concerns about possible mental illness bother you during these years, visit your medical advisor. Life events may certainly trigger temporary mental or emotional issues, but there's a difference between a temporary mental state and a debilitating condition. If your emotional state severely interferes with your daily life for a prolonged period of time, ask your doctor for a referral to a therapist or counselor.

## Finding the link to menopause

You have estrogen receptors all over your brain, particularly in areas associated with memory and mood, because your brain needs estrogen to function properly. So, a dip in your estrogen levels can affect your mental and emotional health. But medications, illness, and physical conditions other than menopause can lead to mental and emotional problems. Ask your doctor to help you tease out what's going on.

The medical establishment didn't recognize hot flashes as an actual physical condition (as opposed to whining) until the late 1970s. If going to the doctor makes you feel as if you've stepped through a time warp into the 1950s ("It's all in your head. It's just stress, dear. Go out and buy yourself something pretty."), then you, the patient, must take that bull by the horns (or by the hormones), and make it clear to your medical advisor that you want him or her to take the subject seriously. The symptoms caused by estrogen fluctuations are at least as common in perimenopause as they are during menopause itself. You may have to insist on a test to check your hormone levels. And if you meet resistance, ask your friends for the name of a more receptive doctor.

We're sure you'll be delighted to know that you can have perimenopausal symptoms and PMS at the same time! Because so many of the symptoms are the same, especially for women who have a hard time with PMS, it can be difficult to tell whether your moodiness, fatigue, headaches, and weight gain are from your PMS or your perimenopause. Keeping a diary can help you tell — PMS symptoms will be more regularly cyclical, occurring in the days or weeks before your period. Perimenopausal symptoms are more unpredictable and can occur at any point in your cycle.

## Separating menopausal symptoms from psychological disorders

The mental and emotional changes that you experience because of hormonal changes shouldn't interfere with your daily life — cause damage to friendships or relationships with the folks at work, make it impossible to manage your normal schedule of activities, or prompt you to abuse alcohol or drugs to help you feel better. If your symptoms do provoke these changes, talk to your doctor, seek out psychological help, or talk to your spiritual advisor.

You typically experience symptoms of menopause over a limited period of time, in episodes that come and go as your hormone levels fluctuate. Although your loved ones may disagree, these symptoms don't completely alter your everyday life. They may make you occasionally unpleasant to be around for a while, but they're not debilitating or irreversible. On the other hand, mental disorders do alter your everyday life.

# Deciding Whether You're Depressed

When we talk about the mental and emotional changes you may experience during perimenopause and menopause, it's important to distinguish between these symptoms and the psychological disorders of the same name. For example, some women experience periods of depression during menopause. How do you know if you're in trouble or if this is just a symptom you have to deal with?

## Understanding the differences

During perimenopause and menopause, experiencing episodes of sadness isn't unusual. During your younger days, you may have felt moody or blue for a few days each month before your period. But most women in their 40s and

50s have to deal with physiological changes (as they did when they were younger) while they're dealing with one or more items from a menu of life-changing events: aging parents, the death of a loved one, marital problems, empty nests, retirement, job loss, and maybe a few unfulfilled dreams.

A hormonal link between depression and menopause seems to exist. Like a lot of issues that pop up at about the same time that your estrogen begins to decline, however, this may (or may not) be another coincidence of timing. Estrogen therapy, for instance, has not been found to be a good treatment for depression. And after you're fully into menopause and your fluctuating hormone levels finally settle down, you may find your blues pack up and leave, too.

This does *not* mean that any depression you're feeling isn't completely real. Lots of things can cause depression, among them:

- **Hormonal imbalances:** Shifting levels of estrogen and other hormones can contribute to depression.

- **Heredity:** If you have a parent or other close relative who suffers from depression, you are much more likely to experience it than is someone with no family history of this problem.

- **Gender:** Women are twice as likely as men to have depression.

- **Prescription medications:** Depression can be a side effect of medication.

- **Seasonal changes:** Seasonal affective disorder (SAD) is a common problem, still not fully understood, in which lack of exposure to sunlight during winter months seems to contribute to depression.

- **Situational events:** Depression can be triggered by loss or by major life changes.

We all feel sad, dejected, or blue now and then. You may become upset when you look in the mirror and see that your face has a few more wrinkles today than it did last year. Or perhaps you haven't yet won the Nobel Prize or published that novel or climbed Mt. Everest. Or you may be in the midst of profound mourning after the death of a loved one. Such sorrow may last for several months. This is a completely normal response to a deeply felt emotional loss. The major difference between sad feelings and a true major depression is that sad feelings eventually pass — depression doesn't.

## Knowing the signs

Are you depressed? If you're even asking yourself the question, it may be time to speak with your doctor, but here are some signs that your sadness is more than just a passing thing:

- Favorite things or activities no longer bring you pleasure
- Your patterns of eating, sleeping, or sexual activity have changed
- Everything seems as though it takes more effort than it used to
- You cry more than you used to or you don't seem to feel much of anything
- You have thoughts about harming yourself

If these descriptions apply to you, talk to a doctor about whether you may be suffering from clinical depression. People who seek help for their depression are likely to find relief from medications or other treatments that can help you to get a handle on depression and feel like yourself again.

# Dealing with the Head Games

Your memory works because *neurons* (nerve cells) talk to each other across special connectors in your brain. It's normal for these cells to wear out over time, but they're also affected by the decreasing amount of estrogen available in your body. Estrogen keeps your brain — like so many other systems in your body — running smoothly. In the case of your brain, it plays a role in stimulating the growth of new neural connectors, and also helps keep blood vessels in the brain nicely dilated so that blood can flow through them without interference. So, a decrease in estrogen makes your brain run, well, not quite as smoothly as before.

## Knowing the symptoms

The mind games associated with menopause are tricky, and they come on gradually — so gradually that you're not sure whether you've always been this way or if this is something new. You think you're going crazy. Your brain just doesn't seem to be working the way it used to! Some of the symptoms you may experience include

✔ **Fuzzy thinking:** Having trouble staying focused at work? Do you feel as though you're walking around in a fog some days? Many women complain of problems concentrating during perimenopause and menopause. Shortened attention spans also seem to be associated with hormonal change.

✔ **Memory lapses:** Not everyone experiences memory lapses, but if you do, they can be annoying, even downright scary. Misplacing your purse or temporarily forgetting how to spell a simple word is aggravating, but not recognizing your husband or child is another story altogether. Just because you occasionally experience this can't-find-my-pencil type of memory loss doesn't mean that you have Alzheimer's disease or that you're going to develop it.

There's hardly anyone who doesn't worry about Alzheimer's when confronted with a frustrating episode of minor memory loss. Remember — losing your car keys, forgetting what you were about to say, or trying to use your office key to unlock your front door at home are all examples of normal forgetfulness. The time to worry is when you can't remember how to *drive* your car, suddenly don't recognize the person you were talking to, or can't figure out how a key works. The old adage about memory is true, too: if you can remember to worry about your memory, you're most likely still okay. If those around you are beginning to be concerned, it's time to speak with your doctor.

## Looking at the research

Since the first edition of this book came out in 2003, the women's health community has almost completely reversed its position on whether hormone replacement therapy (HRT) is effective for maintaining sharp mental functioning and preventing dementia after menopause. Remember how we said that estrogen plays an important role in brain health? It really does, so for years the conventional wisdom was that estrogen replacement would keep your memory sharp and help to ward off Alzheimer's.

But — go figure — the research findings of the Women's Health Initiative Memory Study don't bear this out. Instead, this is what the long-term studies of cognitive functioning and HRT have found so far:

✔ HRT (neither estrogen-alone nor combination therapy using estrogen plus progestin) does not protect women from cognitive impairment associated with aging.

✔ In fact, hormone therapy actually seems to *increase* the likelihood of both general cognitive decline and the development of dementia.

As with any longitudinal study, research will continue and long-term findings may be different. Findings may not apply in the same way to all women in all groups, either — the WHI memory study, for instance, only looked at women 65 and over, so we can't say with certainty what the findings mean for younger women. For now, however, it doesn't look as if seeking protection from dementia or cognitive decline is a good reason to go on HRT. If you're already taking HRT, talk to your doctor about whether this is still the best choice for you, and how long you ought to continue taking hormones.

## Beating the memory game

The least invasive (and very effective) ways to improve your memory during and after menopause are also good for the rest of your health: Stick to a balanced diet and exercise regularly. Also remember (no pun intended; well, okay, it was intended) that your brain needs exercise too. Throughout your life, you need to challenge and exercise your brain to keep those neurons firing and to keep your memory from getting flabby and weak. Here are some things you can do to help manage your memory:

- ✔ **Check your thyroid and ovarian hormone levels.** Checking your hormone levels can help determine whether your symptoms are related to menopause or whether you may have a more serious condition.

- ✔ **Don't smoke.** As if you needed yet *another* reason to quit smoking, those gray clouds suffocate the nerve cells as they restrict the amount of oxygen that gets to your brain.

- ✔ **Exercise your mental muscle.** Do crossword puzzles or sudoku, read, take a class, or try memorizing poems or recipes. Even just traveling, trying new foods, or keeping interesting company helps to build new neural connections and protect existing ones.

- ✔ **Exercise your body.** Get going! Walk or swim, climb mountains or do yoga — just find something you love to do, and do it! Brisk aerobic activity three to five times a week for 30 minutes to an hour keeps the oxygen flowing to your brain, which improves your memory and your mood.

- ✔ **Get enough sleep.** A loss of estrogen can cause disruptions in your sleep. Whether your particular brand of sleep deprivation is due to stress, urinary problems, low levels of estrogen, or your partner's snoring, it can do a number on your memory.

Be careful about using sleeping pills; they interrupt your normal sleep patterns, which in turn, has a negative impact on your memory. You should never use sleeping pills for more than two weeks in a row.

✔ **Limit your alcohol consumption.** Consumed in excess, alcohol damages nerve cells in the brain and depletes your body of vitamins necessary for building neural connections. Ironically, though, a number of studies show that moderate use of alcohol may actually help protect you from dementia and senility.

✔ **Take your vitamins.** Certain vitamins help build nerve cells and the neural connectors that you need to remember things (or to just plain think). Some of the more important vitamins include

- **B vitamins:** This group includes vitamins B1, B2, B6, and B12, and the lack of these can cause memory problems. You can find vitamin B in meat, milk, and eggs, but if you're vegan or vegetarian, you can also find them in enriched flour, cereals, and wheat germ, and in some enriched soy products. If you have a serious B vitamin deficiency, your doctor may even prescribe vitamin B injections.

- **Folic acid:** Good news for veggie lovers, this B vitamin relative is found primarily in vegetables rather than flour and meat. Green, leafy vegetables, such as spinach, collard greens, kale, and broccoli, are rich in folic acid (but it's also often added to enriched breads and cereals, for those of you who still don't like green foods).

- **Antioxidants:** The antioxidants serve as rust protection for your cells. Oxidation of your cells has a similar effect as oxidation of metal (called rust) — it damages and eventually kills your cells. Antioxidants include vitamins E and C, beta-carotene, and selenium.

Take a look at Chapter 18 to find out more about the importance of vitamins during and after menopause. Most women require a multivitamin to get sufficient dosages of these vitamins.

# Straightening Out the Commotions with Your Emotions

As a woman, if you're going to develop depression or an anxiety disorder in your lifetime, it will most likely happen when you're in your late 30s or early 40s. Is there a link between depression and menopause-related hormone changes? More than likely. Aside from this fairly obvious coincidence in timing, some physical characteristics of women with depression point to lower levels of estrogen as a factor: Women with depression tend to have lower estrogen levels, and their estrogen levels go up after they pull out of the depression. Also, women with depression have lower bone density than

## Connecting mental changes and thyroid function

The thyroid is a butterfly shaped gland in your throat right in front of your larynx. It produces the hormone thyroxin, which is responsible for regulating the rate of oxidation in your body, but it also has a profound effect on your moods and your mental functioning. There are two basic forms of thyroid disease: you can be hyperthyroid (in which the thyroid gland produces too much thyroxin) or — and this is more common in women, particularly as we age — hypothyroid (in which it produces too little). Both disorders result in changes, usually subtle but sometimes dramatic, in your overall health.

The kicker is that the symptoms of a thyroid gland on the blink are remarkably similar to the symptoms of menopause. Thyroid disease also tends to occur, when it does, at about the same point in your life as menopause. It's understandable, therefore, that you might go through menopause blaming your symptoms on estrogen depletion without ever knowing your thyroid

is behind some or all of your discomfort. Both are associated with changes in skin, hair, menstruation, and weight, with depression, insomnia, fatigue, mood swings, and memory problems, and with anxiety, heart palpitations, and loss of libido.

At each checkup your doctor should palpate (feel) your throat to check the size and shape of the thyroid gland, but if you or she have concerns about your symptoms she can also order blood and other tests. She will also look for symptoms that are common to thyroid dysfunction but not to menopause, such as tenderness or pain in the throat, swelling in the arms or legs, or loss of eyebrows and eyelashes. Treatment will depend on whether your thyroid levels are too high or too low, and on what your doctor determines to be the cause of the malfunction. Many thyroid problems are treated easily, effectively, and inexpensively with oral medication.

non-depressed women. Low bone density is another common byproduct of low estrogen levels. Estrogen therapy, however, has not been found to be an effective treatment for depression, so the exact nature of the link between hormonal changes and an increase in emotional upsets, if one exists, still isn't well understood.

## *Feeling your way through the symptoms*

Here are the emotional changes you may notice as you approach menopause:

✓ **Anxiety:** You're driving along and all of a sudden you feel panicky. With anxiety, you may experience both emotional and physical symptoms. Emotionally you may be irritable or have trouble focusing. Physically, your heart may start beating as though you've just sprinted a 50-yard dash. You wonder if you should drive straight to the hospital. Heart *palpitations* or a racing heart accompanied by butterflies in your stomach are common during perimenopause and menopause.

✔ **Depression:** If you're dealing with interrupted sleep, hot flashes, or memory lapses, avoiding the blues is hard. If you experienced depression related to PMS or if you had to deal with postpartum (after-childbirth) depression, you're more likely to experience depression during the change (see more about depression earlier in this chapter, under "Deciding Whether You're Depressed").

✔ **Increased sensitivity:** You may feel that life isn't fair or that everything is your fault, or you may find yourself looking for a fight. Performing at any level that falls short of perfection can cause a negative emotional reaction. Or you may experience crying jags — with or without reason.

✔ **Mood swings:** One minute everything is fine, and the next minute you're sad and gloomy. You may find it difficult dealing with family situations, relationships at home, or professional relationships.

## Understanding the physiology and getting relief

When estrogen levels drop, the hormone *serotonin* decreases. Serotonin helps decrease anxiety, so when it drops, you tend to get more anxious. When serotonin drops, it also aggravates adrenaline-inspired irritability and heart palpitations in addition to anxiety. Your doctor may prescribe serotonin-enhancing antidepressants to relieve anxiety during perimenopause and menopause. SSRIs (selective serotonin reuptake inhibitors) can balance certain brain chemicals to help relieve the symptoms of depression.

Keep in mind that, though these symptoms can be annoying, they aren't actually dangerous. Anxiety and depression can also be treated without medication through acupuncture, counseling, biofeedback, yoga, relaxation, herbal remedies, and massage. (See Chapter 17 for more information on alternative therapies.) The decision to take antidepressant medication should be yours, not your doctor's. If you decide to take them, talk with your doctor about possible side effects, and never stop taking them suddenly or change your dosage without medical supervision.

SSRIs are also used to treat depression triggered by an imbalance between estrogen and progesterone in your body. With estrogen levels lower during perimenopause and menopause, progesterone can temporarily overpower the effects of estrogen and testosterone in your brain. You may feel like crying, or you may feel irritable, grumpy, or downright ugly.

Situational stress (not unfamiliar to women in their 40s and 50s) triggers changes in ovarian function. Hormone production can then drop off, causing even more emotional changes. Life events may start your mental and emotional symptoms, but hormonal changes turn up the volume.

# Managing life changes

Going through menopause might be a little easier if you could do it in a social vacuum. You know, maybe take a nice stack of great books, a few bottles of wine, and your favorite comfy clothes and hole up in the mountains (or at the beach or in a luxury big city penthouse apartment — select your favorite scenario) for, oh, say, three or four years. You might still have hot flashes and night sweats and irregular periods, but the aggravation factor in your life would be almost nil.

Instead, though, we all get to go through these life changes in the midst of a crazy, busy world. Menopause seems to get plunked down into your life just at the point at which you still have the concerns of a younger woman but are also beginning to take on the roles of an older one. You might have children still at home when you start taking care of your aging parents or in-laws. Perhaps you're simultaneously dreading and looking forward to having the nest empty out just a bit. You might be wondering when your periods are going to stop and your preteen daughter's are going to start. And you may have reached a position of new responsibility in your job — and here your brains seem to be turning to oatmeal.

Whatever's on your plate, it's going to bring both stress (and, if you're lucky) and joy. Ups and downs. Mood swings and stretches of tranquility. In Chapter 20 we'll talk a lot more about how the changing features of your life affect (and are affected by) your menopause experience.

# Part III
# Treating the Effects

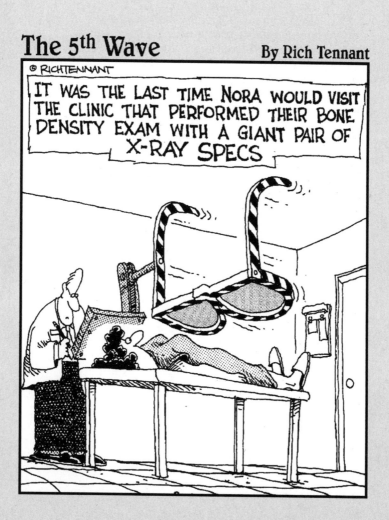

The 5th Wave                    By Rich Tennant

IT WAS THE LAST TIME NORA WOULD VISIT THE CLINIC THAT PERFORMED THEIR BONE DENSITY EXAM WITH A GIANT PAIR OF X-RAY SPECS

# In this part . . .

If you're like most women, the barrage of news flashes and special reports on hormone therapy that seem to pop up a few times a year may leave your head spinning. Flash: "Never take hormones." Report: "Never stop taking hormones." Getting a handle on the risks and benefits of hormone therapy can be challenging. In this part, we attempt to demystify the subject, so that you're in a position to make informed decisions (with the assistance of your medical advisor) about what approach to managing symptoms is right for you.

In the chapters that follow, we present you with the latest information regarding hormone therapy and its relationship to your cardiovascular system, breast cancer, your reproductive organs, your mental and emotional health, and other health concerns. We also provide a bunch of information on non-hormonal treatments (both conventional treatments, such as medications, and non-conventional routes like herbal therapy and acupuncture) for many of the symptoms and conditions facing menopausal women.

# Chapter 11

# The Basics of Hormone Therapy

*H*ormone therapy (HT) may not be right for everyone, but it definitely can relieve many menopausal symptoms and prevent or postpone diseases that afflict women later in life.

Many women are experimenting with hormone therapy to figure out the types, combinations, and dosages that are right for them to maximize the protective effects of HT and minimize the risks. Some women swear by it. Some women fear it. Some women do both. New research findings are announced frequently — sometimes contradicting earlier ones. We make sense of these findings in many chapters of this book, particularly in Chapter 16.

But many women still aren't comfortable enough with their level of knowledge about HT to make up their minds about where they stand on the subject. If you're a member of this group, that's okay. In this chapter, we explain the various hormones and hormone therapy regimens and how they work.

Hormones are powerful, and you should understand what you put in your body.

## Defining Hormone Therapy

*Hormone therapy* is a program of estrogen or estrogen and progestin that are administered to relieve menopausal symptoms. Doctors often prescribe hormones during *perimenopause* (the years before menopause when women experience many of the symptoms — hot flashes, sleeplessness, and so on — associated with menopause). After menopause, you can gradually discontinue use of hormone therapy.

Physicians who recommend that hormone therapy continue *after* menopause do so because it provides some protection against osteoporosis and relieves *urogenital atrophy* (thinning and drying of your vagina or ureter) caused by low levels of estrogen. In many women, the hormone boost also improves mood and the sense of well being. You and your doctor can work together to determine whether hormone therapy is right for you and how long you should remain on it.

Some experts don't like to include the term *replacement* when referring to hormone therapy because *replacement* implies that a *deficiency* exists. Producing lower levels of hormones isn't a disease; it's one of many natural, normal transitions a woman's body makes throughout her lifetime.

Women without a uterus (women who have had a hysterectomy) may take estrogen by itself. When estrogen is used alone, it's called *unopposed estrogen therapy* because progestin isn't included to oppose the effects of the estrogen.

From the 1950s through the 1970s, doctors routinely prescribed *estrogen* (the female hormone responsible for giving you breasts, a curvy figure, a menstrual period, and more) by itself to treat menopausal symptoms. As the incidence of endometrial cancer in menopausal women climbed, researchers noticed that menopausal women were more prone to endometrial cancer if they were taking estrogen therapy. Researchers also found that if you also take *progesterone* (the hormone that causes you to have a period and slough off the endometrial lining during your reproductive years) for a few days, the risk of endometrial cancer drops.

Here's why the addition of *progestin* (the synthetic form of progesterone) reduces the risk of endometrial cancer: Estrogen stimulates growth of the *endometrium* (uterine lining) to make a nice soft nest for a fertilized egg. The uterus is neatly designed to shed the endometrial lining if the egg isn't fertilized. That way you clean out the nest each cycle to get ready for the next ovulation. Shedding the endometrium also serves another purpose because an occasional precancerous cell may be located among the endometrial lining. Stimulated growth month after month causes the occasional precancerous cell to multiply along with the normal cells. If you don't shed these precancerous cells, you're liable to develop endometrial cancer.

So researchers tried giving women progestin (the female hormone that causes changes in the uterus) for a few days. Just like in a natural cycle, when the progestin levels rise and then fall, the endometrial lining sheds — getting rid of any precancerous cells.

Menopausal women who don't take hormone therapy and women who are still menstruating (and shed their endometrial lining each month) rarely have problems with endometrial cancer.

Taking estrogen without balancing (or opposing) it with progestin is referred to as *unopposed estrogen therapy* (check out the section, "Unopposed estrogen therapy," for more information). Women who've had a hysterectomy are really the only women who should receive estrogen alone. Without a uterus (which is removed during a hysterectomy), their chances of developing uterine cancer drop to zero. For most other women who take hormone therapy, a combination of estrogen and progesterone is necessary.

## Slaying the symptoms

For some women, perimenopausal symptoms are so severe that they truly interfere with their relationships, careers, self-esteem, or happiness.

Physicians have routinely prescribed hormone therapy to alleviate symptoms of perimenopause, such as hot flashes, vaginal dryness, disrupted sleep, mood swings, and so on, and it works fabulously. (Check the Cheat Sheet or Chapter 3 for a full rundown of perimenopausal and menopausal symptoms.) Despite studies that suggest that there are health risks associated with hormone therapy, many women don't want to go without hormone therapy because perimenopausal symptoms threaten their enjoyment of life.

People around the world have developed alternative therapies to alleviate the symptoms associated with perimenopause, and women in the Western world have started to choose alternatives to traditional hormone therapy. (Check out Chapter 17 for a rundown of alternative approaches.)

## Preventing serious health problems with hormone therapy

Thanks to improvements in nutrition and healthcare, women living in the United States and Canada today may live into their 80s and 90s. Consider this: In 1900, North American women could expect to live to the ripe old age of 50 (barely into menopause). But today the average life span is about 80 years (way beyond menopause), so you've definitely got an incentive to live a healthier lifestyle. And you may want to consider hormone therapy.

Here's why: Estrogen keeps the engine that is your body running smoothly, and you're going to be driving this car for quite some time (unlike the women in historical times who only drove the car while it was new). Think about how you maintain your car. It's one thing to be a quart low on oil when you're driving a couple miles to the grocery store. But taking a 2,000-mile trip when you're down a quart of oil is a completely different story. Your engine will burn up long before you reach the end of your journey. You may want to intervene with medicine even when you're not sick to keep your body running smoothly.

The health problems standing in the way of staying active and comfortable are related to the fact that women produce lower levels of estrogen after becoming menopausal — which can be 30, 40, or more years of your life. Low levels of estrogen are associated with such health issues as:

- Osteoporosis
- Hardening of the arteries
- Heart disease (including heart attack and angina)
- Increased risk of some cancers
- Memory changes

Preventing some of these debilitating diseases and conditions is one of the reasons women have traditionally elected to take hormone therapy. Now that recent research indicates that hormone therapy is not as effective at dealing with some of these problems as originally thought (and may even make some of them worse — we'll talk more about this later in this and the next few chapters), it's especially important to sort out exactly what's right for you.

Studies such as the Women's Health Initiative also emphasize that whatever you decide to do about hormone therapy, it's critical that you also choose a healthy lifestyle that includes frequent exercise, a healthy diet, and regular medical checkups.

# Ticking Through the Therapies

Every woman's body is different, and you can choose from a variety of regimens and many different types of hormones. We know that trying to get a handle on all the available hormones and therapies on the ever-changing market can be overwhelming. So, in this section, the goal is to help you understand the different types of treatment programs women use and why they use them.

Estrogen plays such a large role in so many of your body's functions that compensating for the decreased production levels that menopause brings is a key component of most hormone therapies.

During menopause and beyond, the perimenopausal symptoms generally begin to subside, and the bigger concern is preventing, delaying, or treating health issues such as bone loss, cancer, and upwardly mobile blood cholesterol levels.

# Unopposed estrogen therapy

*Unopposed estrogen therapy* refers to a treatment program in which you receive only estrogen without any form of progesterone.

Doctors only use unopposed estrogen if you have no uterus (you've had a hysterectomy) because taking estrogen without progestin can lead to endometrial cancer.

Blood-clotting problems are associated with high dosages of estrogen. If you smoke *and* take estrogen, your risk is even higher. Some evidence shows that the estradiol form of estrogen may be less likely to contribute to blood clots than the conjugated types of estrogen. Because patches don't send estrogen to the liver where it stirs up trouble, they may also lower the risk of clotting. Even so, be sure your doctor is aware of any personal or family history you may have of clotting disorders before you use any estrogen products.

If you have an existing problem with liver or gallbladder disease, discuss these conditions with your doctor before using any type of estrogen. Patients with uncontrolled blood pressure shouldn't start on high doses of estrogen. You should also inform your doctor of any history of diabetes, breast cancer, endometriosis or fibroid uterine tumors, pancreatitis, or vaginal bleeding.

## Treatment methods

Your doctor will evaluate your symptoms and hormone levels to establish an appropriate dosage. You may take an estrogen pill every day or use a patch that you apply to your abdomen once or twice a week (the exact timing depends on the brand and your doctor's recommendations). Creams you apply to your skin (like you apply a moisturizer) are also available.

## Benefits

Taking unopposed estrogen boosts the amount of estrogen circulating in your bloodstream. This boost alleviates a variety of symptoms including:

- ✔ **Headaches:** Estrogen increases blood flow by relaxing blood vessels.

- ✔ **Hot flashes, heart palpitations, and anxiety:** A drop in estrogen triggers your brain to release adrenaline, which makes your heart race and your blood vessels dilate.

- ✔ **Interrupted sleep:** This state of affairs is often the result of hot flashes. Estrogen alleviates hot flashes and increases serotonin production, so you're able to sleep through the night.

- ✔ **Mood swings and irritability:** Estrogen increases serotonin production.

- ✔ **Vaginal dryness and atrophy, frequent urination, and urinary incontinence:** Estrogen acts as a moisturizer to your urogenital tissues, keeping them pliable enough to avoid these problems.

Taking unopposed estrogen also eliminates the premenstrual-symptom-like side effects of bloating, breast tenderness, and similar symptoms caused by progesterone. Taking unopposed estrogen also seems to help prevent fractures.

Recent research, however, finds that estrogen therapy is not helpful in preventing many of the problems it was previously associated with relieving. New findings, for example, indicate that it *increases* your risk of blood clots, heart attack, and stroke.

### Side effects

If you take estrogen alone without progesterone or progestin, you won't have periods after menopause as you would with combination hormone therapy (see the "Combination therapy" section later in this chapter). Your *endometrium* (lining of your uterus) will continue to thicken and create quite a buildup. The buildup can lead to endometrial (uterine) cancer.

Another side effect of estrogen includes breast fullness or tenderness. This side effect can often be reduced or eliminated by decreasing the dosage or switching from the pill form of estrogen to an *estradiol* (active estrogen) skin patch.

Sometimes side effects reflect a reaction to a dye or some inert (inactive) ingredient in an estrogen tablet and can be eliminated by switching from the pill to the patch. These side effects may include joint aches, muscle aches, skin irritation, and a burning sensation that accompanies urination. Skin irritation can also be a side effect of patch use.

### Cautions

Have a uterus? Don't use unopposed estrogen therapy (because of the risk of endometrial cancer). If you have a history of breast cancer or you're experiencing undiagnosed vaginal bleeding, your physician won't prescribe unopposed estrogen therapy even if you've had a hysterectomy. If you only have a family history of breast cancer, talk with your doctor about whether unopposed estrogen is an option for you.

Stay away from estrogen therapy if you're pregnant.

# Combination therapy

*Combination therapy* means taking a combination of hormones instead of just estrogen. Combination therapy typically consists of a combination of estrogen and progesterone (or the synthetic form of progesterone called *progestin*). Some women who experience low libido also take a small dose of testosterone in their "hormone cocktail."

Combining progesterone with estrogen provides the benefits of estrogen while reducing the risk of endometrial cancer that taking unopposed estrogen can heighten. The only bad part is that progestin/progesterone may slightly reduce some of the benefits of estrogen. The sole purpose for including progestin in hormone therapy is to reduce your risk of endometrial cancer. If you have a uterus and you elect hormone therapy, your doctor will put you on some form of combination hormone therapy.

## Treatment methods

Choosing combination therapy gives you several options, as long as your medical history doesn't rule it out. Combination hormone therapy comes in two basic forms: cyclic and continuous combination therapy. And cyclical combination therapy has a few different options you can choose from. Each form has its own set of indications that make it the right choice.

✔ **Cyclic combination therapy:** With this form, you're taking estrogen and progestin in a cycle — estrogen in the first part and progestin in the second. The progestin tells your uterus to shed the endometrial lining, so you'll have periods.

"But I thought menopause meant that you don't have a period," you say (with justifiable indignation). Okay, you're not technically having a *menstrual* period; you're having vaginal bleeding. Drugs, not ovulation, trigger this bleeding. Cyclic hormone therapy causes most women to have predictable vaginal bleeding, sometimes for years.

There are two common cyclic combination programs:

- In one, you take estrogen every day of the month and estrogen and progestin together for the last 10 to 14 days of every cycle.

- In the other cyclic combination regimen, you take estrogen every day for 25 days of the month and progestin for 10 to 12 days, then no medication for 3 to 6 days each month (expect bleeding on these days). Some people refer to this regimen as *sequential combination therapy* because you take the estrogen and progestin in a sequence.

✔ **Continuous combination therapy:** With this form of therapy, you take estrogen and progestin together every day. This approach is associated with these benefits:

- Lower risk of endometrial cancer

- Cessation of periods after six months or a year

- Slightly reduced risk of colorectal cancer

- Fewer fractures

- A slightly diminished risk of mild cognitive impairment

- Fewer progestin-related side effects in some women (see the following "Side effects" section), especially bleeding

Pills and patches on the market today combine the two hormones, making them easy to take. But some women who are sensitive to progestin experience fewer side effects when using a progestin cream and taking estrogen as a pill or patch. If you're bothered by side effects, talk with your doctor about experimenting with different dosages or forms to make you more comfortable.

Some women on combination therapy don't like the side effects they feel on the days they take progesterone. Don't stop taking progesterone/progestin without consulting your doctor, and take it for the exact length of time prescribed by your doctor. Taking estrogen without progestin/progesterone can lead to endometrial cancer. (For more information, see the "Unopposed estrogen therapy" section earlier in this chapter.)

Certain progestins are derived from testosterone and can help women who complain of low libido (sex drive) during and after menopause. The generic name for this progestin is *norethindrone.* Although norethindrone reduces many of the progestin side effects, it's not recommended for women with high LDL-cholesterol or triglyceride levels. Like estrogen, you can take testosterone via creams, regular pills, pills that dissolve under your tongue, and vaginal suppositories. Doctors most commonly prescribe low-dosage skin creams and pills because these forms cause your body to absorb the testosterone more slowly, helping you avoid side effects caused by rapid shifts in your hormone levels.

## Benefits

Combination therapy should give you the best of all worlds — the benefits of estrogen (and perhaps testosterone) without the risks of endometrial cancer.

Continuous hormone therapy causes fewer side effects in older women (several years beyond menopause) than in younger women. Continuous hormone therapy also causes fewer PMS-type symptoms than cyclic hormone therapy does. The good news for those of you who are tired of tampons is that one-third of women stop bleeding when they start the continuous combination therapy, many others stop monthly bleeding after two to three months, and most have stopped monthly bleeding after one year of therapy. Another bonus: women who have problems with their libido often find that a bit of testosterone in their hormone mix gives it a boost.

### Side effects

Some women have a hard enough time tolerating either human progesterone or synthetic progestin. Proper dosages and delivery forms can help to curb the side effects of progestin, which can include acne, bloating, depression, and weight gain.

### Cautions

Women with a history of breast cancer should not take hormone therapy, and those with a family history of breast cancer should seek their doctors' advice. Women who have heart disease, uncontrolled diabetes, high blood pressure, high triglyceride levels, fibromyalgia, or depression should make sure their doctors are aware of their history of these conditions before they prescribe a specific HT regimen.

Contrary to what researchers believed just a few years ago, combination therapy does not prevent coronary artery disease or reduce the risk of heart attack. Recent women's Health Initiative findings show that combination therapy users are at increased risk of

- ✔ Heart attack
- ✔ Stroke
- ✔ Blood clots
- ✔ Breast cancer
- ✔ Dementia (study included only women 65 and older)

## Selective Estrogen Receptor Modulators (SERMs)

Meet the stealth bombers of the hormone therapy world. SERMs are manufactured designer drugs that provide the benefits of estrogen to specific parts of the body while blocking its effects in parts of the body it has the potential to harm (your breasts and uterus, for instance). SERMs don't contain estrogen itself, but they act to stimulate estrogen receptors where the effects of estrogen are desired, and to block its effects where they aren't wanted. The U.S. Food and Drug Administration (FDA) has approved two SERMs for use in the United States:

✔ **Tamoxifen:** Though it was designed to prevent further recurrence for women with a history of specific types of breast cancer, research showed that Tamoxifen is also effective at improving bone density.

✔ **Raloxifene:** Approved by the FDA for treatment and prevention of osteoporosis, Raloxifene also seems to be associated with a decrease in the incidence of breast cancer among its users.

A breast cancer drug that's effective against osteoporosis and an osteoporosis medication that's effective against breast cancer? The need to find the one most effective drug led to a showdown of sorts — but in the Study of Tamoxifen and Raloxifene (STAR), sponsored by the National Cancer Institute and other groups, and not in the OK Corral. Recently STAR began releasing findings from their two-year study comparing the effectiveness of these two drugs. It's likely that more results will trickle in, but the main findings so far indicate that

✔ Both drugs cut breast cancer risk in half.

✔ Study participants who took Raloxifene had 39 percent fewer uterine cancers than those taking Tamoxifen.

✔ Both drugs increased the risk of blood clots, but Raloxifene users had 29 percent fewer blood clots than Tamoxifen users.

✔ Both drugs were equally effective at preventing bone fractures.

✔ Both are associated with menopausal side effects, but Raloxifene takers experienced fewer of these.

### Treatment methods

Both Tamoxifen and Raloxifene are available in pill form and should be taken as directed by your physician.

### Benefits

SERMs may reduce bone loss in menopausal women, but not as well as estrogen. SERMs reduce the risk of breast cancer in women if taken for no more than five years. Unlike combination hormone therapy, SERMs have no negative effects on blood lipids, so they won't raise your triglyceride or LDL-cholesterol levels.

A lot of research is still ongoing, and new types of SERMs are on their way. Targeting specific estrogen receptors for enrichment seems to be a very promising way to help women stay comfortable and healthy during and after menopause.

### Side effects

Unfortunately, SERM use brings some side effects, but STAR found fewer of these with Raloxifene:

- Insomnia
- Slight increased risk of endometrial cancer (with Tamoxifen)
- Significant hot flashes

SERMs are beneficial to your blood cholesterol, but they do increase the risk of blood clots in your veins and lungs and may lead to strokes.

### Cautions

Anyone at risk of cardiovascular problems should avoid SERMs. Also note that if you have hot flashes, SERMs have the potential to make them worse.

# Prescribing Pills, Patches, and Pomades

Over the years, scientists have worked hard to provide hormone therapy that maximizes the benefits and minimizes the side effects and inconveniences. Basically, you have three hormone therapy paths to choose: your mouth (pill), skin (patch or cream), or vagina (cream, gel, or ring).

In the following sections, we list the types of delivery systems available and the benefits and drawbacks of each. We also go through the different types of hormones used in hormone therapy one by one and indicate how they can be delivered. You and your doctor can experiment to find the delivery methods and dosages that are most effective for you.

## Popping pills

Taking pills by mouth is the easiest and most traditional way of taking medicine. Getting the exact dose that the doctor ordered is also simple because the prescribed dosage is already loaded in the pill; plus the frequency is written on the label. For older women who may already be taking several medications, an additional pill in the parade can be a pain.

## Pasting on a patch

Patches deliver drugs that are absorbed through the skin. In the old days (five or six years ago), the alcohol in the original bulky patches often caused skin irritation. In today's thinner, smaller *matrix* patches the hormone is actually incorporated in the adhesive that holds it on.

Patches have some significant advantages:

- ✔ You put them on once or twice a week.
- ✔ They deliver a steady and consistent supply of hormone.
- ✔ They're easier on your liver and digestive tract than pills are because the medication they release bypasses these areas of your body and goes straight into your bloodstream.

Exposure to heat can increase the amount of medication released by your patch (leaving less for later). Doctors don't recommend exposing it to direct sunlight (or tanning lamps) or hot environments such as saunas or hot tubs.

Location, location, location. You may experience different results depending on where you apply the cream or wear the patch. If your patch falls off, or if you have bad side effects, talk to your doctor about using a different location (for example, hip instead of abdomen) before trying a different medication.

Because HT has been associated with an increase in the risk of heart disease, a five-year study was launched in 2005 at eight medical centers in the United States to look at whether delivery of HT by patch, rather than in pill form, is less likely to contribute to cardiac problems. The study, called Kronos Early Estrogen Prevention Study (KEEPS), will follow younger perimenopausal and menopausal women than those being followed by the Women's Health Initiative.

## Applying creams

Vaginal lining responds very quickly to treatments applied directly to the area as a remedy for dryness or atrophy. Some women like vaginal creams because they deliver the hormones localized in a small area. They won't, however, treat your hot flashes, mood swings, bones, or blood cholesterol.

If you're treating vaginal dryness or atrophy yet worry about breast or endometrial cancer, a cream may be a good choice, even though its measurement may be somewhat imprecise. For example, an estrogen cream relieves vaginal dryness and atrophy but doesn't increase your risk of breast cancer because the dosage is low and the estrogen stays put. Vaginal estrogen suppositories or tablets are another option. These are neater than creams, easy to insert, and give a precise dose. You insert them high into the vagina with an applicator similar to one you'd use for a tampon, only narrower.

Don't expose a male sexual partner to the medication in hormone creams or suppositories. The active ingredients can be absorbed through the skin of his penis. Don't use them right before intercourse. Also, some estrogen creams contain oils that can weaken latex condoms.

A *compounding pharmacy* is one that will make up prescriptions in a custom-tailored dosage (stronger or weaker), formula (a cup of estrogen, a few teaspoons of progestin, a pinch of testosterone), or form (cream, gel, even — though probably not for HT — lollipops or gummy bears). If you just can't find the right balance of hormones to keep your risk low and your symptoms at bay, talk to your doctor about working with a compounding pharmacy to make up just the right prescription for you. Though not regulated by the Food and Drug Administration, these are closely regulated by individual states. If there's not one near you, ask your doctor to recommend one who does mail order.

## Slipping on a ring

This ring doesn't go on your finger; you place it in your vagina. Rings are fairly new in the United States, but women in Europe have been using them for quite a while to address vaginal and urinary symptoms of menopause. The doctor usually inserts the flexible, hormone-containing ring initially; after that you can change it — usually every 90 days. The ring slowly delivers an even supply of hormones to your bloodstream.

Don't worry: The ring won't get in your way during sex. But some women do have a problem tolerating the ring because they have short or narrow vaginas. Also, you can pop it out if you're straining on the potty. But, if you're okay with a diaphragm, the ring isn't that much different.

A ring is a great option for women with vaginal and urinary tract menopausal symptoms, but it doesn't provide all the other health benefits of estrogen such as relief of perimenopausal symptoms and improved bone maintenance. The ring's risk factors for endometrial cancer have not been systematically compared with those of other estrogen-delivery methods. The Food and Drug administration, though, warns that this may be a risk if you still have a uterus.

## Rejecting injections

Although hormones are available in a fourth form (all other forms are described in the section, "Prescribing Pills, Patches, and Pomades," earlier in this chapter), as shots, they're not used in routine hormone therapy. Physicians generally prescribe hormone shots just prior to surgery for patients who are about to have their ovaries taken out. Injections keep the hormone levels in the patient's bloodstream from crashing after the surgery.

# Searching for Sources

For those of you who like to exchange recipes, here's a quick overview about how drug companies make these hormones. In the following sections, you can see that those folks in white lab coats have been very resourceful in finding ways to create hormones.

## Synthetic versus natural hormones

Deciding what's *natural* when it comes to hormone therapy can be difficult. Like beauty, natural (hormone therapy) is in the eye of the beholder. You can look at *natural* a couple of ways:

- Natural can mean similar to what you already have in your body. In the laboratory, scientists can replicate the exact molecular structure of human hormones. The results are identical to human hormones but without the stray bits that exist in all animal hormones. So these hormones have the same structure as natural human hormones, but they're made in a lab, so they're synthetic.

- Natural can also mean coming from nature (you know, plants and animals). Some hormones are derived from plants but need to be modified to produce a beneficial effect in our bodies. Other hormones come from animals. So, these natural hormones come from nature, but they're not *natural* to humans.

So, *natural* isn't really a good term for describing the hormones used for hormone therapy. In the next section, we give you the source of the hormone — you get to decide whether you consider it natural or not.

## Estrogen

Some really clever scientists have found a variety of sources from which to make estrogen. Over the years, trying to get the right type and amount of estrogen into your body has been quite a challenge for the guys and gals in lab coats.

Before we get started with the recipes for hormone therapy, a quick reminder about the ins and outs of estrogen may be in order. Three types of estrogen exist: estrone, estradiol, and estriol. We mention this fact because all types of estrogen are not created equal. Here's a brief estrogen primer (the whole story is in Chapter 2):

✔ **Estradiol** is the biologically active type of estrogen and the most potent form of human estrogen. It's a player in hundreds of bodily functions.

✔ **Estrone** isn't the workhorse that estradiol is; estrone is more like the warehouse variety of estrogen that's stored in your body fat. It can be turned into estradiol, but only in premenopausal ovaries.

✔ As for **estriol,** fuggetaboutit — in this context anyway. Estriol is mostly found in pregnant women.

All right. Now that that's taken care of, here are the sources of estrogen that scientists have come up with:

✔ **Conjugated equine estrogen:** Made from the urine of pregnant horses. (If you're a vegan or lean toward animal rights activism, this one might not be right for you.) Some of the most-prescribed estrogens used in hormone therapy are conjugated equine estrogens. This type of estrogen has the least amount of estradiol, but it delivers lots of estrone and a significant amount of *equilin,* an estrogen used by horses. Although equilins are great for female horses, doctors occupy both sides of the fence on the subject of whether equilin is beneficial to human females. Conjugated equine estrogen is available in pill, injection, and cream form.

✔ **Estradiol estrogen:** Derived from soybeans and/or wild yams. These estrogens are chemically identical to human estradiol estrogen. Estradiol estrogen is available in every delivery method — pill, cream, ring, and patch. (Check out the "Prescribing Pills, Patches, and Pomades" section earlier in this chapter for more info.) In fact, it's the only type of estrogen used in the patch.

✔ **Esterified estrogen:** Made from soybeans and/or wild yams (sometimes referred to as Mexican yams). Esterified estrogen provides high levels of estrone and much lower levels of estradiol estrogen, but it has been shown to help maintain bone and improve perimenopausal symptoms and lipid profiles in the blood. Esterified estrogen is available as a pill.

✔ **Estropipate:** Also known as *piperazine estrogen sulfate.* Available as a pill or cream, this synthetic form of estrogen is chemically similar, but not identical, to human estrone. A drawback of estropipate: It may actually aggravate pain in women who have muscle- or bladder-pain syndromes.

✔ **Micronized estradiol:** *Micronization* means that the particles are small enough to be absorbed into your bloodstream before your digestive system destroys them. So here we go with the "What's natural and what's not?" discussion. Micronized estradiol is made from a "natural" plant, but technicians tweak it in the lab so that your body can use it. You take this estradiol as a pill. Provides women with the same type of active estrogen (estradiol) that the ovaries produce naturally. The estradiol is produced synthetically (in the lab) from soybeans.

Some doctors claim that using a form of estrogen that's molecularly similar to human estradiol is no more beneficial to women than estrogen products derived from pregnant mares; others claim that it makes all the difference in the world.

## Progestin

Most of the side effects attributed to hormone therapy are the result of the progestin, but progestin protects you from developing endometrial cancer. Because every woman's body is different, you may need to do some experimenting to figure out which progestin is right for you.

Adding progestin to the hormone therapy mix does seem to reduce the benefits estrogen can have on your cholesterol levels and increase changes to your mood.

There are three types of progestin on the market:

- **Progesterone:** Identical to the human hormone produced by the ovary in premenopausal women. Progesterone is available as a pill and as a vaginal gel.

- **Medroxyprogesterone acetate (MPA):** Originally used to regulate menstrual cycles. Doctors now prescribe it in hormone therapy to slough off, or thin, the endometrial lining at the end of a course of estrogen, thereby reducing the risk of endometrial cancer.

- **Progestin derived from testosterone:** Includes norethindrone and norethindrone acetate progestin. They seem to have fewer side effects than MPA and offer a boost to the libido in some women. These progestins aren't recommended for women with high cholesterol or low HDL (the "good" cholesterol) levels. Norethindrone and norethindrone acetate are available either as pills or patches.

## Combinations of estrogen and progestin

For the sake of convenience, you may want to combine estrogen and progestin into a single pill or patch.

A couple brands on the market combine conjugated estrogen with a progestin called medroxyprogesterone acetate (MPA). The U.S. Food and Drug Administration approved MPA for women having trouble with their periods. MPA helps prevent the *endometrium* (uterine lining) from thickening too much and helps regulate periods. Because it inhibits over-thickening of your endometrium, MPA can lower your risk of endometrial cancer.

Conjugated estrogen and MPA is a commonly prescribed combination therapy and can be administered as either sequential courses of estrogen followed by progestin or as continuous combination therapy (see the "Combination therapy" section earlier in this chapter).

Today, new combination therapies use a progestin derived from testosterone, *norethindrone acetate,* instead of MPA because it causes less vaginal bleeding. You can get a combination therapy in both patch and pill forms. The combination patch administers the estradiol form of estrogen and norethindrone acetate. Many women like the patch because you don't have to remember to take a pill and it's convenient to have both hormones delivered in a single patch.

## Androgens

REMEMBER

When we talk about *androgens* (male hormones), we're mainly talking about testosterone.

You may need to include androgens (most likely testosterone) in your hormone therapy for a couple of reasons. If you've become menopausal due to surgery (removal of your ovaries), your androgens may take a nosedive very quickly. You may want to bump your androgens up because they help bone maintenance and libido. Women who experience natural menopause may need androgens in the regimen because estrogen supplements may decrease the amount of physiologically active testosterone in your bloodstream (which could lower your libido and lessen muscle tone).

Using too high a dose of testosterone has some side effects: acne, oily skin, hair loss, unwanted hair, and a deeper voice. Rest assured that prescribed dosages are rarely high enough to trigger these side effects.

# Doing the Dosing

The guideline that every doctor uses is this: Use the smallest dose possible to alleviate symptoms and health risks while minimizing the side effects. That said, individual women react to hormone supplements very differently. No one knows why a particular regimen causes one woman to experience side effects and another to sing its praises from the rooftop. Hormone therapy should be an ongoing process, and a responsible doctor will work *with* you to find the dosage that works *for* you.

Your doc will review your personal medical history, your family medical history, and the results of your physical examination and lab work. He'll also want to consider what conditions or problems you're trying to overcome or prevent. (For example: Are we talking about lessening perimenopausal symptoms or preventing osteoporosis after menopause? Could your libido use a little boost?) Share your personal preferences and prejudices with your doctor at this time as well. (Do you have a hard time swallowing pills? Do you forget to take medicine? Are you determined to turf the tampons as soon as possible? These kinds of issues.) Convenience and cost are also legitimate issues to raise.

So just how much active estrogen do you need pulsing through your body to keep you healthy and comfortable for the years to come? With new information from the Women's Health Initiative about the potential risks of hormone therapy — particularly for women over 65 — many doctors are prescribing hormones for shorter periods (no pun intended) than they used to, but every case is different. You and your doctor may conclude that continuing hormones for some years will be beneficial enough for you to outweigh any risk factors you have.

If you have issues with your libido, your doctor takes it into the equation when prescribing hormone therapy. Convenience is also an issue. Convenience considerations include how many other medications you take (do you really want to take more pills or use a patch), the cost, and how anxious you are to quit bleeding every month. As far as the last issue goes, *sequential/cyclical therapy* (taking estrogen for part of the month and progestin another part of the month) results in continuing your periods for some time, but *continuous combination therapy* (taking both estrogen and progestin at the same time every day) generally stops your periods. SERMs also eliminate your periods.

# Chapter 12

# Understanding Hormone Therapy and Your Heart

*U*ntil the results of the Women's Health Initiative (WHI) study were released early in 2002, most medical folks thought that the one certainty in hormone therapy (HT) was the benefits it brought to your heart. Although there's still no question that the estrogen produced naturally in your body lowers your risk of heart disease and keeps your blood cholesterol healthy *during your reproductive years,* HT (which doesn't use precisely the same type of estrogen your body naturally produces) turns out not be the cure-all for menopausal women that most experts had hoped it would be.

You need to take cardiovascular issues seriously. Whether you're talking about stroke, high blood pressure, or heart attack, more women die of cardiovascular disease than men do.

This chapter shows you the risks and benefits of hormone therapy as it affects your cardiovascular system. We also take you through the major findings of the Women's Health Initiative and other large studies of heart health as they apply to menopausal women. With this info in hand, you can make better long-term decisions about how to cope with cardiovascular risks that increase with age, and how to live a healthy life now and in the future. (But, before you make any decisions, check out the other HT chapters in this book, too — Chapter 11 and Chapters 13 through 17.)

# Meeting the Players: Hormones and Your Heart

It seems appropriate that your own natural sex hormones should play a role in keeping your heart healthy. The jobs they do in your cardiovascular system before menopause aren't so different from the ones they play elsewhere in your body. They keep you supple, strong, and vigorous, so it makes sense that they'll do the same in promoting heart health.

## The star: Estrogen

Because estrogen protects the cardiovascular system, women have about a ten-year grace period for developing heart disease when compared to men. In fact, most of the cardiovascular benefits attributed to hormone therapy are due to the protective nature of estrogen:

- ✔ Keeps triglycerides low, and increases HDL ("good") cholesterol
- ✔ Keeps fibrinogen, a protein which can cause blood clots, at healthy levels
- ✔ Relaxes artery walls to help dilate blood vessels, improve blood flow, and avoid spasms
- ✔ Reduces the buildup of plaque in your coronary arteries
- ✔ Helps prevent dangerous enlargement of the heart

For years hormone therapy — at first just estrogen, and later on, estrogen with progesterone, to mimic your natural hormonal cycle — was routinely prescribed for women. Hormone therapy was given not only to limit menopausal symptoms, but also with the idea that it will keep your heart strong and healthy. Doctors eventually figured out that estrogen can be a tricky thing to replace, though. It serves up a few pretty serious potential side effects along with its benefits. These can include

- ✔ Blood clots (deep-vein thrombosis) at high levels
- ✔ Increased triglyceride levels (when given as a pill)
- ✔ Uterine cancer, in women with a uterus

Continually reviewing your hormone-therapy regimen throughout your life is very important. Your health conditions can change, which may lead you to make a change in your program.

# The supporting actor: Progesterone

Progesterone's main function is to prepare your body for pregnancy. When progesterone levels peak, most women feel bloated and ravenously hungry. Your breasts often feel tender and enlarged. If your egg isn't fertilized, progesterone levels drop, you have your period, and these symptoms go away.

With all the uncomfortable symptoms progesterone causes, why in the world should anyone knowingly take this hormone after they finally rid their systems of it? Doctors have added *progestin* — synthetic progesterone — to nearly all HT programs to lower the risk of endometrial cancer. (Women who have their uterus surgically removed don't receive progestin because they no longer have to worry about uterine cancer, so they can take estrogen alone, or unopposed estrogen.)

Although progestin reduces the risk of endometrial cancer, it has some negative effects on your cardiovascular system. In particular, progestin

- Lowers HDL ("good" cholesterol) levels.
- Increases triglycerides (very-low-density lipid — nearly all fat).
- Lowers your sensitivity to insulin, which affects your ability to process glucose. This effect is of great concern to diabetics.
- Tends to make women's bodies store fats instead of breaking them down.

# The assistant: Testosterone

Women's bodies naturally produce testosterone, a so-called male hormone. When given with *estradiol* (the active form of estrogen), testosterone helps to relax and dilate the blood vessels, improving the flow of blood. If testosterone is given on its own with no estradiol, it seems to have the opposite effect, promoting plaque buildup on vessel walls. Testosterone is tricky stuff, so if you're taking it, ask your doctor to keep an eye on your blood cholesterol and modify treatment as needed.

# Understanding the Difference Between Hormones and Hormone Therapy

The *Women's Health Initiative* (WHI) study, the one that stirred the HT debate early in 2002, recruited over 160,000 volunteers to make sure the study's findings would be applicable to a wide range of women. The WHI put together four large studies, one of them specifically about hormones.

---

# Living in "The Big Study" era

You know how there was a Big Band era, right? Well, you're fortunate enough to live in the "Big Health Study" era . . . at least when it comes to studies on hormones and menopause. In addition to the WHI, these long-term studies are making hormone headlines:

- ✔ The Framingham Heart Study (FHS) is the longest-running study of health in America, with data on three generations in one Massachusetts town.

- ✔ The Heart and Estrogen/Progestin Replacement Study (HERS) collects data on the effects of hormone therapy on 2,763 women with a history of heart disease.

- ✔ The Nurses' Health Study (NHS) has studied menopause and other health issues since 1976.

- ✔ KEEPS (Kronos Early Estrogen Prevention Study) is the new kid on the block, still in the early stages of a study of hormones and the heart in women 40 to 50.

In most cases, other heart researchers reported similar findings to those of the WHI. In the HERS, women who were taking unopposed estrogen did not experience any protection from heart disease or deaths from heart disease, and experienced a greater incidence of blood clots. In the first year of this study there was an increased incidence of heart disease (but again, the HERS participants had a prior history of heart disease). In the Framingham study, after 24 years of follow-up, women who had been taking unopposed estrogen reported twice the levels of coronary heart disease that they had experienced prior to menopause.

---

The WHI researchers focused their look at hormones on two clinical trials: one on unopposed estrogen (remember, that's estrogen all by its lonesome, with no progestin), and one in which participants took conjugated equine estrogen combined with MPA, or medroxyprogesterone acetate (this type is often called combination therapy).

Remember, estrogen — at least in its homegrown state in your own body — is good for the heart and blood vessels. The WHI folks were surprised, then, when they found no protective function for cardiovascular health in either the unopposed estrogen or the estrogen plus progestin group. In fact, in some cases, particularly among study participants taking estrogen and progestin, the hormone therapy was actually having some detrimental effects. In this section, we tackle the differences that the WHI study uncovered.

## Using estrogen plus progestin

Compared with those taking a placebo, the group taking the estrogen and progestin therapy experienced more

- ✔ Breast cancer
- ✔ Heart attacks and an overall increase in coronary heart disease

✔ Stroke

✔ Blood clots (deep vein thrombosis — clots in the lower body and legs — and pulmonary embolism — clots that broke off and traveled to the lungs)

There was no protective effect against either heart disease or peripheral artery disease.

The Food and Drug Administration (FDA) has placed a warning on estrogen products, advising against their use to prevent coronary heart disease.

## Taking unopposed estrogen

In the estrogen group, and, again, compared with the women who took placebos, the group taking the actual estrogen therapy experienced

✔ More strokes

✔ A slight trend toward a greater risk for blood clots

The only good news: Marginally fewer women (those at the younger end of the 50- to 79-year-old group studied) from the unopposed estrogen group required procedures to open clogged arteries.

# Identifying the Heart Disease Culprit

Does your risk of heart disease increase over time because of menopause, or just because you're older? Is the culprit age, or is it menopause itself? Doctors say that our "absolute risk" of many diseases more or less doubles with each passing decade (encouraging, huh?). Your risk for a given disease in your 60s, then, is about twice what it was when you were in your 50s. And yet, most of us know vital, healthy women who make it to their 70s, 80s, even 90s and beyond without getting cancer, or heart disease, or lung disease, or any of the other serious conditions we often associate with aging. This is why studies such as these large ones, that follow individuals for years or even decades, are an important means of figuring out what factors differ between the people who get sick and the people who stay remarkably healthy for their ages.

## Considering the age of menopause

The age at which you reach menopause seems to be one of the heart disease risk factors worth looking at. The Nurses' Health Study found that

✔ The risk of heart attack for women who experienced early menopause after their ovaries were surgically removed increases with younger age at menopause.

✔ Entering menopause in your early 40s instead of your 50s increases the risk of heart disease, hardening of the arteries, and death from certain types of heart disease.

The WHI studied women of normal menopause age and older (50 to 79), but the Framingham and Nurse's Health Studies include younger women as well. Younger women are the *primary* focus of the KEEPS initiative. Studies such as these will help us learn more about the relative effects of age and of menopause.

## Factoring in other factors

Of course, things are never simple in research. Simply looking at age at menopause and heart disease will probably not tell us much. Good research teases out the likely effects of age plus other risk factors, including

✔ Genetics

✔ Lifestyle

✔ Health history and health habits

All of these factors interact so that every woman's situation — and thus her risk of heart disease — is unique. The Nurses' Health Study, for example, shows that if you entered menopause early, after ovary removal, and you're a smoker, you are at increased risk for coronary heart disease.

Given the lack of a definitive answer about which of several answers puts a middle-aged woman at risk for heart disease, we can only suggest that you take care of the variables you can control:

✔ Eat a diet low on the food chain, high in fruits and vegetables, and low in animal products (see Chapter 18, "Eating for the Change," for more suggestions.

✔ Don't smoke!

✔ Use alcohol in moderation or not at all.

✔ See your doctor regularly and follow her advice about keeping your cholesterol and blood pressure at a healthy level.

✔ Exercise regularly.

# Skimming the Fat: Hormone Therapy and Your Blood

In general, what's good for your blood is good for your heart. Age and bad habits can contribute to the accumulation of fats and calcifications in your arteries, clogging them up just like old plumbing, and raising your risk of a whole host of dangerous events and conditions, including hypertension, heart attack, stroke, and angina. In this section we'll talk about some of these risks, and the role that hormones and hormone therapy play in their development and their management.

## Combating hypertension

Hypertension (high blood pressure) is often caused by hardening of the arteries or coronary artery disease. Over the years, lipids and cholesterol can get deposited on the walls of your blood vessels. This process, called *atherosclerosis,* causes your arteries to thicken and impedes the flow of blood through your veins. This can raise your blood pressure, forcing your heart to pump harder. Hypertension can lead to stroke, heart attack, heart failure, and other serious health problems such as kidney disease and vision problems.

### Recognizing the signs

One of the scariest things about hypertension is that about 30 percent of people who have it never have any symptoms at all — only a blood pressure check will reveal the condition. Some women, though, have warning signs like these:

- Vision problems
- Severe headaches
- Blurred vision
- Shortness of breath

Smoking, being older than 35 (need we add that most menopausal women are?), overweight, African American, or eating fatty foods or too much salt also put you at greater risk of hypertension; so does a family history of the condition.

Once upon a time it was thought that higher blood pressure was a normal part of aging, the body's way of helping blood through stiffening veins and arteries. Now we know, of course, that high blood pressure (hypertension) is a danger sign at any age, and is associated with heart, kidney, and eye diseases, as well as an increased risk of stroke.

### Determining the role of hormones

By helping maintain healthy triglyceride and cholesterol levels in your blood, estrogen lowers your risk of developing atherosclerosis, which is a major cause of angina, heart attacks, and other problems. Estrogen can help prevent atherosclerosis in two ways:

- ✔ **It decreases LDL levels:** Estrogen helps get rid of some of the "bad" cholesterol in your blood by increasing the amount of LDL your liver breaks down, so that more LDL gets purged from your arteries. Estrogen pills are more effective than patches at this job, but both work over time.

- ✔ **It increases HDL levels:** HDL cholesterol is the type of cholesterol that can carry excess fat out of your bloodstream and back to your liver for reprocessing.

In spite of the role estrogen plays in regulating cholesterol, neither unopposed estrogen therapy nor combination (estrogen plus progestin) therapies have been found to protect women against heart disease, peripheral artery disease, or coronary death. The WHI found that among the younger women in their 50- to 79-year-old study group, there was a slight hint of lowered risk of cardiovascular disease among those using unopposed estrogen. Even so, the FDA warns against the use of any type of HT to prevent heart coronary heart disease. If you feel you need HT for the relief of menopausal symptoms, take the smallest effective dose for the shortest possible amount of time needed to treat your symptoms.

You can only use unopposed estrogen if your uterus has been removed.

## Cleaning out clots and clogs

A chunk of the *plaque* (the goop formed by fat, and other substances) can break off and clog an artery, causing a heart attack or stroke. A stroke can also be caused by blood clots forming unexpectedly because of the presence of a greater-than-necessary level of clotting chemicals in your blood. These clots can get stuck in a blood vessel that feeds your brain (stroke), in a deep vessel the feeds your heart (deep vein thrombosis) or lung (pulmonary embolism), or in your heart itself (heart attack). All in all, the blood, blood vessels, and heart comprise your *cardiovascular system,* and a problem in one area means trouble for another. To avoid blood problems that can lead to heart disease, keep your total cholesterol, LDL ("bad" cholesterol), and triglyceride levels low and keep your HDL ("good" cholesterol) levels high.

### Recognizing the signs

As with hypertension, blood clots can sneak up on you without giving you any obvious symptoms. Pulmonary embolism can cause shortness of breath, or it may not. Early signs of a stroke may include some or all of these:

✔ Numbness or weakness on one side of your body

✔ Sudden blurring or dimming of vision

✔ Difficulty speaking

✔ Sudden dizziness or severe headaches with nausea and vomiting

✔ Sudden confusion or loss of consciousness

Rapid treatment is critical in stroke treatment. If you even *suspect* that you or someone with you is having a stroke, call for emergency care immediately!

### Determining the role of hormones

WHI findings indicate a strong association between unopposed estrogen therapy and stroke. The increased risk was so great that the researchers halted the treatment portion of the study on unopposed estrogen and heart health in 2002. Again, keeping your triglyceride and cholesterol levels normal is the most important way to lower your risk of blood clots and the damage they can do. Your body's own home-grown estrogen does this naturally, but estrogen — with or without progestin — HT has been associated with an *increased* risk of stroke and blood clots. Keep your doctor aware of any history of blood clots or stroke in your family. If you are at risk, your doctor may decide you are not a good candidate for hormone therapy.

Another large study, the Nurses' Healthy Study, also found that hormone therapy (estrogen and progesterone) increased the risk of stroke in the first two years of use. After two years, the risk seemed to drop back down to a risk level corresponding to the risk women not using hormone therapy face.

In women, maintaining this balance is even more important than your total cholesterol number.

---

## Deciphering the diet data

Findings from the WHI Dietary Modification study confused a lot of folks, because, women who followed a low-fat diet did *not* have significantly less heart disease than those following their normal diet. Does this give you the green light to replace fruits with French fries? Um . . . no. First, women on the low-fat diet did exhibit small improvements in LDL ("bad") cholesterol levels, blood pressure, body weight, and levels of a blood clotting factor called Factor VII C.

Second, the study looked only at *total* fat intake, so good fats such as those containing omega-3 acids (in Chapter 18 we fill you in on these) were lumped in with saturated and trans fats. Third, many of the women in the low-fat group hadn't stuck closely to the study's low-fat guidelines. Women who did so had better individual outcomes. Bottom line? Restricting your consumption of saturated fats and trans fats plays an important role in keeping you healthy.

The Food and Drug Administration (FDA) has placed warnings on estrogen products against their use to prevent coronary heart disease.

# Oiling the Pump: HT and Your Heart

The changes that menopause brings have a large impact on your heart, so it makes sense that hormone therapy has a large effect also.

## Slowing the pace

A fluttering heart doesn't always signal new love. Many women experience heart *palpitations* (a pounding, racing heart) for the first time during the change.

Palpitations can indicate a variety of cardiovascular problems and should be taken seriously. Check these symptoms out with your primary care physician.

The effects of hormone therapy on heart palpitations aren't really on the radar screen of scientists investigating the benefits and harms of hormone therapy. When your estrogen levels drop, as they do during the change, your brain sends out adrenaline in an attempt to spur on estrogen production. Your heart responds to this adrenaline surge by pounding.

## Keeping angina away

Angina can feel like you have a weight on your chest. Although some women feel angina even when they do nothing, most women feel the pressure only when they exercise. You feel pressure because your heart isn't getting enough blood. When you exercise, spasms cause your coronary arteries to tighten, which restricts the flow of blood to your heart. In response, your heart screams to get your attention, and you feel chest pain.

Estrogen, prior to menopause, has a soothing effect on blood vessels and reduces spasms. The WHI, however, found an increased risk of heart attack among participants in the estrogen plus progestin study.

Ironically, there was some hint in the findings of the WHI study of women taking unopposed estrogen, that women at the younger end of their group of 50- to 79-year-old participants *may* actually have experienced a slight decrease in cardiovascular risk.

# Avoiding the big one

The medical name for a heart attack is *myocardial infarction* (sometimes abbreviated as MI). A heart attack is caused by a blockage (usually from a blood clot or a plaque deposit) in one or more of your coronary arteries. Blockages can restrict blood flow to your heart and cause either a heart attack or the death of heart tissue (heart disease).

A woman having a heart attack may experience the symptoms men do — pain in the chest, jaw, and right arm, sweating, and shortness of breath. But you may also have nausea, abdominal and/or back pain, nausea, vomiting, and extreme fatigue. It still takes longer for a woman's heart attack to be diagnosed in the emergency room than it does for a man's, so don't delay. Seek emergency help immediately if you even *think* it's a heart attack.

### Women's Health Initiative findings

The WHI study found that heart attacks actually increased 24 percent for women using conjugated estrogen and MPA progestin, and an 81 percent rise in the risk of coronary heart disease. But, although the risk of having a heart attack increased, the incidence of dying from one didn't. Based on this information, some doctors are removing patients from hormone therapy. Others are taking more of a wait-and-watch attitude, especially given that these results are out of whack with a number of other studies.

### Unopposed estrogen

Estrogen improves blood flow in your coronary arteries by dilating the blood vessels, helping your body continue to eliminate plaque inside the vessels, and maintaining healthy clotting. Estrogen therapy, however, provides no protection from heart disease for women older than 60. Among younger study participants there was a hint of lowered cardiovascular risk and a possibility of lowered rates of procedures to open arteries.

### Estrogen plus progestin

The WHI study found an increased risk of heart attacks in this group, and no suggestion of protection against cardiovascular disease or peripheral artery disease.

# Chapter 13

# Checking Out Hormone Therapy and Breast Cancer

*In This Chapter*

▶ Recognizing your breast-cancer risks

▶ Debating the benefits of HT and the risk of breast cancer

▶ Choosing an HT regimen with breast cancer in mind

*I*s hormone therapy (HT) risky business in terms of increasing your risk of developing breast cancer? Reports place hormones at the scene of the crime time and again, and it is clear now that long-term exposure to estrogen plus progestin therapy is strongly associated with breast cancer. Questions remain, though, about who is at greatest risk, and what guidelines exist to help you make informed decisions about hormone use. In this chapter, you can find out what researchers know for sure and what they're still studying about HT and the risk of breast cancer.

## Beginning with Breast Basics

Breast tissue and fat are the two main components of the breast. You no doubt already know about fat, so that subject needs no further explanation. But breast tissue is slightly more complex.

Breast tissue is composed of sections called *lobes.* Lobes are made up of *lobules,* which produce milk when you breastfeed. *Ducts* carry milk from the lobules to the nipple. Cancers tend to form either in the lobules or in the ducts. Figure 13-1 illustrates the parts of a breast.

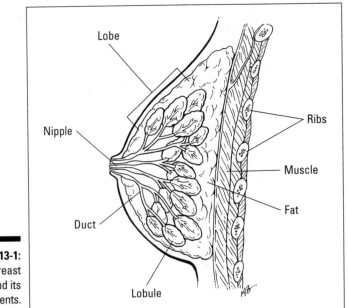

**Figure 13-1:**
The breast
and its
components.

Labels in figure: Lobe, Nipple, Duct, Lobule, Ribs, Muscle, Fat

# Defining Breast Cancer

Whether breast cancer forms in the lobules or the ducts, it begins when cells divide and grow at an abnormally fast rate. The cells morph into odd shapes and start clumping together to form cancerous (*malignant*) tumors.

What triggers this process? Researchers know that it takes a *mutation* (a freak act of nature that affects the basic building blocks of cells) to get things going, but no one knows how the initial cells become mutated. Most researchers feel that a *carcinogen* (a cancer-causing agent) in the environment serves as the trigger. There are two main types of breast cancer and one condition that can lead to cancer:

✔ **Ductal carcinoma *in situ* (DCIS):** Technically, this is cancer, because the cells are abnormal and grow very quickly. It's called *in situ* (which means *in place*) because the cancer cells haven't spread beyond a very restricted area (usually a breast duct or lobule). Carcinoma *in situ* is sometimes called Stage 0 cancer. Although your doctor will likely recommend removing such a cancer, your treatment will probably not be as aggressive as it would for an invasive cancer.

- **Lobular cancer in situ (LCIS):** Though contained for now in the lobules, this is not considered a true cancer. Your doctor may advise a "watch and wait" approach or a hormone treatment (more on these in the section on "Using Hormones as Therapy" later in this chapter).

- **Invasive ductile cancer:** This type of cancer starts in the ducts and spreads to surrounding tissues.

- **Invasive lobular cancer:** This type of cancer starts in the lobules and spreads to surrounding tissues.

Both invasive ductile and invasive lobular cancers can move through the breast tissue into your blood vessels, thereby gaining access to your entire body. When this happens, the cancer is said to have *metastasized,* or spread.

Early detection means you can treat cancer before it spreads.

# Taking Care of Your Breasts

You probably already know about the importance of performing a monthly breast self-exam and getting a regular mammogram. The following sections tell you why these two simple tests are so vital to your breast health.

## Examining your breasts every month

The American Cancer Society recommends that you examine your breasts for lumps and bumps every month after you reach the age of 20. And your doctor should do a breast exam as part of your yearly gynecological visit.

The American Cancer Society even offers self-exam guide cards you can hang in your shower that show you how to perform a breast exam and what you should look and feel for. Ask your gynecologist for a card, give the American Cancer Society a call (phone: 800-ACS-2345) and ask a representative to send you one, or request one at www.cancer.org.

The most common symptom of breast cancer noticeable during a self-exam is a hard, immovable lump in your breast, which may or may not be painful. Sometimes the skin that stretches over the lump looks thick or indented; sometimes it looks dimpled like an orange peel. You may also notice that your nipple leaks a dark fluid or turns inward. If you notice any of these signs, contact your doctor.

Sometimes a lump you feel in your breast isn't cancerous. Breast lumps can occur as the result of several breast conditions. (For more information on breast conditions, take a look at *Breast Cancer for Dummies,* Ronit Elk and Monica Morrow published by Wiley Publishing, Inc.)

## *Making time for mammograms*

Although you may see articles every year or so questioning the necessity of mammograms, most medical folks say, "Just do it." Mammograms are relatively painless, cost effective, and fast.

Have your first mammogram around age 35 so your doctor has something with which to compare future mammograms. If you're between 40 and 49, you should have a mammogram every year or two. If you're over 50, do it every year. At your annual checkup, make sure your medical practitioner gives you a clinical breast exam, too (essentially a more expert version of your self-exam).

Here's a fact: The best chance of surviving breast cancer comes from early detection. Individuals who downplay the importance of annual screenings question whether mammogram screenings actually decrease the *death rate.* The more useful measure of the effectiveness of mammograms is whether regular mammograms increase the *detection rate* of new breast cancers — and they do!

If you're a woman in your 40s, having mammograms on a regular basis can reduce your chance of dying from breast cancer by about 17 percent. For women between the ages of 50 and 69, regular mammograms can reduce deaths by about 30 percent. Early detection can reduce the numbers of women who have to undergo drawn-out and painful treatments for breast cancer. With today's mammogram technology, healthcare providers can identify cancer at an early stage, before it invades the bloodstream and gains access to other parts of your body. Early detection allows doctors to treat breast cancer with a shorter and less invasive course of treatment.

Medicare pays for a yearly mammogram for all women over 40, plus a baseline mammogram for women between 35 and 39.

# *Determining Estrogen's Role*

Although a great deal of controversy surrounds the why's and how's, nearly everyone agrees that estrogen plays some role in the development of breast cancer. Even the natural estrogen in your body during your reproductive years increases your risk of breast cancer because it stimulates cell reproduction in your breasts. When it comes to estrogen and menopause, here are the things most experts agree on:

✔ Estrogen is a key promoter of breast-cancer development. So controlling estrogen levels in breast tissue should lower your risk of breast cancer.

✔ The earlier you begin perimenopause and the shorter your reproductive cycle is, the lower your risk of breast cancer because these factors decrease you total lifetime exposure to high levels of estrogen.

✔ Being overweight (gaining 45 pounds or more after your 18th birthday or being 20 percent over your target weight) after the onset of menopause increases estrogen levels in your body and can increase the risk of breast cancer. (Check out Chapter 18 for more information on determining your ideal weight.)

This risk doesn't apply to perimenopausal women who are overweight (though extra weight does put you at risk for other health problems).

# Checking the Link between HT and Breast Cancer

Findings from several parts of the Women's Health Initiative (WHI) study address the relationship between hormone therapy and breast cancer. The major findings were:

✔ Women taking estrogen plus progestin began to show an elevated incidence of breast cancer after four years of use, so much so that the treatment portion of the study was actually stopped early.

✔ Women taking estrogen plus progestin also tended to have larger, faster-growing tumors than did the women taking placebos in this study.

✔ Out of every 10,000 women, 38 taking estrogen plus progestin were diagnosed with breast cancer, as opposed to 30 women out of every 10,000 who were taking placebos.

✔ Women taking estrogen alone did not have an elevated risk of breast cancer after seven years of hormone use. In fact, this therapy actually seemed to have some protective effect against breast cancer. In the group of roughly 5,000 women taking estrogen, 129 got breast cancer. In the same sized group of women taking placebos, 161 got cancer.

Outcomes from other large studies of hormone use have their own findings, only some of which are consistent with what the WHI found:

✔ In the HERS study of 2,763 women with a history of heart disease, women taking estrogen plus progestin were at increased risk for breast cancer.

- ✔ In the Nurse's Health Study (of over 120,000 participants), the duration of hormone use was significant. Breast cancer incidence was higher in women taking estrogen plus progestin (compared with those taking placebos), but only after 20 or more years of hormone use.
- ✔ Women in the Nurse's study taking estrogen alone had an increased risk for breast cancer after only five years of use.

All of these studies found that taking estrogen plus progestin was associated with an increase in breast cancer. In some cases, this increased risk was only apparent after a number of years of hormone use, but in the WHI study risk was apparent after only four years and increased with each additional year of hormone use.

These results of the WHI estrogen-alone study sound like good news for women who have had a hysterectomy (remember, only women without a uterus can take estrogen alone), but were somewhat surprising to researchers. Estrogen has for so long been associated with an *increased* risk of breast cancer, and other studies seem to support an estrogen-breast cancer link. The Nurse's study found that women taking estrogen only had an elevated risk of breast cancer. Doctors are continuing to follow up on the women in the estrogen-only study, to find out whether lifetime risk of breast cancer is consistent with this initial WHI finding.

The risk of breast cancer for any given woman is still small, and we still don't know what the effects of hormones on younger women will be (the WHI study also focused on the use of hormones by women between 50 and 79), so we don't know what outcomes for younger women would be. Other studies, such as the Kronos Early Estrogen Prevention Study (KEEPS), is still (as of this writing) collecting data on the effects of hormone use in younger women and in those receiving their estrogen from a patch instead of by mouth; which may have a lowered risk of side effects. In the meantime, the WHI findings are significant and will likely help to shape the way most doctors approach recommending estrogen to their patients.

# Assessing Your Risks

The two biggest risks for breast cancer are being female and being over 40. Both risks are realistically unavoidable, and they both present you with a whole bunch of positives. So who would want to avoid them?

# Recognizing risks you can't control

As frustrating as it is, some breast-cancer risk factors are out of your control. Even your own estrogen appears to heighten your breast-cancer risks (see the "Determining Estrogen's Role" section earlier in this chapter). This section lists the risks you can't do anything about, but you can control other factors (which we cover in the "Recognizing risks you can control" section later in this chapter):

- ✔ **Age:** Of course it's not fair, but the older you get, the greater your risk of breast cancer. That's an important fact to keep in mind. When you're younger than 40, your risk is quite low. But, after 40, your breast cancer risk increases until you're about 80. The good news is that when you hit 80, your risk of breast cancer actually decreases a bit.

- ✔ **Breast density:** Breasts with more breast tissue than fat tissue are comparatively denser, and detecting small tumors in dense breast tissue is more difficult than detecting them in fatty tissue. At least one study has found a correlation between greater breast density and an increased risk of breast cancer.

- ✔ **Ethnicity:** In North America, Caucasian women have the highest risk of breast cancer. Ashkenazi Jews are at greater risk of breast cancer than women from other cultures too (it appears that they have a higher rate of the genetic mutation known as BRCA1, which we'll discuss momentarily). Hawaiian and African-American women have the next highest risk of breast cancer, while Latinas, Asian Americans, and Native Americans have the lowest rates of breast cancer in the United States.

- ✔ **Genetics:** If someone in your immediate family has breast cancer, your risk of breast cancer almost doubles. If both mom and sis have breast cancer, your risk is about 2½ times greater than the risk of a woman without breast cancer in her family.

If you're worried about your family history of breast cancer, you may want to take genetic tests that look for two genetic mutations — BRCA1 and BRCA2 — that leave you more susceptible to breast cancer. However, only about 10 percent of breast cancers come from inherited genetic mutations.

The letters BRCA stand for *breast cancer*. BRCA1 is a genetic mutation found in people with a family history of ovarian and breast cancer. BRCA2 is a genetic mutation found in people with a family history of male and female breast cancer. Your lifetime risk of getting breast cancer if you carry one of these genetic mutations is between 50 percent and 85 percent. The presence of one of these (especially BRCA1) also increases your risk of developing ovarian cancer.

✔ **Location of fat on your body:** If you wear your fat high in your body (around your midsection), your risk of breast cancer is about six times as high as that of a woman who wears her fat around her hips, thighs, and buttocks.

✔ **Menstrual history:** The later you begin menstruating and the earlier you begin menopause, the lower your risk of breast cancer, presumably because you generate less estrogen over your lifetime.

✔ **"Precancerous" breast tumors:** Receiving a diagnosis of abnormal cell growth, carcinoma *in situ,* for example, increases your risk of breast cancer. (Check out the "Defining Breast Cancer" section earlier in this chapter for more on carcinoma *in situ.*)

*Fibrocystic condition of the breast,* a condition in which you develop little lumps in your breast tissue (usually seven to ten days before your period), does *not* increase your risk of breast cancer.

## Recognizing risks you can control

The very thought of breast cancer may make you feel panicked and helpless, but there are risk factors you can control. If a look at the list below shows that you're already following a "breast healthy" lifestyle, give yourself a pat on the back:

✔ **Alcohol consumption:** Having more than three drinks a week raises your risk of breast cancer. This fact holds true whether you're taking hormone therapy (HT) or not, but it's especially true if you take the conjugated equine form of estrogen. Alcohol raises the level of estrogen (the estrone type) in your body.

✔ **Antioxidants:** Vitamins A, C, E, beta-carotene, selenium, and glutathione are antioxidants that protect the body from premature aging and cancer (see Chapter 18 for more on antioxidants). When taken by menopausal women, these antioxidants lower the risk of breast cancer.

✔ **Dietary fat:** Dietary studies yield mixed results, but most indicate (or at least strongly suggest) that a diet high in fat, especially saturated and animal-derived fats, increases your risk. Animal fats also introduce pesticides and antibiotics into your diet.

✔ **Exercise:** Multiple studies associate regular exercise with a lowered risk of getting an initial cancer or a recurrence.

✔ **Pregnancy:** Women who have at least one pregnancy have a lower risk of breast cancer during their *lifetime* than women who have never been pregnant. But you have to read the fine print that accompanies this risk factor because you actually have a slightly higher risk of breast cancer during the ten years immediately following the birth. After ten years or so, your risk of breast cancer drops so that women with one child have a lower risk of breast cancer than women who have never borne a child. In general, the more babies you have, the lower your lifetime risk of breast cancer.

✔ **Weight gain/obesity:** Gaining more than 45 pounds at any point increases your risk of breast cancer. Breast cancer is linked to higher levels of estrogen (especially the *estrone* type of estrogen found in fat). (Check out Chapter 18 for additional information on weight-related issues.)

# Using Hormones as Therapy

A special class of artificially created hormones has the potential to treat or help to prevent certain breast cancers in some women. Many cancer cells are classified as *hormone receptor positive* — that is, they seek out and link up with hormones that promote their growth. Estrogen or progestins connect with these cancer cells much as two puzzle pieces fit together; this linkage promotes or accelerates the cancer's activity. Hormone therapy (sometimes called anti-estrogens or anti-progestins) work in different ways to prevent your body's hormones from making this cancer connection.

## Knowing for sure: Tests for breast cancer

If you find a lump in your breast, there are several ways to examine it to see if the lump is something to be concerned about. The type of test your doctor uses depends on the size of the lump and its location:

✔ **Fine needle aspiration:** Right in the office, the doctor sticks a tiny needle into the lump, drains some fluid, and sends the fluid off to the lab to check for cancerous cells.

✔ **Needle core biopsy:** The doctor performs this test in the hospital as an outpatient procedure, and uses a local anesthetic. The doctor sticks a needle into the suspected problem area, removes some breast tissue, and sends it to the lab to be checked.

✔ **Open biopsy:** This surgical procedure is performed in the hospital using anesthesia. The doctor makes a small incision and removes part or all of the lump, which he then sends to the lab for analysis.

✔ **Noninvasive procedures:** Non-surgical technologies such as PET scans, MRI, and ultrasounds are sometimes used for screening following an abnormal mammogram, but studies show that they miss too many cancers to be a standard replacement for biopsy.

## Counting the ways

If tests reveal that your cancer is hormone receptor positive, there are basically four classes of hormone treatment that your doctor might recommend:

- ✔ **SERMs (selective estrogen receptor modulators).** These man-made hormones work by blocking the cancer cell's hormone receptors. It's a little like using an outlet plug to keep your child from sticking her finger in the socket and getting hurt. Two SERMs have been prominent in the cancer news of late: Tamoxifen (designed to fight breast cancer) and Raloxifene (an osteoporosis medication that turned out to have cancer-fighting potential). The STAR study found them to be equally effective at fighting cancer, but Raloxifene has fewer side effects (see Chapter 11 for more information about SERMs).

- ✔ **ERDs (estrogen receptor down-regulators).** ERDs are a lot like SERMs, except that instead of merely blocking cancer cells' receptors to keep them from getting a green light from hormones, they actually destroy the cancer cells' estrogen receptors so they can't communicate with your hormones at all.

- ✔ **Aromatase inhibitors.** No, these don't have anything to do with keeping you from smelling the cookies baking. Remember that after your ovaries throw in the towel, your body's fat cells continue to make a certain amount of estrogen that can feed growing cancers. Aromatase inhibitors keep a lid on how much estrogen your body can make after menopause.

There's one more way doctors can manipulate your hormones to help prevent cancer or the recurrence of cancer, or to try to inhibit a cancer that's already there. Remember when we talked about how premature menopause can result from surgical removal of your ovaries, from the use of certain medications, or from exposure to radiation treatments? Doing any of these things on purpose can have the same effect: shutting down the working of your ovaries. This results in less estrogen being available to promote cancer growth. The down side, of course, is that doing these will put you into menopause.

Most of these hormone therapies are administered by mouth, as a daily pill. Remembering to take your pill and adhering to the routine your doctor recommends is very important.

## Reviewing the risks and benefits

The benefits of using these kinds of hormone therapies are obvious. They can help to prevent an initial breast cancer in women at greatest risk, work toward preventing a recurrence in those who have had breast cancer already, help to shrink tumors before or after more traditional treatment, or augment each other, because one type of hormone therapy is sometimes prescribed when another has done the best work it can and still needs some help. Hormone therapy doesn't typically take the place of traditional therapies such as surgery, radiation, or chemotherapy, but it can support and enhance these, or, when before them, give them a head start by shrinking the size of a tumor.

Hormone therapies of this kind, alas, are not without unpleasant side effects. You may experience hot flashes, moodiness, vaginal dryness, and weight gain. Some therapies increase your risk of uterine cancer (the breast cancer-fighting element outweighs the small less-than-one percent increase in risk, though), weaken your bones, increase the risk of blood clots, and cause upset stomach.

# Choosing Your HT Regimen

If you're a woman concerned about breast cancer (and aren't we all?), you will find conflicting information and advice at every turn about the use of hormone therapies. When the first edition of this book was released, the type of HT believed to have the greatest correlation with breast cancer risk was estrogen-alone. New information from the WHI seems to implicate estrogen plus progestin, while the estrogen alone trial actually found a hint that estrogen use might have a small *protective* effect when it comes to breast cancer. Findings like these don't make decision-making that much simpler.

Take a close look at yourself when you answer the question, "Is HT right for me?" The role of HT in breast cancer is still unanswered. Despite lots of research, all we can say is, "We don't know." You need to review all the available information on breast cancer and HT and then consider your own medical issues and family history.

# Chapter 14

# Reviewing Reproductive Cancers and Hormone Therapy

Hormone therapy (HT) has been linked to all kinds of reproductive cancers. In some cases, HT is thought to lower the risk of cancer. In other cases, it may increase the risk of cancer. And, in others, it's thought to have absolutely no effect.

In this chapter, we look at cervical, colon (or more accurately colorectal), endometrial (uterine), vaginal, vulval, and ovarian cancers. In each case, we introduce you to the particular cancer and its symptoms, review the screening procedures and tests, discuss the role (or lack thereof) HT plays in connection with each cancer, and perform a quick risk-benefit analysis.

What about breast cancer? Well, because of all the issues that surround that topic, — it gets its very own chapter — Chapter 13.

## Colorectal Cancer

The colon and the rectum are the last stops on the digestive tract before waste moves out of the body. The first six feet or so of the large intestines is called the *colon;* the last six inches is called the *rectum*. If you're wondering how your body holds six feet of tubing, take a look at Figure 14-1, which shows the location of the colon and rectum.

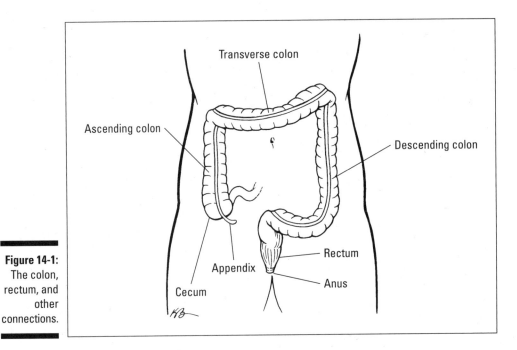

**Figure 14-1:**
The colon, rectum, and other connections.

Though commonly known as colon cancer, the proper name for this type of cancer is *colorectal cancer* because it can occur in either the colon or the rectum. And yeah, we know these aren't *really* reproductive organs, but they're in the same neighborhood, and are often checked as part of your regular gynecological exam, so they're along for the ride in this chapter.

Colorectal cancer is a slow-growing cancer that begins as a *polyp* (a small growth) on the mucous lining (*mucosa*) of the colon, as shown in Figure 14-2. Polyps can show up in the colon and be perfectly harmless (asking why is like asking cats why they pounce; they just do). But some polyps have the potential to become cancerous.

One of the most common cancers, colorectal cancer is the third leading cause of cancer death in American women (behind lung and breast cancer). Over 90 percent of cases are found in people over 50 years of age. Colorectal cancer is easily detectable, and you can easily prevent it by making a few healthy lifestyle choices and having regular checkups.

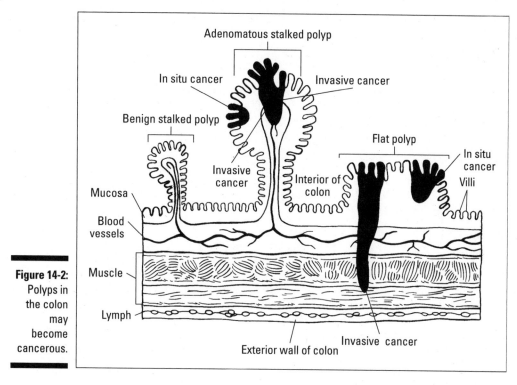

**Figure 14-2:** Polyps in the colon may become cancerous.

## Recognizing the signs

Rectal bleeding and bloody stools are the most common symptoms of colorectal cancer. Additional symptoms include diarrhea, constipation, skinny stools, frequent gas pains, and feeling as though you can't completely pass the stool. Some people with this disease lose weight, feel fatigued, or become *anemic* (a condition in which you don't have enough red blood cells to carry oxygen around your body).

## Finding out for sure: Screenings and tests

A number of screening procedures reduce your risk of colon cancer. Having an annual screening, in fact, is *the number-one way* to reduce your risk of colorectal cancer if you're a woman over age 50. When your doctor checks you out for colorectal cancer, she can look for cancer *and* polyps on the lining of your colon that may become cancerous. Removing any polyps removes some of your cancer risk as well.

Here's why catching polyps early is so important: When colorectal cancer is found before it spreads to other areas of the body, the survival rate is 96 percent. When colorectal cancer spreads, long-term survival rates drop dramatically. So getting annual screenings after you turn 50 is well worth the effort.

Generally doctors start out with minimally invasive screening procedures, such as the digital exam and fecal occult test, and move to more invasive procedures only when initial results warrant additional tests. The following tests are generally your first line of defense:

- ✓ **Digital rectal exam:** Your doctor inserts a gloved finger into your rectum to check for lumps, bumps, or other changes in the rectum. Not the most pleasant part of your annual checkup, but important all the same.

- ✓ **Fecal occult blood test:** This test is a bit messy, but it really must be done. Some of the newer tests look like some home pregnancy tests — a piece of paper turns a different color if the sample has blood in it. Your doctor takes a sample during your exam and places it on a test card. You know the results immediately. There's a home version, too, that you use in the privacy of your own bathroom and return to the doctor.

If blood is found in your stool or the doctor feels something suspicious during the digital exam, the doctor may perform one of these procedures to further check things out:

- ✓ **Colonoscopy:** While you're under mild sedation, your doctor inserts a scope into your colon, which allows her to carefully examine the walls of your colon and rectum (yes, all six feet or so). She can even take pictures of your colon walls, and any polyps can be removed on the spot and examined by a lab for evidence of cancer.

- ✓ **Sigmoidoscopy:** Doctors normally sedate patients before performing this test. Your doctor inserts a thin scope about 10 to 12 inches into your rectum through which he can see any polyps or damaged areas in your colon and take a sample if necessary.

- ✓ **Barium enema:** You may hear folks refer to this test as a *lower GI series*. It's not used very often; colonoscopies and sigmoidoscopies are more common. This procedure involves a barium enema and a technician taking a series of x-rays of your colon and rectum. The barium highlights your colon — particularly any polyps or growths. If you have growths, your doctor will probably follow up with a colonoscopy or sigmoidoscopy.

A colonoscopy is now recommended as a routine screening procedure for people 50 and over.

## Determining the role of hormone therapy

For reasons unknown (though most researchers suspect estrogen plays the role of the heroine here), hormone therapy actually lowers your risk of colon cancer. In fact, you reduce your risk of colon cancer by more than one-third while you take hormone therapy. The Women's Health Initiative findings on hormone therapy and colorectal cancers were a bit complicated, though. Women taking estrogen plus progesterone therapy had fewer colorectal cancers, but they were more advanced cancers than the ones found among participants taking placebos.

The risk reduction only exists while you stay on hormone therapy; the protection diminishes after you stop taking it.

## Assessing your risks

Some of the factors that raise your risk of colorectal cancer are

- ✔ **Age:** Over 90 percent of colorectal cancer patients are over the age of 50. With each decade after 50, your risk doubles.

- ✔ **Diet:** Diets high in fat and low on fiber-rich vegetables are associated with more colon cancer. Eating red meat frequently (once a day) can double your risk. Animal fat not only is the saturated, unhealthy variety of fat, but also is the place in which toxins gather. If the animal you're eating was exposed to pesticides or other toxins before it became dinner, you get those poisons when you chow down.

- ✔ **Family history:** Genetics play a role in colorectal cancer (and many other cancers as well). If you have one or more family members with colon cancer, your risk doubles.

- ✔ **Lifestyle:** If going from the couch to the freezer to grab a bowl of ice cream is your idea of a brisk walk, you can cut your risk of colorectal cancer in half by putting down the spoon and exercising. Whether you bike, jog, or simply walk (not to the fridge), you lower your risk. Turn to Chapter 19 for the skinny on exercise.

# Endometrial (Uterine) Cancer

Cancer of the uterus is usually referred to as *endometrial cancer* because the cancer usually starts in the *endometrium* — the lining of the uterus. Take a look at Figure 14-3 to see the uterus and nearby organs.

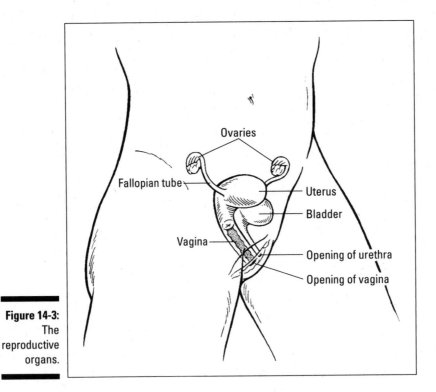

Endometrial cancer is one of the most common reproductive cancers in North America, but it's readily detected — 75 percent of cases are caught before the cancer moves beyond the pelvic region — and treatment is very effective.

The endometrium is very responsive to changes in hormone levels. Too high a level of estrogen or continued high levels of estrogen over a sustained period of time cause cells in the endometrium to continue to multiply. If a mutant cancer cell or two are among those normal endometrial cells, the estrogen will stimulate cell growth and allow the cancer cells to multiply along with the normal cells. The occasional cancer cell is usually not a problem because it gets flushed away during your period, so it doesn't have a chance to proliferate. But, with high levels of estrogen (stimulating cell growth), these cancer cells can multiply.

If you don't have a uterus because you've had a hysterectomy, you don't need to worry about endometrial cancer because you don't have endometrial tissue.

## Recognizing the signs

Most cases of endometrial cancer are caught and caught early enough to cure because the symptoms are so obvious. Any of these symptoms are a signal to see your doctor:

- ✔ Bleeding after menopause
- ✔ Irregular vaginal bleeding
- ✔ Unusual spotting between periods during perimenopause

Pain and cramping are generally *not* an early symptom of this type of endometrial cancer. (But, after endometrial cancer develops, it can invade the blood vessels and spread to other organs causing this type of pain.) Sometimes there are no symptoms at all.

## Finding out for sure: Tests

A number of tests can identify endometrial cancer:

- ✔ **Ultrasound:** Using sound waves, the doctor is able to create images of the uterine lining with this test. Ultrasounds are done in the doctor's office, and they're relatively painless. An ultrasound wand is inserted into the vagina so the technician can get a clear view of the uterus and lining.

- ✔ **Saline infusion sohohysterogram or SIS:** This specialized form of ultrasound is increasingly common these days because it gives us far better and useful pictures of the endometrium and intrauterine cavity. It is performed in the doctor's office.

- ✔ **Endometrial aspiration or biopsy:** In this test, the doctor removes a tissue sample from the lining of the uterus for examination. Endometrial aspirations can be done in the doctor's office. Usually there's no need for painkilling medication beyond ibuprofen.

- ✔ **Dilation and curettage (D & C):** While you're under anesthesia, your doctor will gently scrape tissue from the lining of the uterus for examination.

- ✔ **Hysteroscopy:** This test — now routinely used at the same time that a D & C is performed — involves the doctor inserting a special microscope into the uterus to examine the lining (while you're under anesthesia in the operating room).

# Determining the role of hormone therapy

This one is pretty simple. The higher the dose of estrogen and the longer the duration of high estrogen levels, the higher the risk of developing cancer in your uterus.

In the 1970s, after women had been taking estrogen replacement therapy without a *progestin* (a term that encompasses both synthetic and natural forms of progesterone) for years, medical folks noticed that the incidence of endometrial cancer was three to eight times higher among women taking estrogen compared to women not taking it.

After studying the problem, doctors realized that without a progestin, the lining of the uterus continued to thicken unchecked. So now hormone therapy includes a progestin to routinely flush the lining of the uterus through vaginal bleeding (cyclical hormone therapy) or to keep the lining from growing (continuous hormone therapy). For more information on the different types of hormone therapy, turn to Chapter 11.

If you don't have a uterus because you've had a hysterectomy, you don't need progesterone in your hormone therapy (as women with a uterus do) to balance the estrogen to avoid endometrial cancer.

# Assessing your risks

Because an imbalance in hormones (particularly estrogen and progesterone) increases your risk of this type of cancer, things that alter your hormone levels can raise your risk:

- ✔ **Age:** Over 95 percent of women with endometrial cancer are over 40 years of age. The rate of endometrial cancer rises between the ages of 40 and 70 and then drops around age 80.

- ✔ **Estrogen:** Taking estrogen replacement therapy without progesterone increases the risk of endometrial cancer, so estrogen alone therapy is not recommended for women who still have a uterus.

- ✔ **More years of menstruation:** The earlier you began menstruation and the later you reach menopause, the more periods you have in a lifetime. More periods mean more estrogen, and that means greater risk.

- ✔ **Obesity:** Women who are 20 percent over their ideal weight walk around with sustained, high levels of estrogen because their body fat produces it. (For more on weight-related issues, see Chapters 18 and 19.)

  If you're obese, losing weight reduces your risk of endometrial cancer.

Birth control pills actually *lower* your risk of endometrial cancer. Women who use the pill for more than two years reduce their risk by about 50 percent, and women who use the pill for more than five years reduce it by 80 percent.

# Ovarian Cancer

The *ovaries* hold your *oocytes* (seeds that develop into eggs over the course of a woman's reproductive years) and produce sex hormones throughout your life. Take a look at Figure 14-3 to locate the ovaries. Ovarian cancer originates from cells in the ovary — both the egg-making cells and the lining of the ovary.

Cancer of the ovaries (known as *ovarian cancer*) kills silently, with no early, predictable warning signs. Few tangible symptoms warn women of this disease until the tumor has spread beyond the ovary. Ovarian cancer is deadly, but fortunately, it's very rare.

Some researchers suggest that ovarian cancer is related to frequency of ovulation during your lifetime. Every time you ovulate, you get a little tear in the ovary wall. The cells of your ovary repair the tear by dividing rapidly. This wear and tear in connection with the rapid cell division needed to repair the damage may be the source of ovarian cancer. Given this explanation, women who have taken birth-control pills (either the old-time high-dose pills or the current low-dose pills) may actually lower their risk of ovarian cancer because the pill suppresses ovulation.

If you've had no pregnancies, you may have a higher risk of ovarian cancer than women who have been pregnant simply because you've never experienced prolonged periods of time during which you haven't ovulated.

## Recognizing the signs

Most of the symptoms of ovarian cancer seem unremarkable because they can apply to any number of conditions, many of them harmless. Many women first notice bloating in their abdomen. Other women experience nausea, vomiting, or gas that doesn't respond to changes in diet. Frequent urination and constipation are also possible symptoms as are abdominal or pelvic pain. The problem is that the symptoms usually aren't present until the disease has entered an advanced stage.

## Finding out for sure: Tests

If you experience any of the symptoms listed in the "Recognizing the signs" section directly above, consider getting a pelvic exam and then a blood test that looks for the presence of CA125. *CA125* is an ovarian cancer *antigen*, meaning that it's a substance that causes the body to fight ovarian cancer. If your CA125 levels are high, you may have ovarian cancer. Unfortunately, determining the meaning of high CA125 levels is tricky. Sometimes elevated levels show up if you have endometriosis, ovarian cysts, or fibroids or if you're pregnant. Because this test produces a lot of false positives, most doctors don't use it very often. But you should discuss this test with your doctor during your annual gynecological screening after you turn 50.

Just because your CA125 levels aren't elevated doesn't necessarily mean you definitely don't have ovarian cancer — 20 to 30 percent of women with ovarian cancer don't have elevated CA125 levels. Likewise, having elevated CA125 levels doesn't mean that you absolutely have ovarian cancer, but it's a reason to further explore the cause of the results.

Because CA125 screening can result in either a false positive or a false negative, doctors also rely on other tests to rule out ovarian cancer:

- ✔ **Pelvic ultrasound:** With this exam, a technician inserts a sounding device into your vagina so he or she can view an image (a *sonogram*) of your ovaries. Tumors can be identified with the sonogram.

- ✔ **CAT scan:** The *CAT* in *CAT scan* stands for *computerized axial tomography*. This procedure lets your doctor get a graphic image of your ovaries to check for tumors.

- ✔ **Laparoscopy:** This is a minor surgical procedure in which the doctor makes a tiny incision in your belly button and inserts a scope to get a better view of your ovaries. This exam is done under a general anesthesia in an operating room on an outpatient basis.

### Determining the role of hormones

Hormone therapy doubles your risk of dying of ovarian cancer. The good news is that this risk is very low to begin with, so doubling it raises it from about 1 percent to 2 percent. In a study of over 200,000 women, those who had used unopposed estrogen (estrogen without the protective effects of progestin) for ten years or more increased their risk of ovarian cancer.

Birth-control pills may reduce your risks of ovarian cancer, mainly because they suppress ovulation, not because of the estrogen or progesterone levels in your bloodstream. Using birth-control pills for two years reduces your risk by 40 to 50 percent. Using birth-control pills for five years reduces your risk by 60 to 80 percent a risk reduction that can last for as long as 10 years from the time you take your last pill.

*Fertility drugs* that increase the number of eggs released during ovulation or increase the number of ovulations you have over a lifetime can increase your risk of ovarian cancer. Again, it doesn't seem to be the blood hormone levels that create the problem so much as the physical wear and tear of ovulation.

### Assessing your risks

Ovarian cancer is fairly rare. It only affects 4 percent of women, most of whom are over 50 years of age. But this form of cancer is quite deadly because it usually goes unnoticed until the advanced stages of the disease.

Certain factors increase your risks for ovarian cancer:

- ✔ A family history of ovarian cancer (mother, sister, or daughter) or breast cancer (mother or sister). Having the BRCA1 or BRCA2 gene that increases breast cancer risk also increases your risk of ovarian cancer (you can read more about this gene in Chapter 13, "Checking out Hormone Therapy and Breast Cancer").

- ✔ The use of fertility drugs that stimulate the ovaries to release multiple follicles during a single ovulation

- ✔ Being over the age of 50

- ✔ Being of Ashkenazi Jewish genetic heritage

- ✔ Taking hormone therapy for a number of years

- ✔ Having never been pregnant

# Cancers Unaffected by Hormone Therapy

We're including information on a couple of other cancers of the female persuasion even though hormone therapy has no known effects on a woman's risk of developing these cancers or her ability to recover from them.

So why are they here? We primarily include them so we don't leave you wondering how hormones affect these reproductive organs. After all, only women have these organs, so questioning the effects of hormone therapy on them is natural.

Also, we think a book that addresses health issues facing menopausal women would be incomplete without at least discussing these cancers.

## Vaginal and vulvar cancers

Although cancers of the vagina or the vulva are rare, they occur with greater frequency in midlife. Of women diagnosed with vulvar cancer, for instance, 85 percent are over 50. Fifteen percent, though, are under 40, so it's important to be aware of the risks at any age.

One risk factor for vaginal cancer is having been exposed to the drug DES while your mother was pregnant with you (DES was given in the 1950s to prevent miscarriage, but has since been associated with a number of cancers among both the women who took it and their daughters). Others include having HPV (human papilloma virus), and being 30 or younger or 60 or older.

The main risk factor for vulvar cancer is HPV infection. Having a large number of sexual partners (or having partners who have themselves had many partners) increases your risk.

Using hormone therapy has not been found to increase the risk of vaginal or vulvar cancers.

## Cervical cancer

*Cervical cancer* (cancer of the cervix) can be detected early with a Pap smear. Because human papilloma virus is associated with cervical cancer, practicing safe sex can help to prevent it (but not with 100 percent certainty). Over 100,000 cases of cervical cancer are diagnosed in the United States every year, but the five-year survival rate after treatment is over 90 percent.

HT is not known to have any impact on cervical cancer.

# Chapter 15

# Considering Hormone Therapy and Other Health Conditions

*I*n Chapters 12 through 14, we detail the relationships (positive, negative, and neutral) between hormone therapy (HT) and cardiovascular disease and several types of cancer. This chapter reviews a number of conditions you may hear discussed in the same breath as HT.

In this chapter, we define each of these conditions, discuss the signs and symptoms, and review how the conditions have been linked to HT. We discuss the symptoms because, whether they're linked to HT or not, these conditions usually affect folks who are over the age of 40, so you may want to be aware of them.

## Dealing with Deep Vein Thrombosis

*Deep vein thrombosis* (DVT) is probably not a phrase you use everyday, and if you do hear it, we hope it's from a doc on a TV drama and not from your own doctor. *Thrombosis* is a five-dollar word for a *blood clot* (a lump of coagulated blood) that forms in a deep vein and impairs the flow of blood through the vein.

To find deep veins, you have to look no farther than your upper arms, your legs, and your pelvis, but 95 percent of DVTs occur in your leg. These veins lie deeper under the skin than surface veins and return more blood to the heart. A clot in one of these veins can cause more complications than a clot in surface veins.

Blood is designed to clot, right? Sure. When you cut yourself, normal clotting keeps you from bleeding to death. But a clot forming *inside* a vein is up to no good. If it breaks free from the wall of the vein and travels through your bloodstream, it can travel to your lung. Here it can form a blockage called a *pulmonary embolism* — *pulmonary* meaning it's *in the lungs* and *embolism* meaning *a part of a blood clot*. If the diagnosis is missed, pulmonary embolism is fatal about 33 percent of the time.

## Recognizing the signs

By far, the most troublesome and common cases of DVT occur in the leg. It's a good idea to acquaint yourself with possible symptoms:

- **Pain or tenderness** in your calf or thigh
- **Redness:** Your leg may look red as though you bumped it.
- **Swelling** in your whole leg or along a blood vessel
- **Warmth:** Your leg may feel warm to the touch.

These symptoms may signal a blood clot in your lung (pulmonary embolism):

- Chest pain that gets worse with a deep breath
- Cough that may bring up blood
- Sudden shortness of breath, even if you're not exercising

About half of all blood clots come without any warning at all. If you do have any of these symptoms, treat them as an emergency and seek medical attention immediately. Prompt treatment may save your life.

## Determining the role of hormones

Deep vein thrombosis has long been linked to estrogen (that's why you might have heard blood clot risk warnings in connection with the use of birth control pills).

A growing body of evidence exists (including that from the Women's Health Initiative [WHI] study) that shows a correlation between the use of conjugated estrogen therapy and blood-clotting problems. The risk was found to be greater for women taking estrogen plus progestin (women on the hormone had double the blood clot risk of women on placebos). Study participants taking unopposed estrogen (with no added progestin) also had a somewhat elevated (but not statistically significant) risk of blood clot.

Both of the WHI hormone studies were stopped early because of increased health risks associated with hormone therapy, so it's unknown whether these patterns would have gotten stronger or changed with longer hormone use. Clearly, though, hormones are associated with increased risk of DVT. The risk is greatest during the first year of use.

Determining the reason behind the clotting connection is more controversial. Some researchers believe that *not all forms of estrogen* would have this effect on women. They believe that the *type* of estrogen (conjugated estrogen) is responsible for the increase in clotting. Research in the future may show that hormone therapy using natural estradiol (which the body uses more easily than conjugated equine estrogen) won't increase the risk of DVT or pulmonary embolism.

The method of hormone delivery may also affect DVT risk. The WHI studied only women taking hormone therapy by mouth. Some evidence suggests that the skin patch, which delivers the medication more directly into the bloodstream, bypassing the liver, may be safer. The Kronos Early Estrogen Prevention Study (KEEPS) was formed to examine this and other questions about the safety of hormone therapy. A future edition of this book may be able to answer this question. In the meantime, carefully consider the risk of DVT and other blood-clotting problems, particularly if you're taking or thinking of taking estrogen plus progestin therapy.

Women with a history of blood-clotting problems should approach hormone use with extreme caution. Many doctors will not prescribe hormone therapy for women who have already had one or more blood clots, especially if they have a genetic defect linked to clotting disorders. If you have had a blood clot, and tests show that you have such a genetic predisposition to clots, you should not use any estrogen-containing products.

# Dissecting Diabetes

*Diabetes* is characterized by high levels of *glucose* (sugar) in the blood. These high concentrations of glucose are the result of the body's inability to absorb the sugar a person eats.

*Insulin* is a hormone that acts as the great facilitator in the blood-to-tissue glucose-transfer process. When the glucose levels in your blood get relatively high, your pancreas releases insulin to help your cells absorb the sugar in your blood and use it for energy. When the pancreas produces insufficient insulin, diabetes is the result. This can occur because either the body can't make enough insulin or the tissues quit responding to insulin and won't take in glucose.

Two main kinds of diabetes exist:

- ✓ **Type-1 diabetes:** No one knows what causes Type-1 diabetes, but the condition is genetic. (It was once called *juvenile-onset diabetes* because the majority of sufferers are diagnosed before their 20th birthday.) In Type-1 diabetes your pancreas doesn't produce enough (or, in some cases, any) insulin.

- ✓ **Type-2 diabetes:** This form of diabetes, in which your body produces enough insulin but still cannot metabolize sugar properly, is the most common and is most often diagnosed in people over 40 years of age. Eighty percent of people with this form of diabetes are overweight. Excess weight in combination with age is the greatest risk factor for Type-2 diabetes.

## Recognizing the signs

Over 18 million people in the United States live with diabetes. The American Diabetes Association says that more than 5 million of these are people walking around with the disease who haven't yet been diagnosed. Symptoms include:

- ✓ Extreme thirst (causing you to drink an unusual amount of fluids)
- ✓ Frequent urination
- ✓ Constant hunger
- ✓ Unexpected weight loss
- ✓ Fatigue
- ✓ Itchy skin or genitals
- ✓ Pain or numbness in your extremities
- ✓ Slow-healing wounds

## Determining the role of hormones

No one has yet demonstrated that hormone therapy actually leads to diabetes. Some very small and short-term studies suggest that hormone therapy could slightly increase your blood-glucose levels, but most other studies have found absolutely no increase in risk of diabetes for women who take HT. Similarities between diabetic and menopausal symptoms may contribute to a delay in diagnosis. Menopausal hormone changes can also increase the likelihood of low blood sugar episodes and contributing to vaginal and urinary-tract infections. If you're a diabetic and are also approaching or going through menopause, work extra closely with your doctor to help you keep your blood sugar under control (and read more about menopause and diabetes in Chapter 18).

# Facing the Facts about Fibromyalgia

Ever heard of this one? Well, nearly 80 percent of the people who suffer from fibromyalgia are women, and most of them are over 40 years of age. The laundry list of symptoms may make you say, "You've gotta be kidding," but we're not fibbing about fibromyalgia.

*Fibromyalgia* is not a disease, but a chronic condition in which you experience a broad group of symptoms including muscle and soft-tissue pain, tenderness, and fatigue. Fibromyalgia is normally first diagnosed between 30 and 50, but it can be later.

## Recognizing the signs

Fibromyalgia symptoms are intensely felt and varied. They can include

- Stiffness and soreness, especially in the morning.
- Extremely tender places on your body, especially where tendons and muscles meet (on the inside of your elbows and in your hips and knees, for example). Pain in 11 of the 18 tender points is usually the threshold doctors look for in diagnosing this condition.
- Difficulty getting a full night's sleep.
- General fatigue.
- Irritability, mood changes, and depression.
- Problems with eye muscles. (Your eye may turn inward or close slightly.)
- Numbness, burning, or cold sensations in your hands and feet.

Some people with fibromyalgia also experience problems with their memory or concentration, difficulty hearing, sensitivity to certain sounds, and may suffer migraine headaches.

If you have or think you may have fibromyalgia, you may want to check out *Fibromyalgia For Dummies* (Roland Staud with Christine Adamec, Wiley Publishing, Inc.).

## Determining the role of hormones

The cause of fibromyalgia isn't well understood. Most scientists believe that some type of hormonal imbalance causes the condition, but they can't agree on which hormones are unbalanced. Researchers are focusing their attention on these areas:

- Brain chemicals that control mood and the sleep cycle
- Hormones released by the pituitary gland (which are also found in the brain and are sensitive to estrogen)
- Deficiencies in growth hormones

A link to the female sex hormones also seems likely because fibromyalgia is most likely to occur

- In women approaching menopause or who have gone through menopause
- In women who have just had a baby (especially women over 35)
- A few years after women have had a tubal ligation or a hysterectomy

# Getting the Goods on Gallbladder Disease

The gallbladder is a warehouse for *bile,* a greenish liquid that helps digest fats. The gallbladder is supposed to take the bile from the liver and inject it into the intestines (where it goes to work) via a bile duct. When too much cholesterol is present in the bile, the cholesterol hardens, forming crystals inside the gallbladder. The crystals then come together to form *gallstones.*

## Recognizing the signs

Most people don't even know they have gallstones. They experience no symptoms and only find the stones when they're tested for some other condition (such as ulcers or kidney stones). Any pain is usually like a dull ache or cramping. But large or numerous gallstones can cause strong pain, vomiting, or nausea lasting from 30 minutes to several hours. You feel it in your upper abdomen under your ribcage. Sometimes the pain radiates, moving all the way down your lower back or up to your right shoulder. If gallstones cause other infections, doctors usually remove your gallbladder, but gallstones themselves are rarely life threatening.

If you have a high fever or chills, your *bile duct* (pathway to the small intestine) may be inflamed or blocked. A blocked bile duct can also cause urine to be dark yellow, stool to be light in color, and skin to take on a yellow cast. The symptoms often occur at night or after eating (especially a high-fat meal).

## Determining the role of hormones

Estrogen is believed to promote gallstones. Because estrogen, taken by mouth, has to be processed in the liver before entering the bloodstream, it tends to increases the level of LDL cholesterol (the bad stuff) in the bile. Raising the level of cholesterol in the bile can increase the risk of gallstone formation.

Using estrogen in patch form means estrogen doesn't go through the liver. This avoids adding cholesterol to the gallbladder and limits gallstone formation.

# Thinking about Your Thyroid

Many of the 11 million or more Americans who have thyroid disease — either an over- or an underactive thyroid gland — are women over 50. The thyroid, a butterfly shaped gland at the base of your throat, is responsible for helping to regulate growth and metabolism throughout the body.

## Recognizing the signs

Symptoms of hypothyroidism (an underactive thyroid) include unexplained weight gain, depression, memory loss, hair loss, heart palpitations, fatigue, feeling cold all the time, and dry skin. If you have hyperthyroidism (overactive thyroid), you may experience fatigue, insomnia, weight loss, intolerance to heat, and jittery or nervous feelings. Both disorders may cause enlargement of the thyroid gland.

The symptoms of thyroid disease mimic those of other diseases and changes. In fact, among women at midlife, symptoms are so similar to some menopausal symptoms that you may dismiss them as just a normal part of the change. Doctors recommend a thyroid function check (a simple blood test) every five years.

## Determining the role of hormones

Remember that the thyroid gland is a part of your endocrine system, just as your ovaries are. So it's no surprise that estrogen and thyroxin interact with each other, especially as your hormone levels begin to shift. Unopposed estrogen can interfere with the working of thyroxin, leaving you in a hypothyroid state (remember, *hypo* means too little). The addition of progesterone often eases the situation. If your thyroid functioning is perfectly normal, estrogen therapy shouldn't cause a problem. If you're already taking thyroid medication to help balance your thyroxin levels, though, work closely with your caregiver to keep both thyroid hormones and estrogen at healthy levels.

# Looking at Lupus

*Lupus* is the short name for a disease called *systemic lupus erythematosus.* Although lupus is a fairly rare disease, it's much more common among women than men — particularly women between the ages of 15 and 45.

Because lupus is a disease of the immune system, it attacks nearly every organ in your body. The immune system normally protects your body from infections. However, with lupus, the immune system starts attacking "friendly" tissues in your own body. This wreaks havoc in your body, causing tissue damage and illness.

Lupus is a complex disease, and researchers have yet to determine the cause. The likely scenario is that no single cause exists. Instead, a combination of genetic, environmental, and possibly hormonal factors may work together to cause the disease.

The hormone connection is curious. If you look at the U.S. population in general, only 1 out of 2,000 people have lupus. But, if you only consider women between the ages of 14 and 45 years old, 1 in 250 has the disease. This leads scientists to conclude that the female sex hormones are somehow involved.

# Recognizing the signs

Lupus can affect many parts of the body, and it often attacks the joints, skin, kidneys, heart, lungs, blood vessels, and brain. Although people with the disease may have many different symptoms, some of the most common symptoms are

- Extreme fatigue
- Kidney problems
- Painful, swollen, inflamed joints (arthritis)
- Skin rashes and inflammation
- Unexplained fever

Many women who have lupus initially think that their swollen or stiff joints are simply caused by arthritis. In fact, some researchers believe that lupus is related to rheumatoid arthritis. If left untreated, lupus can cause many complications.

# Determining the role of hormones

Given that women of childbearing age are at greatest risk of this disease, it's not surprising that researchers have found an increase in lupus among women taking hormone therapy. The complicated nature of lupus and the suggestion that estrogen replacement could trigger or exacerbate lupus has led many doctors to be wary of prescribing it to women who have the disease.

One large study found that women taking hormone therapy had double the risk of developing lupus compared with menopausal women not taking hormone therapy. The longer women used estrogen, the greater their risk of developing the disease. Some of these findings, though, may have been complicated by other factors in the women's health histories, so some researchers are uncertain about whether estrogen is uniformly bad for women with lupus. Research is ongoing, but if you have a personal or family history of lupus, work with your doctor to keep abreast of news about the disease and, if needed, to identify alternatives to traditional hormone therapy for menopausal symptom relief (check out Chapter 17 for information on alternatives).

# Monitoring Migraines

Roughly 10 to 11 percent of people in the United States and Canada suffer from migraines, and 70 percent of them are women. Most women who have them are between the ages of 30 and 49; many have a family history of migraines.

## Recognizing the signs

Migraines are not like everyday headaches. They're a whole lot worse, but they also have many qualities that distinguish them from more garden-variety headaches. Migraine pain can be intense enough to cause nausea and vomiting. Your head may throb and you may feel hot at the site of the pain, or might feel pain on only one side of the head, and sensitivity to light, noise, and strong odors. Some people also see *auras,* flashing lights or blind spots in their field of vision.

## Determining the role of hormones

Fluctuations in estrogen levels are one of the most common migraine triggers. A sudden drop in estrogen brings on a migraine in many women. It's also worth noting that

- Menstrual migraines generally occur during the part of the cycle when estrogen levels drop.
- Women often report that migraines go away during pregnancy and after menopause.

Many women first suffer these headaches during their reproductive years, specifically a day or two before or on the first day or two of their period. Other women get migraines around the time they ovulate, when estrogen levels again drop.

Headaches with other causes can feel a bit like migraines. A sudden headache that's significantly more painful than any you've ever had warrants an emergency call to the doctor. Such pain may indicate a stroke or brain aneurysm.

The active form of estrogen in HT relieves the symptoms associated with migraines. Women on a cyclical hormone therapy regimen (one in which you quit taking estrogen for a few days each month) are more likely to have migraines because of rapid drops in estrogen. Continuous hormone therapy may prevent the headaches.

# Considering Cognition

Menopause moments. That's what many of us call those brief episodes of forgetfulness that seem to occur more and more often as we get older. We've all been there: forgetting why we went into the other room, or buying a bag full of groceries but forgetting the milk we went to the store for in the first place. A certain amount of memory loss is a normal part of aging. For years, hormone replacement was touted and prescribed for, among other things, its ability to keep us mentally sharp in our perimenopausal years and beyond. New findings, though, have turned this notion around 180 degrees.

## Recognizing the signs

We'd bet there's scarcely a person reading this who hasn't secretly feared that losing her keys or coming up blank on an acquaintance's name heralds the onset of Alzheimer's disease. There's a big difference, though, between mild cognitive impairment (a little trouble with memory, concentration, calculations, word retrieval, and the like) and dementia:

- Losing your car keys is normal; forgetting how to drive is not.
- Forgetting a friend's birthday is normal. Not recognizing your friend when you run into her isn't.
- It's normal to forget to put the milk away. It's not normal to put the milk away in the oven.

There are many causes of mild cognitive impairment, but there are also many things that contribute to normal everyday forgetfulness: fatigue, insomnia, poor nutrition, thyroid imbalances, depression, stress, and some medications can all contribute to forgetfulness. So can simply having too much to do or keep track of. It's no wonder many of us end up calling one kid by the other one's name or forgetting the dry cleaning.

## Determining the role of hormones

The Women's Health Initiative Memory Study (WHIMS) looked at whether hormone use had an effect on mild cognitive impairment (forgetting your keys) and on dementia (not knowing what a key is). The unofficial expectation was that estrogen would have a protective effect against cognitive decline, but the findings surprised and dismayed the researchers:

✔ Women taking unopposed estrogen and those taking estrogen plus progestin both experienced poorer cognitive functioning than did women taking a placebo. The effect was strongest on women who had poorer cognitive functioning to begin with.

✔ Both unopposed estrogen and estrogen plus progestin therapies were associated with sharp increases in the risk of dementia. Almost half of the dementia in both groups was due to Alzheimer's disease.

It's important to note that the WHIMS participants were all 65 or older. No one can say for certain yet what the effects of hormones on the cognitive functioning of younger women would be. Unless additional research yields more positive outcomes, though, doctors are no longer prescribing hormone therapy just to prevent cognitive decline or dementia.

# Chapter 16

# Making the Decision about Hormone Therapy

*W*e want to start this chapter by encouraging you to return to it periodically over the next few years. Your decisions about coping with perimenopause and menopause will probably change as your health issues evolve, your priorities shift, and new options for controlling menopausal symptoms (check out Chapter 4) and conditions such as osteoporosis (more on this in Chapter 5) become available. This evaluation process doesn't end with a one-time pronouncement about whether to use or not use HT that you have to follow for the rest of your life. You can (and should!) revisit your alternatives periodically.

# Outlining Attitudes about HT

Women have a lot of different feelings about hormone therapy (HT):

✔ "Natural is beautiful. I don't need estrogen replacements to age gracefully."

✔ "I tried to go the natural route, but living with these symptoms is a nightmare."

✔ "I'd like to take advantages of the benefits of hormone therapy, but what I hear about the risks really scares me. It feels like a no-win thing."

✔ "You can have my hormones when you pry them out of my beautiful, youthful hands!"

✔ "I've tried hormones, and they were awful. I guess I can put up with hot flashes for a couple of years."

It's certainly possible to hold two (or more) beliefs about hormones at the same time, and your opinions and concerns may shift as you learn more or your symptoms wax and wane. Your ideas will also be influenced by what you hear on the news about hormone research, your doctor's approach to prescribing them, and experiences your mom, sisters, and friends have had with them.

Don't be surprised if your friends and relations try to influence your decisions about hormone therapy. You may feel pressured to use — or not use — HT, depending on who's doing the talking and what her experience was. If your sister found happiness in using HT, or your next door neighbor had a bad reaction to it, they may just assume you'll have the same experience. Keep in mind, too, that the controversy surrounding the use of HT may make some women feel better if you do what they are doing. You may feel pressured when you run up against an over-the-top cheerleader for HT, or someone who insists its use is the root of all evil. If this is the case, acknowledge their experience ("I'm so glad the hormones made your hot flashes less of a problem"), thank them for their advice ("It's great to be able to learn what worked for other people"), then quietly slip off and make the decision that's best for *you*.

No two women will have the same set or severity of symptoms, the same personal or family medical history, and the same beliefs and expectations about menopause. That means that what will work best for you might not be the same approach that worked for your mom or your friend at work.

# Taking Everything into Consideration

The purpose of HT is to bring your hormones into a "healthy" balance after your ovaries quit producing enough estrogen. This balance can help to keep discomfort and anxiety in check.

## Revisiting WHI answers — and questions

Early results from the Women's Health Initiative (WHI) study, released in 2002 when the first edition of this book was being written, seemed to put the kibosh on hormone therapy (HT). Not only did a combination of estrogen and progestin *not* lower the risk of cardiovascular disease, it actually increased the risk of breast cancer, heart attacks, strokes, and blood clots. Another part of the study found that taking estrogen alone led to an increase in stroke. Based on these findings, the National Institutes of Health, the sponsor of the study, terminated both parts of the hormone trial several years ahead of schedule. Although the participants were told to stop taking their hormones, researchers are continuing to follow up on women in both groups to assess any long-term effects of hormone use.

The WHI study was designed carefully to minimize the risk of coming up with outcomes that were due to chance or coincidence. It was designed to study a huge number of women (more than 161,000 of them) over a 15-year period. No study, however, is perfect or will come up with results that are universally applicable to all women. Clearly, the findings of this study raise big and bright red flags about the use of hormone therapy. Concerns are great enough that the Food and Drug Administration (FDA) has mandated that a warning be incorporated into the packaging of hormone therapy products (see the later sidebar "Heeding the warnings").

That said, there are a few legitimate questions the WHI findings can't answer:

✔ What are the risks and benefits of hormone use for younger women? Thee WHI studied women between the ages of 50 and 79, but many women begin to take hormones during their perimenopausal years, often well before the age of 50. At least one WHI finding, a hint of lower risk of cardiovascular disease among women taking unopposed estrogen, applied only to women at the younger end of the study's age spectrum, so age may well be a factor. This may be an especially important question for women who go through menopause at an extremely early age. Women in this group almost always begin hormone therapy at a young age and may stay on it for decades.

✔ What do the WHI findings tell us about the effects of taking hormones other than the ones studied? In a word, nothing. This isn't through negligence on the part of the research group. It made sense for them to study the forms of hormones most often taken by women in the United States: conjugated equine (*equine* means they were derived from horses, specifically from the urine of pregnant mares) estrogen plus MPA progestin. Other major studies performed in the 1980s and 1990s showed that horse-derived estrogens might produce higher risks of heart disease than the natural estradiol form of estrogen. Some experts believe that treating menopausal symptoms with estrogens more closely matching those of actual human women might yield quite different results and fewer risks. Bottom line? We just don't know yet.

✔ What are the risks of short-term use of hormones? Women in the WHI studies took their hormones for seven or eight years. The FDA now recommends taking hormones — if at all — for only as long as is necessary to ease women past the stage in which menopausal symptoms are most troublesome. Granted, the study did, in some cases, discover risks (for a rise in the incidence of coronary heart disease, for example) occurring within the first year of use. We still don't know much about the use of hormones for brief periods of time.

✔ Would the potential risks be as severe if hormones were taken in a different form? The answer (so far) to this question is a resounding "maybe." Women in the WHI took their hormones orally, in pill form, so the medication was processed by organs in the body (especially in the liver) instead of being delivered more directly to the bloodstream. But we know that estrogen administered vaginally, for instance, seems to ease vaginal atrophy without a rise in the risk factors associated with oral estrogen use. The Kronos Early Estrogen Study (KEEPS) is, as this edition of the book is being written, looking at the benefits and risks of administering hormones through a transdermal patch you wear on your skin (for the record, they're also looking at a participant age range that includes younger women than the WHI did).

But taking hormone therapy does present health risks. Estrogen encourages the growth of some breast cancers and may also be a problem for women who have or are at risk for gallbladder or liver problems, blood clots, or undiagnosed vaginal bleeding.

So how do you decide? The information in this chapter (and other HT-related chapters in this book) can help you perform a cost-benefit analysis that includes your personal concerns, habits, and health profile.

If you have a family or personal history of osteoporosis or colorectal cancer, this may be a mark in the "pros" column as you weigh the benefits of hormone therapy against its potential risks. (Check out Chapter 17 for information on treating osteoporosis without hormones.)

As with any personal decision, you also have to consider your values, lifestyle preferences, and personal preferences. Also, look at your medical history and that of your family. You may eventually face the same medical problems that affect your parents, siblings, or grandparents. We help you sort through these issues, too.

# Weighing the Benefits and Risks of HT

Most women consider hormone therapy (HT) chiefly because their symptoms make them uncomfortable. Only you can decide whether this disruption warrants use of a medication that might have other effects on your health. (Check out the "Figuring out just how bad it really is" sidebar later in this chapter to get an objective look at your symptoms.) It's important, though, to know what other potential benefits and risks are associated with taking hormones. Later in this chapter we'll give you the dirt on how hormones can affect your heart health and your risk of breast cancer.

## Rounding up the benefits

First, though, here's a quick overview of some other hormone-related health findings.

Controlling perimenopausal symptoms — in both its unopposed estrogen form and combination (estrogen plus progestin) form — relieves perimenopausal and menopausal symptoms and protects your body. HT has been found to be quite effective at relieving

- Hot flashes
- Insomnia and fitful sleep due to hot flashes or night sweats
- Vaginal dryness and *atrophy* (thinning and shrinking)

Some evidence points to the fact that menopausal symptoms are actually worse during perimenopause than after you're officially menopausal. The wild hormone fluctuations are probably the culprit. But that means that, if you're like most women, your symptoms will subside eventually. If your symptoms are driving you crazy now, though, or if you are in the small group of women who continue to have some symptoms after menopause, work with your healthcare provider to find a level of hormone or alternative treatment (read up on other treatments for symptoms in Chapter 17) that brings relief.

### Avoiding bone breaks

WHI results indicate that taking HT (estrogen plus progestin *or* estrogen alone) dramatically reduces the risk of osteoporosis and the debilitating results of the disease in Caucasian and Asian women. Evidence from the WHI shows that hormone therapy (estrogen plus progestin) has a beneficial effect on women's bones. Specifically:

- ✔ Women taking combination hormone therapy experienced 24 percent fewer overall fractures and 33 percent fewer hip fractures during the years of the study.

- ✔ Bone density, measured in the hip, increased 3.7 percent after the first three years among women taking combination hormone therapy (and only 0.14 percent among women taking a placebo.

- ✔ Women taking unopposed estrogen were also at decreased risk for fractures.

- ✔ Findings applied both to women felt to be at high risk of osteoporosis and those judged to be at lower risk.

The protective effects of HT on your bones only last as long as you take hormones. So when you stop — wham — you begin losing bone mass quickly.

### Keeping colon cancer at bay

Here's another one of those "we don't know exactly why, but it does" benefits of HT. While you take HT, you have a slightly lower risk of developing colon cancer. After you discontinue using hormones, the protection gradually disappears. Specifically, findings for women taking estrogen plus progestin included:

- ✔ A 44 percent decline in the risk for colorectal cancer

- ✔ Among the cases of colorectal cancer that were found in the hormone and placebo groups, there was no difference in the characteristics of the cancers

Strangely, though, the tumors found among the women in the hormone therapy group were more likely to be advanced when first discovered (more likely to have spread to the lymph nodes and other parts of the body). The spread (metastasis) of cancer in this way is more likely to indicate a poorer outcome. So far, researchers are unable to explain this finding.

## Corralling the risks

HT also presents some additional risks to women:

- ✔ **It increases your risk of endometrial cancer if you take estrogen without also taking progesterone.**

- ✔ **It increases your risk of gallbladder problems.** HT increases your risk of gallstones. The risk can be lowered by using a patch instead of a pill.

- ✔ **It increases your risk of breast cancer.** Recent WHI findings indicate that taking combination HT (estrogen plus progesterone) increases your risk for breast cancer by as much as 24 percent. The evidence is stacking up on this issue (see Chapter 13).

- ✔ **It increases your risk of deep-vein blood clots.** Women who took HT during the WHI combination therapy trials had two times the risk of blood clots as women taking placebo. Among women taking estrogen alone, there was also a pattern suggesting greater risk for blood clots that cause pulmonary emboli (blood clots that travel to the lungs). Chapter 15 talks about the relationship between clots and HT.

- ✔ **It increases your risk of dementia.** In the WHI trials, this was true both for the estrogen plus progestin study and the estrogen alone trial. Risk was greater for women who already had some degree of cognitive impairment.

# Getting to the Heart of Cardiac Health

One of the most dramatic changes in the way researchers and healthcare providers think about hormone therapy in the past few years is the change in our understanding of heart disease. Because heart disease is the most common cause of death among women, this is no small matter. For years doctors assumed that estrogen (and thus hormone therapy of both major types — with and without the addition of estrogen) provided a significant level of protection against heart disease. This assumption was so strong that many healthcare providers routinely prescribed hormone therapy to help prevent heart disease.

The WHI findings on hormone therapy and heart disease have helped us to rethink our former assumptions. In fact, the Food and Drug Administration now recommends that HT (in either form) should no longer be prescribed for the prevention of heart disease. There are some differences, though, in findings related to combination therapy use and the use of unopposed estrogen. Read on to find out about research that applies to your situation.

# Going along on estrogen alone

Just a few years back, most experts would have said that taking hormone therapy provided a strong measure of protection against coronary heart disease and related concerns, such as stroke, peripheral artery disease (PAD), and deaths from heart attack. Since then, information from the WHI has raised serious concerns about the link between coronary heart disease and HT. Here are the major heart-related findings from the WHI for women (who have had hysterectomies) taking estrogen alone:

- ✔ The WHI results show that estrogen provided *no* protection against coronary heart disease, heart attack, or coronary death, especially among women 60 and older.

- ✔ For women in the younger end of the study group only, there was a non-significant suggestion of lower rates of heart attack and a decrease in the need for procedures for clearing arterial blockage.

The WHI study included women between the ages of 50 and 79. Though more age-specific research is needed, there are a few suggestions that the use of HT may have different outcomes for women at different ends of this age range.

Based on these findings, the jury is still pretty much out on the issue of estrogen use for women who can use the unopposed version (that is, women who no longer have a uterus and are thus free of the endometrial cancer risk associated with estrogen use). If you're in this group, especially if you are younger than 60, talk with your doctor about whether the benefits of short-term use of estrogen therapy might not outweigh the risks.

If you still have a uterus and thus the only form of hormone therapy available to you is estrogen plus progestin, the FDA recommends that you not take hormones for the prevention of heart disease. Given the increased risk of heart disease, whether you want to consider them at all will probably depend on the severity of your menopausal symptoms and your level of risk for other diseases, such as colorectal cancer and osteoporosis.

Hormone therapy shouldn't be used to prevent or treat heart disease or heart attack. You should also discuss with your doctor any plan to use hormone therapy if you have a history of heart disease or heart attack. The first line of defense against heart disease and heart attack should be a healthy diet, regular exercise, and an overall healthy lifestyle.

What about other types of cardiovascular disease such as high cholesterol and triglyceride levels and *hypertension* (high blood pressure)? Glad you asked. Estrogen is a mixed bag as far as cholesterol and triglycerides are concerned:

✔ Estrogen lowers LDL levels (by as much as 15 percent in one study).

✔ Some forms of estrogen raise HDL ("good" cholesterol) levels.

✔ Oral estrogen seems to increase triglycerides (boo), but the patch tends to lower triglycerides (yeah).

If you have a problem with blood cholesterol and triglycerides, you need to find the right type of estrogen to keep them in check.

Estrogen's benefits are clearer in relation to high blood pressure. It helps dilate blood vessels and improve blood flow, both of which lower your blood pressure.

The WHI unopposed estrogen study was stopped because of the high incidence of stroke in the group taking estrogen (compared with that of the group taking a placebo).

### Adding progestin to the mix

Now, when you add *progestin* (synthetic forms of the hormone progesterone) to the hormone therapy, everything changes. Progestin seem to dull the positive effects of estrogen on your cardiovascular system.

For women taking combination therapy (estrogen plus progestin):

✔ There was an overall 24 percent increase in the risk of coronary heart disease

✔ There was an 81 percent increase in the risk of coronary heart disease in the very first year of taking hormones

Your risk of heart attack increases while taking combination HT (estrogen plus progestin), but you're not more likely to *die* of a heart attack while taking HT (compared with women who don't take any form of hormones).

Here are the findings related to the combination HT (estrogen plus progestin) on your blood:

✔ It lowers HDL cholesterol (when taken in pill form).

✔ It raises triglycerides (when taken in pill form).

It's important to note that researchers stopped the WHI study, but they didn't put the breaks on because participants were in grave danger of dying from a heart attack or heart disease. (Although use of hormone therapy seemed to increase the risk of heart attack, it didn't increase the risk of dying from a heart attack.) Researchers halted the estrogen plus progestin study because of the increased risk in breast cancer.

Before the WHI study, most doctors agreed that women could lower their risk of cardiovascular problems by using HT. Most doctors now agree that combination HT shouldn't be the first line of defense against cardiovascular disease. Here's what we know:

- The risk of stroke doesn't increase during the first year of HT use, but it increases over time — after the first year for about five years (even in healthy women).

- Your risk of suffering a heart attack increases while taking HT, but you're not more likely to *die* of a heart attack while taking HT.

# Assessing Your Personal Risk

As you approach menopause, the risks and rewards of HT may look different to you. The pros and cons may become more balanced; you may even throw up your hands and say, "Damned if I do, damned if I don't." What can you do to sort through the decision-making process? Read on. While you're reading, take your family medical history and personal health concerns into account. And keep in mind that you can always take a fresh look at the situation next month or next year.

Some studies indicate that use of HT slightly increases your risk of breast cancer (other studies show no effect whatsoever — so it's still controversial). If you're worried about your risk of breast cancer, take an objective look at your personal risk factors for the disease.

It's important to realize that *risk* is not the same as *certainty*. We all know people who smoked and drank and lived a long life and others who lived healthy and exercised and died of a heart attack well before their time. But, in between these unlikely extremes, you can evaluate your risk factors and try to take some steps to improve your chances of preventing disease.

Many women choose to weigh their risk of osteoporosis and cardiovascular disease against their risk of breast cancer because HT protects you from osteoporosis but may raise your risk for breast cancer, and depending on what form of HT you take, it may or may not help protect you from heart disease.

If you are at great risk of osteoporosis but have few risk factors for breast cancer or cardiovascular disease, HT may be for you. If you're at great risk for breast cancer, you may want to consider other alternatives for protecting your bones and heart. Chapters 17 through 19 give you some great ideas about alternatives.

Some of the risk factors for each of the conditions are things that you can control by modifying your lifestyle, eating habits, or other behaviors. You can lower these risks immediately by making some changes now.

# Summing Up the Studies

If you've made it this far through the chapter, you've digested a lot of information, and your plate is probably still full. We thought we'd included a little synopsis at this point to help you separate your peas from your potatoes, regroup, re-energize, and re-weigh the risks and benefits associated with hormone therapy.

You should realize that the best-studied type of HT is the regimen in which women take a daily pill that contains both conjugated equine estrogen and MPA progestin. Studies of other regimens are more scattered in terms of the size of the study group and the types of HT investigated. So these results are heavily biased toward the benefits and risks of combination therapy using conjugated estrogen and MPA progestin. (For more information on all the different types of therapies and hormones, check out Chapter 10.) For now, Table 16-1 provides a rough summary of the benefits and risks of HT.

### Table 16-1   Evaluating HT Risks and Benefits: Just the Facts Ma'am

| Benefits | Risks |
| --- | --- |
| Decrease in hot flashes | Increase in breast cancer |
| Improved sense of well-being | Increase in gallbladder disease |
| Decrease in sleep interruption | Increase in heart attack |
| Decrease in *urogenital atrophy* (atrophy of the vagina and urinary tract) | Slight increase in stroke |
| Decrease in mood swings | Significant increase in deep-vein clots |
| Increased bone density | Increase in heart attack |
| Reduction of colon cancer | Increase in dementia |
| Reduction of spinal fractures | |
| Reduction of hip fractures | |

## Heeding the warnings

The strongest statement the federal Food and Drug Administration (FDA) can make about potential dangers associated with a medication (other than withdrawing a product from the market) is the issuing of what they call a "black box" warning. Early in 2003, the FDA mandated the use of these notices on hormone medication packaging. The warnings vary according to the specific product, but they all include statements to the effect that

✔ Estrogens increase the risk of getting uterine cancer.

✔ Hormone therapy, with or without progestins, should not be used to prevent heart attacks, heart disease, blood clots, or strokes.

The warnings on your package may vary, depending on which specific type of HT you take. Read any black box notice carefully, take its warnings seriously, and discuss with your healthcare provider any part of the warning you don't understand. As with any hormone medication, have regular checkups and discuss with your doctor on a regular basis whether you continue to need to take the product.

# Presenting the Options for Perimenopause

In the following sections, we present several ways that women deal with perimenopausal symptoms. Even though we group them into individual options, you may want to mix and match. For example, we discuss diet and exercise, herbal solutions, and HT in separate sections. But adopting better eating and exercise habits can only enhance the positive aspects of herbs or HT.

## Option 1: The lifestyle solution

If you're perimenopausal and your symptoms annoy you but rarely interfere with your life, some lifestyle changes may be enough to alleviate them. Many women find that some of the symptoms of perimenopause fade with a renewed focus on getting or staying fit.

Eating a healthy diet and exercising regularly, as described in Chapters 18 and 19, will boost your immune system, help maintain bone density, and keep your blood lean so you lower your risk of cardiovascular disease and reverse some of the effects of low estrogen levels that define menopause. A healthy diet and exercise trim you down and improve your state of mind.

## Option 2: The herbal solution

For most women, perimenopausal symptoms are not life-threatening so using drugs and hormones to relieve symptoms may seem like using a shotgun to kill mosquitoes. You may want to consider some non-HT alternatives to alleviate your symptoms. These alternatives can be as diverse as herbs, relaxation techniques, and vaginal lubricants. Herbs of interest for relieving perimenopausal symptoms include black cohosh, soy, dong quai, and ginseng. We cover herbal solutions and relaxation techniques in detail in Chapter 17.

## Option 3: The HT solution

Maybe you aren't wild about taking medication, but your symptoms are interfering with your quality of life; HT may be the answer. HT has been shown to relieve hot flashes because estrogen helps regulate body temperature. In addition, estrogen improves sleep and lowers anxiety by increasing the production and extending the action of *serotonin* (a brain chemical that regulates mood and activity level). Serotonin boosts concentration, improves pain tolerance, enhances memory, and regulates adrenaline so you avoid heart palpitations. Progesterone has been added to the HT regimen to reduce the risk of endometrial cancer that estrogen-only HT would present.

Many women choose to take HT to get rid of their annoying perimenopausal symptoms and may get added protection for their bones and hearts.

If you decide that HT is for you, remember that perimenopausal symptoms eventually subside for most women. You may decide to limit your use of HT to perimenopause.

Remember that many types of estrogen and progesterone (and combinations thereof) are available. It may take time to try some different formulas to find the correct therapy for you. When it comes to HT, one size does not fit all.

## Quitting HT

Most experts now recommend taking HT at the lowest dose possible and for the shortest time available. If you're taking HT when you hit menopause, it may be a good time to re-evaluate your situation and consider the benefits you want to gain from hormone therapy. As you reconsider your decision, talk to your doctor. *Do not* simply stop taking HT. If you elect to quit taking HT, your doctor is the person in the best position to guide you.

Differences exist between the benefits and risks of long-term HT use and short-term HT use (see Table 16-1 for a summary). The risks you're most worried about may not be a problem (or as big a problem) if you're taking HT for the short term — just long enough to get through the perimenopausal symptoms. With the recent study results in from the Women's Health Initiative, preventing cardiovascular disease no longer seems like a good reason to begin HT. To reduce heart disease and cardiovascular risks, start by improving your diet, getting more exercise, and quitting smoking. These methods are absolutely safe and proven to reduce your risk of cardiovascular problems (including heart attack and stroke). After you make it through the hot flashes (with or without the use of HT) and you stop having periods, it's time to consider what you want to do about preventing health problems associated with sustained, low levels of estrogen. This is a good time to re-evaluate your regimen and consult with your healthcare advisor.

# Recognizing Whether HT Is for You

Making the decision to take HT should only come after you've studied all the issues: your personal risk factors, medical history, and priorities. Are you primarily interested in reducing hot flashes and other menopausal symptoms? In maintaining a youthful appearance? In keeping the va-va-voom in your sex life? In reducing your risk of osteoporosis? In the end, only you — in consultation with your doctor and taking all of these variables into consideration — can decide what is right for you.

No one facet of your health history and lifestyle can point you with certainty to the right answer about whether to use HT. You can, however, use the statements in the sections below to help you identify your greatest concerns and priorities. Knowing what these are can help point you in the right direction.

## Deciding that HT may not be for you

Read the following statements and see if you agree with them. If you're in agreement with a lot of these statements, you may want to try HT alternatives including a healthy diet, exercise, herbal alternatives, and other preventative treatments:

I've had breast cancer.

My mother, sister, or daughter has had breast cancer.

I have coronary heart disease.

I don't have or can live with my menopausal symptoms.

I have a history of blood clots, DVT, or pulmonary embolism.

I hate taking medication and believe herbs can do a better job than drugs.

I typically eat a healthy, balanced diet.

I exercise regularly, and I'm successful at maintaining my target weight.

I think physicians and pharmaceutical companies are just out to make money from women going through menopause.

I haven't gone to a doctor in years and don't plan on starting now.

My mom had an easy menopause and I think I will, too.

I have few risk factors for osteoporosis or colorectal cancer.

## Thinking you may be ready for HT

No one wants to take medicine just to take it. Women who take HT during menopause are concerned about preventing disease or eliminating discomfort. To find a successful HT regimen, you must have confidence in your doctor and understand why you're making this decision. Even if you decide to try HT, you may have to experiment for a while (under your doctor's guidance) to find the right hormone regimen.

---

### Figuring out just how bad it really is

Just how bad are your perimenopausal symptoms? This is a pretty subjective area. One woman may say hers aren't that bad while another who has precisely the same number of hot flashes in a week might call hers unbearable. A recent poll (sponsored in part by a pharmaceutical company that makes women's healthcare medications) says that the vast majority of women find their menopausal symptoms to be much worse than they expected, but an independent study published at about the same time says most menopausal women describe their quality of life as good. This little quiz is designed to help you decide whether perimenopausal symptoms are interfering with your quality of life. There are no right or wrong answers and all of these are normal — you decide how bothersome your own symptoms are for you.

**How often do you experience hot flashes or night sweats?**

✔ Never — cool as a cucumber here.

✔ Four or five times a month, but I can cope. This, too, will pass.

✔ Daily — my boss is going to fire me if I adjust the office thermostat one more time.

✔ Constantly — I'm thinking of having central air conditioning installed in my bra.

**How often do you experience interrupted sleep or insomnia?**

✔ About the same as I have in the past; sleeping is one of the things I do best.

✔ I get a full eight hours — in two-hour blocks.

✔ Often enough that I have the TV schedule between midnight and 4 a.m. memorized.

✔ Sleep? Who sleeps?

**Do you feel irritable, anxious, or apprehensive?**

✔ Nah, I'm my usual charming self.

✔ Irritable? Anxious? Why? Do I seem anxious to you? No, really, tell me!

✔ I'm mostly okay, but telephone company ads make me cry.

✔ WHY?! WHAT MAKES YOU ASK? NONE OF YOUR DARN BUSINESS!

**Are you experiencing vaginal dryness, burning, or itching?**

✔ Hadn't ever crossed my mind — things are fine.

✔ Hmm, now that you mention it . . ..

✔ Is this what they meant when they said, "love hurts?" Not tonight, honey. Probably not tomorrow night, either.

✔ Even during everyday activities I feel dry and uncomfortable.

**Do you experience any other perimenopausal problems, such as headaches, prickly skin, leaking urine when laughing or exercising, forgetfulness, a fluttery heart . . .**

✔ Uh . . . no. Do you?

✔ No, not me. Well, okay, once in a while.

✔ You kidding? Where do I trade in my panty liners for some Depends?

✔ Yes, yes, yes, yes, and yes. What else is on that list?

If you experience many of these symptoms but they appear at about the same time each month — prior to your period — and then go away for some length of time during each menstrual cycle, you probably have premenstrual syndrome rather than perimenopausal symptoms.

If you find yourself agreeing with some of these statements, you may want to consider HT:

I have a lot of osteoporosis in my family.

My mother or grandmother broke her hip.

My hot flashes and mood swings are driving me crazy.

I've been taking HT for a year now and haven't had any trouble.

I'm a junk-food junkie and I hate to exercise.

My sex life is a huge problem because I'm not in the mood for it and intercourse is painful.

Given my risk factors, I think that I'm at greater risk for osteoporosis than breast cancer.

I think there are a lot of HT options, and I'm good at sticking to a medical plan.

I'm not big on herbal remedies to prevent or treat serious diseases.

I have a good rapport with my doctor, and I'd like to give HT a try.

If you still have concerns or questions, talk to your physician. Don't simply stop a therapy you're presently taking. Your medical advisor may be able to help you interpret the information you read about a study. Don't base your decision about HT — or any medication, for that matter — on TV commercials or newspaper articles.

# Chapter 17

# Taking an Alternate Route: Non-Hormone Therapies

. . . . . . . . . . . . . . . . . . . . . . . . . . . . . . . . . . . . . . . . . . . . . . . .

## In This Chapter

▶ Seasoning your therapy with herbs

▶ Subduing your symptoms with biofeedback, acupuncture, or yoga

▶ Soothing your privates with lubricants

▶ Beefing up your bones without estrogen

▶ Heading toward a healthy heart without hormones

. . . . . . . . . . . . . . . . . . . . . . . . . . . . . . . . . . . . . . . . . . . . . . . .

*W*e'd hate for you to go away thinking that, when it comes to treating menopausal symptoms, your choices are hormones or nothing. At least one-third of perimenopausal and menopausal women in the United States use some form of *nonconventional therapy* (medical therapies not commonly used or previously accepted in conventional Western medicine) to treat their symptoms.

There are a number of alternatives to hormone therapy for women seeking help coping with perimenopausal symptoms such as hot flashes or vaginal dryness. There are also plenty of women who — because they can't or prefer not to take hormones — look for alternative treatments for concerns common among women in their menopausal years. There are, for instance, things you can do to lower your risks of osteoporosis or heart disease.

If you're using (or considering using) nonconventional therapy, let your physician know what you're taking or planning to take. Natural supplements are still medicines — they can affect the way your body functions, just as conventional medications can. Treat these nonconventional approaches as seriously as you treat other medications — maybe even *more* seriously, because there are few FDA controls on them, and typically they haven't undergone safety studies.

One way to approach nontraditional therapy is to use it in conjunction with traditional medicine. We devote a number of chapters in this book to hormone therapy (HT) and traditional approaches to dealing with the symptoms of perimenopause and menopause, but in this chapter we talk about the use of herbs, mind-body therapies, and acupuncture.

If eliminating the annoying symptoms of perimenopause were all that it took to keep women healthy during their menopausal years and beyond, (and if the alternative therapies worked reliably and effectively on all women), alternative therapies would be a good bet (though lack of controlled studies on most of them mean we can't adequately compare their complications and risks to those of hormone therapies. But staying healthy during perimenopause and menopause requires the prevention of more serious health issues that begin when your body starts producing lower levels of estrogen. That means we'll also be covering non-hormonal ways to help protect the health of your bones and cardiovascular system.

# Weighing the Pros and Cons of Herbs

Interest in nonconventional therapy is growing. Some women enjoy taking a more holistic approach to their lives, menopause included, and others have made the choice to avoid at least some forms of conventional medicine (possibly including hormone therapy) for various reasons. In this section, we detail why more doctors are coming around to considering some herbal therapies as an acceptable treatment for some patients.

*Complementary* and *alternative medicines* are the names we use to refer to nonconventional therapies in this chapter: *complementary* if you use them in addition to conventional medicine and *alternative* if you use them in place of conventional medicine. Though we sometimes think of them as fringe or new-age therapies, many have long been part of a traditional way of health care in a much older sense of "traditional." In the days before it was possible to run to the corner drugstore to get a prescription filled, many people relied successfully on plant-based medicines to help heal what ailed them.

Some therapies that were once considered nonconventional may be adopted by conventional medicine after years of research and treatment success. Nonconventional courses of treatment have become so popular that the National Institutes of Health now has a branch devoted to studying them. The National Center for Complimentary and Alternative Medicine (http://nccam.nih.gov) conducts research and supports public information on the pros and cons of many alternative therapies. Today, safely exploring these types of treatment is becoming easier and easier.

# *Considering conventional concerns*

Conventional medicine's concerns about herbal treatments deal largely with the lack of scientific studies of the plants. Some herbs have been studied in controlled experiments (especially in Germany, where herbs are better studied and integrated into conventional medicine than they are here), but many have not, so researchers aren't sure whether they work any better than a sugar pill.

Because any plant therapy sold as medicine in the United States must go through a rigorous approval process involving testing and clinical trial, most manufacturers of such processes opt instead to market their products as dietary supplements. The FDA has no authority over the sale of these products unless they have been demonstrated to cause harm. This lack of oversight means there is no guarantee that a given product contains what the label says it does, contains the strength indicated on the packaging, or is free from contaminants such as dirt, other herbs, lead, or traces of prescription drugs. Whenever possible, look for standardized supplements that have been verified by private programs such as U.S. Pharmacopoeia, NSF International, ConsumerLab.com, or Good Housekeeping's Seal of Approval.

Conventional medicine is also concerned about dosage: how much of a given herb to take. Even if the packaging lists a recommended dose, it will certainly not be tailored to your specific concern, body size, or symptom severity. A given package may even contain more or less of the product than is advertised on the label. In 2006, for example, a consumer testing laboratory that discovered several popular brands of ginseng contained far lower concentrations of the herb than promised (even though at least one of them was advertised as being "extra strength").

# *Seeking safety in herbal therapy*

Throughout this book, we often recommend that you seek the advice of a healthcare expert before embarking on a course (or change of course) of treatment. When it comes to herbs, though, it's not always clear who the expert is. Your regular doctor or gynecologist is a good first choice. Many conventional practitioners are open to discussing complementary and alternative medicines with you. Chances are your doctor has many patients taking these products, and will be happy to advise you in this regard. Your pharmacist, too, may be able to answer questions about herbs.

You may want to speak with an herbalist. Here, however, some caution is called for. There are currently no national standards or licensing requirements for people wishing to call themselves herbalists. Anyone could hang out a shingle advertising their services as an herbalist — such a person might be learned and wise, or . . . not. That said, there are many schools and universities that teach herbal medicine, and the American Herbalist's Guild certifies herbalists who meet their rigorous qualifications for membership (look for "AHG" after a practitioner's name). Your physician may be able to recommend an herbalist to you, but so might the clerk at your local natural food's store. You can also check directly with an organization such as the AHG (www.americanherbalistsguild.com). Just be discriminating.

Germany has relatively strict guidelines for regulating herbal supplements. Their health authorities use the guideline of *reasonable certainty,* which means that they consider the experiences of general practitioners — not just clinical trials — in evaluating a plant drug. *The Complete German Commission E Monographs: Therapeutic Guide to Herbal Medicines* (by Mark Blumenthal, published by Integrative Medicine Communications) is an English translation of the German "safe herb" list (the Commission E report). For more information on herbs, you can also check out *Herbal Remedies For Dummies* (Christopher Hobbs, Wiley Publishing, Inc.).

# Relieving Your Symptoms with Plants

Herbal treatments for the mental, emotional, and physical symptoms associated with perimenopause and menopause abound. (A lot of these herbal treatments also relieve similar premenstrual-syndrome symptoms as well.) Herbalists use a number of botanical therapies that are mild, effective, and reliable. Some therapies have been tested in clinical trials; others have been proven helpful during years of use. Still others have both up- and downsides you might want to consider. We'll give you more information about the most commonly used of these (including their scientific names) in the section later in this chapter, "Getting the scoop on individual herbs."

## Cataloging herbal therapies by symptom

If you're wondering what herbal therapy can do for you, here are some of the symptoms that perimenopausal and menopausal women look to herbs to relieve, and the herbs that may be effective:

- **Depression and anxiety:** angelica Siberian ginseng ginkgo, licorice root, St. John's Wort, motherwort, Asian ginseng, ashwaganda or Indian ginseng

- **Heart palpitations:** black cohosh, hawthorn, motherwort

- **Heavy bleeding:** yarrow, lady's mantle, shepherd's purse, bayberry or wax myrtle

✔ **Hot flashes and night sweats:** black cohosh, motherwort, Asian ginseng, common sage

✔ **Insomnia:** Siberian ginseng licorice root, lavender, motherwort, passion flower or maypop, kava or kava kava, *scullcap*, valerian, ashwaganda, or Indian ginseng

✔ **Memory problems:** bacon, Asian ginseng, ginkgo, and rosemary

✔ **Vaginal dryness:** black cohosh, marigold, licorice root, American ginseng, *and red clover*

We don't claim to be herbalists, but we do know that women in Europe and Asia have used some herbs for years to treat the symptoms of peri-menopause and menopause. However, we give no advice as to dosage for a couple of reasons:

1. The quantity of active ingredients varies from brand to brand.

2. You should always seek help from a physician or a *qualified* herbalist before taking herbs.

Herbs are natural, but natural doesn't mean that they're always without side effects. Lots of things — sunshine, poison ivy, fresh tomatoes, rattlesnake venom — are natural, but not all of them are good for you.

## Getting the scoop on individual herbs

Many of the herbs used to treat perimenopausal and menopausal symptoms are phytoestrogens (*phyto* means plant, and you know what estrogen is). *Phytoestrogens* are plant estrogens — natural sources of estrogen that act in your body as weak estrogens and seem to produce estrogen effects in menopausal women. In other words, they reduce perimenopausal and menopausal symptoms.

If you take phytoestrogens without a progestin, you're at a higher risk for endometrial cancer. Phytoestrogens are natural, but they are still mild forms of estrogen and cause your uterine lining to continue to thicken. If you use these herbs, simply mention it to your doctor. He or she can monitor your bleeding and perform tests or recommend therapy as needed. (For more information on unopposed estrogen therapy, see Chapter 11.)

Always tell your doctor if you're taking any of these herbs. Some of them interfere with the effectiveness of other medicines. Mention them when your doctor asks you, "What medicines are you taking?" This is especially important if you're being treated for cancer, clotting disorders, high blood pressure, antidepressants, hormone therapy, diabetes, heart or liver disease, or if you're planning to have surgery soon.

### Ashwagandha or winter cherry (Withania somnifera)

Much like ginseng, eleuthero, and licorice, ashwagandha is said to reduce stress and depression and aid sleep with long-term use. The sedative effects of ashwaganda may be heightened if you drink alcohol or take barbiturates.

### Black cohosh (Actaea racemosa, Cimicifuga racemosa)

Even though current studies yield mixed results on whether black cohosh is effective at relieving menopausal symptoms, women have used it for hundreds, maybe thousands, of years. (Early Native Americans used black cohosh, and other folk medicines made use of it.) Today it's one of the more commonly used phytoestrogens in the battle against perimenopausal symptoms because it relieves hot flashes, vaginal atrophy, tension, elevated blood pressure, restless sleep, and stress.

Again, black cohosh is a phytoestrogen, so talk to your doctor before using it if you have breast cancer or if you plan on using it for more than three or four months.

If you're going to give black cohosh a try, you can find it sold under the brand name Remifemin. Remifemin is the extract approved in Germany to treat menopause, and it seems to have fewer side effects than other formulas. The German recommendation is to use it for six months or less (to avoid thickening of your endometrium).

### Dong Quai (Angelica sinensis)

Also known as *tang gu*. Be careful with this one. This herb has been used for hundreds of years in traditional Chinese medicine to "strengthen the blood," but its possible side effects are numerous and significant enough to warrant a thorough discussion with your doctor prior to use. Dong quai is the natural form of Coumadin (generic name: warfarin), a "blood-thinner" drug doctors often prescribe for women who have *arrhythmia* (irregular heartbeat) because it dilates the blood vessels and decreases clotting to improve blood flow to your heart. It also seems to eliminate hot flashes.

Possible drawbacks? Dong quai has been implicated in promoting the growth of breast cancer cells, even in women not taking estrogen therapy. It also interferes with blood clotting, so if you're having surgery be sure to let your doctor know beforehand that you've been using this herb. You should stop using it two weeks before surgery. Also, don't use dong quai if you've had unexplained vaginal bleeding. Try to avoid aspirin and other drugs that serve to thin your blood while using this herb.

### Ginkgo (Gingko biloba)

Here's one that's been in the news quite a bit. This herb is said to improve your memory and feeling of well-being, and one study of 200 women showed that it increased sexual desire.

Don't use it with abandon. Ginkgo interferes with blood clotting so be sure to let your doctor know that you're using this herb. If you're scheduled to undergo an operation, quit taking ginko at least two weeks before surgery. And don't take it if you're taking other blood thinners such as the drug Coumadin (or the herb dong quai). It can also cause skin rashes, headaches, nausea, and diarrhea.

### Ginseng (Panax ginseng, Panax quinqafolium, Eleutherococcus senticosus)

People all over the world consume a variety of different types of ginseng to increase vitality, improve memory, relieve anxiety, and kickstart low libido. Historically, menopausal women have used ginseng to relieve depression, fatigue, memory lapses, and low libido. It doesn't seem to raise your estrogen levels or cause your endometrium to thicken, as some of the phytoestrogens tend to do.

Do not use ginseng if you're taking medications for depressions, anxiety, diabetes, or blood thinners. It's been known to cause mania when combined with certain antidepressant medications.

### Kava or kava kava (Piper methysticum)

Herbalists use kava to reduce anxiety and chronic pain and to promote sleep and relaxation. However, even herbalists recognize a need for further tests to determine if this herb is potentially toxic to the liver.

There is a risk that kava may cause severe liver damage. Talk to your doctor before taking it.

### Motherwort (Leonorus cardiaca)

The Chinese have used motherwort for a long time. Western herbalists make use of it to treat menopausal anxiety, insomnia, heart palpitations, and vaginal atrophy.

Do not use motherwort if you're being treated for a thyroid condition.

### Peony (Paeonia lactiflora)

Peony helps dilate the blood vessels so that blood flows more smoothly through your cardiovascular system. Some folks claim that it also improves your mental focus and reduces mental lapses.

Peony has been associated with liver toxicity. Only use this herb under the supervision of a physician.

### Red clover (Trifolium pratense)

Menopausal women often find that this herb, historically used to treat skin and breathing problems, relieves vaginal dryness and lowers their LDL ("bad" cholesterol) levels while increasing their HDL (the good stuff) levels. Red clover contains *isoflavones* (the chemicals that make phytoestrogens work like estrogen), so it acts as a mild estrogen.

As with all phytoestrogens, don't use red clover if you're being treated for migraines, liver or kidney problems, or cancer.

### Sage (Salvia officinalis)

Sage is said to relieve hot flashes, but the claim hasn't been widely researched.

### Saint John's wort or goat weed (Hypericum perforatum)

The popularity of Saint John's wort for treating depression has grown tremendously in recent years, but people have used this herb since the Middle Ages. During perimenopause and menopause, women use it to treat mild depression. Research on its effectiveness yields mixed results.

This herb can cause sensitivity to light, anxiety, gastrointestinal symptoms, dizziness, and other symptoms. It also interferes with a variety of other medications, so as with any herb; tell your doctor that you're taking it.

### Soy

Soy is a plant estrogen (phytoestrogen), so it has the same pluses and problems as other phytoestrogens. It's reported to relieve hot flashes, interrupted sleep, anxiety, and other perimenopausal symptoms. However, too much soy has the same effect as unopposed estrogen (unfettered thickening of the uterine lining).

Although many advertisements for soy products point to the health of women in Japan and China as evidence that they work, women in these cultures start eating soy early in life, and they eat mostly fermented-soy products, such as *miso* (soybean paste) and *tempeh* (a chicken-like soybean food), rather than soy-protein drinks and milk. But studies have shown that soy can clean up your blood by reducing your total cholesterol, LDL cholesterol (the bad cholesterol), triglycerides, and blood pressure while raising your HDL (the good cholesterol) levels. (Read more about soy in Chapter 18.)

### Vitex or chasteberry (Vitex agnus castus)

Vitex, or *chaste tree,* acts like progesterone by helping to reduce perimenopausal stress and depression. (Some women have found that it does just the opposite, but reports of vitex causing stress and depression are rare.) Because it acts like progesterone, vitex may help stabilize the uterine lining.

Side effects associated with vitex are not severe, but may include spotting between periods, headache, and hair loss.

## Avoiding problems with plants

As we state throughout this chapter, just because herbs are natural doesn't mean they're always safe. Many of them can cause unwanted side effects (but, remember, so can hormones). If you decide to use herbal therapies to alleviate menopausal symptoms, be especially wary of

✔ Exaggerated claims. If a product purports to be able to completely cure your symptoms, improve your sex life, prevent heart disease,

and give you sparkling kitchen floors, it's time to be skeptical.

✔ Any product containing ephedra (*ma huang*). Banned in 2004 after being linked with heart attacks and deaths, ephedra can still be found in a number of herbal products.

✔ Mixtures of different herbs. It's hard enough to tell what's inside when you buy single herbs.

If any herbal therapy gives you heart palpitations or anxiety, stop using it immediately.

# Getting Touchy about Acupuncture

*Acupuncture* is a form of Chinese medicine in which an acupuncturist inserts long, thin needles into specific points along critical energy pathways in your body, to treat pain or disease. The acupuncturist is trained to identify and insert needles into the points on your body corresponding to your symptoms. For the doubters out there, acupuncture has been around for thousands of years and isn't all that far out. Asian doctors have successfully performed surgeries using acupuncture as the anesthesia.

Acupuncture stimulates your body's ability to resist or overcome menopausal symptoms by correcting energy imbalances. Acupuncture also prompts your body to produce chemicals that minimize pain and discomfort. Acupuncture is widely recognized as a legitimate form of complementary or alternative medicine, and many insurance plans cover this type of therapy. If you're interested in trying this therapy, ask your doctor for a referral to a qualified specialist. Most states regulate and license acupuncturists, so you can get names of acupuncturists from your state department of health.

# Soothing Symptoms with Mind-Body Therapies

Stress can be great if it motivates you to do your best — as in a race. But, if you're continually harried and worried, stress can actually do damage to your mind and body. It can lead to changes in your eating and sleeping patterns, anxiety, depression, and irritability. (Sounds a bit like menopause, huh?) Continued stress can also affect your immune system, making you more susceptible to cancer, hypertension, heart problems, and headaches — the medical concerns women worry about after menopause. Take a look at some of these non-medical therapies that can help you relax and reduce the stress in your life.

## Tuning in to biofeedback

Biofeedback, which relies on the interconnectedness of mind and body, has been around in a high-tech form since the 1960s, but it uses some of the mind-body lessons embraced by ancient martial arts. Biofeedback uses monitoring instruments to provide you with physiological information (feedback) about things such as your breathing or your pain level. By watching the monitoring device, and through trial and error, you learn to adjust your thinking to control your body in ways that folks used to think were involuntary.

Some of the menopause-related conditions you can treat with biofeedback are hypertension, migraine pain, insomnia, stress, and urinary incontinence.

## Getting your yoga groove on

Now here's a great way to address a whole host of potential problems at once. Yoga can help you improve both strength and flexibility (two things that may begin to decline after you've been on this planet for about 35 years) and relieve stress. Staying flexible and strengthening the muscles in your torso contribute to better balance and reduce your risk of falling and breaking a bone. A regular yoga practice that combines exercise, stretching, meditation, and mindful breathing also promotes oxygen flow, improves posture, reduces stress (and may thus strengthen your immune system), and improves your overall quality of life.

# Slip Sliding Away with Topical Treatments

Many perimenopausal and menopausal women experience *vaginal atrophy* (drying and thinning of the vagina). In addition to using herbal therapies, you can treat this condition in several ways without using hormone therapy.

You can buy lubricants without a prescription in the grocery store that will help relieve the day-to-day discomfort of vaginal dryness. Replens is one of the more popular brands of lubricants and has been shown to be as effective as vaginal estrogen cream in relieving vaginal dryness in tests. Replens comes in a tube with an applicator, and works best if you use it once a week.

If vaginal atrophy is causing painful intercourse, we have a prescription-free solution for you. A number of lubricants are designed to help you get slippery. In fact, you may find that sex is more fun when you "butter up" than it was before. K-Y Jelly has been around for years. Hospitals and doctors' offices use it for lubricating thermometers when taking temperatures rectally and for many other purposes. It also works well as a lubricant before intercourse. Astroglide is another terrific product that can make you more slippery. You can rub all of these products on your vagina prior to intercourse.

# Offering Options for Bone and Heart Health

Prolonged periods of low estrogen levels can promote bone deterioration and cardiovascular conditions. The latter is of special concern, because new research doesn't give hormone therapy the credit it once did for offering protection against heart disease. Although many women may still choose to use hormone therapy (HT) to prevent osteoporosis, other medications and therapies that directly treat both of these issues are available.

## Battling bone loss with medication

If you entered midlife with a history of strong bones, you're ahead of the game. In any case, you can minimize your risk of osteoporosis by taking calcium supplements and vitamin D — and it's never too late to begin practicing a form of weight-bearing exercise, a critical component of keeping your bones healthy. If you are at high risk for osteoporosis, your doctor may also prescribe medication to help you keep your bones strong.

### Talking bisphosphonates

A group of drugs called *bisphosphonates* are among the most effective medications for halting and reversing bone loss in menopausal women. Remember the tearing-down and strengthening through rebuilding we talked about in Chapter 5? These drugs work by slowing down the destruction phase of this process. The following list (brand names followed by generic names in parentheses) contains some examples of bisphosphonates.

Actonel (risedronate), Fosamax (alendronate), Aredia (pamedronate), Boniva (ibandronate sodium), and Zoneta (zoledronic acid) are among the most commonly used bisphosphonates. Approved by the Food and Drug Administration for use in the United States in 1995, for instance, Fosamax prevents bone material from breaking down. Women who are taking hormone therapy can use this drug to get even more protection from fractures.

Evidence is growing that links bisphosphonate medications (such as Fosamax) to an increased risk for osteonecrosis of the jawbone, a rare but extremely dangerous disease in which bone in the jaw actually dies. As of this writing there is no cure for this disease. Discuss your potential risk for this side effect with your doctor. If you are already taking a bisphosphonate medication, bring this up with your doctor well in advance of any invasive dental procedures you may need, because dental extractions or surgery have been implicated in triggering this side effect in susceptible individuals.

### Introducing calcitonin

Miacalcin (calcitonin) is a nasal spray that uses a different technique to slow down bone loss than the bisphosphonates use. Calcitonin is actually a hormone that occurs naturally in your body. It helps regulate your calcium levels by slowing the rate of bone deterioration and promoting rebuilding. It also relieves bone pain caused by osteoporosis. Calcitonin can be administered either as an injection or a nasal spray, and is typically only prescribed for women who have been in menopause for at least five years.

### Ranging in on Raloxifene

Raloxifene (Evista) fights osteoporosis by increasing bone mass and slowing bone loss. A SERM (selective estrogen receptor modulator), one of Raloxifene's side effects is that it helps to prevent breast cancer. (Read more about Raloxifene and other SERMs in Chapters 11 and 13.)

## Controlling cardiovascular disease

*Cardiovascular disease* includes conditions that affect the blood, blood vessels, or heart (otherwise known as the cardiovascular system). (For more information on how this system works, see Chapter 6.) Because heart disease is the top cause of death of women in the United States, it's important to do what you can to control your risks for problems in this area. Reducing the risks of cardiovascular disease was thought to be one of the biggest benefits of HT, but the results of the Women's Health Initiative study have called all that into question. (See Chapter 12 for the lowdown on this issue.)

### Reducing your risk of heart attack with drugs

Half of all heart attacks occur in people with normal cholesterol levels, so a healthy cholesterol profile doesn't mean you're out of the woods. Of course, the other side of that story is that half of all heart attacks occur in people with lousy cholesterol profiles. So try to maintain a healthy diet and exercise program and take your cholesterol medication if your doctor recommends it.

*Arteriosclerosis* (clogged arteries) isn't the only problem that triggers a heart attack. Many other conditions can lead to a heart attack as well:

✔ Angina (blood vessel spasms)

✔ Arrhythmia (irregular heartbeat)

✔ Blood clots

✔ High blood pressure

To reduce your risk of heart attack, be sure to maintain a healthy diet, exercise regularly, and take the medication your doctor prescribes to treat high cholesterol and any of these cardiovascular conditions. There are more than a dozen classes of medication used to control or prevent heart attacks, but these are among the most commonly used:

✔ **ACE inhibitors:** ACE *(angiotensin-converting enzyme)* inhibitors are used both for the prevention and treatment of heart attacks. If used within 24 hours of the start of heart-attack symptoms, ACE inhibitors can keep you from dying of the heart attack and prevent heart failure stemming from the heart attack.

✔ **Aspirin:** By keeping your *platelets* (special blood cells responsible for clotting) from sticking together and forming blood clots, one or two daily "baby" (81 mg) aspirin can lower your risk of heart attack.

Even though aspirin is an over-the-counter medication, it can have dangerous side effects. Read the warning label on the bottle and discuss possible side effects with your doctor. Be sure to tell your doctor that you're taking aspirin regularly if you're facing surgery.

✔ **Blood thinners:** Coumadin (warfarin) is another drug doctors use to prevent blood from clotting. Coumadin, a prescription drug is more effective than aspirin in preventing blood clots, so you must use caution and have your blood monitored regularly when taking it.

- ✔ **Thrombolytics:** Thrombolytics can dissolve a clot and restore blood flow to the heart. These drugs must be administered within six hours of the heart attack (before heart tissue begins to die from lack of oxygen) to be effective.

- ✔ **Vasodilators:** These drugs help blood vessels relax and dilate (widen) so that your heart doesn't have to work as hard to get oxygen-rich blood in. *Nitroglycerin* is a common vasodilator given to women who suffer from angina. Take these drugs as directed by your doctor.

Other classes of medications used to treat or prevent heart attack include antiarrhythmia medications, calcium channel blockers, beta-blockers, diuretics, and others. Each type works differently and will be prescribed according to the nature of your risk or heart disease. Some focus on keeping your blood pressure at a normal level, while others keep your blood lean and mean — that is, they boost your good (HDL) cholesterol, lower the bad (LDL) cholesterol, and keep both of these and your triglycerides in balance.

### Living a hearty lifestyle

Clean living will put you on the right road to heart health, too. Cardiac specialists recommend taking these steps:

- ✔ Get your blood cholesterol levels checked every year (total cholesterol, LDL, HDL, and triglycerides). For more information on blood cholesterol tests see Chapter 5.

- ✔ Visit your doctor regularly to assess your risk of cardiovascular problems.

- ✔ Read the labels on your foods and choose foods that are low in saturated fat and cholesterol.

- ✔ Eat at least five fruits and vegetables each day to reduce your risk of heart disease (and cancer).

- ✔ Keep your weight in check (turn to Chapter 18 for more on weighty issues).

- ✔ Exercise regularly (see Chapter 19 for recommendations).

- ✔ Don't smoke and avoid second-hand smoke.

A life full of anger, anxiety, depression, and isolation also increases your risk of cardiovascular disease. If one or more of these emotional conditions rule your life, it's not healthy, especially for your cardiovascular system. Having a network of friends or relatives who can offer you emotional support can lower your risk of cardiovascular disease. Try meditation or physical activity to reduce anger, depression, and anxiety. You may want to share your symptoms with a healthcare provider in order to begin treating them.

# Part IV
# Lifestyle Issues for Menopause and Beyond

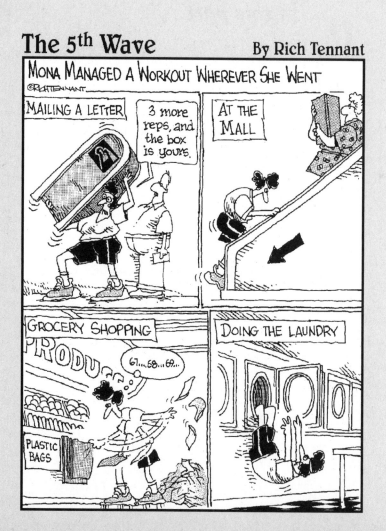

## In this part . . .

Your body is changing. That's a fact. Your body is less forgiving about things like the dish of ice cream you just couldn't resist. That's a fact too. With all the changes going on, now is a perfect time to subscribe (or renew your subscription) to healthy habits like balancing your diet, getting a bit of physical activity, and breaking those bad-health habits. A few slight modifications in your daily routine can ensure that your body is living up to its potential. In this part, we offer practical advice that makes getting or staying fit before and after the change relatively easy. (And dare we say fun?) We even talk about how life after menopause can be the richest and most rewarding part of your life so far.

# Chapter 18

# Eating for the Change

. . . . . . . . . . . . . . . . . . . . . . . . . . . . . . . . . . . . . . . . . . . . . . . . . . . .

## In This Chapter

▶ Eating well to prevent and manage health problems

▶ Healthy eating for the long run

▶ Understanding why a healthy weight is important now

. . . . . . . . . . . . . . . . . . . . . . . . . . . . . . . . . . . . . . . . . . . . . . . . . . . .

**Y**ou've probably noticed that your body is less forgiving these days. That extra glass of wine hits you a little harder than it might have when you were in your 20s, going to your head now and then disturbing your sleep later. Today you may find it tougher to start exercising, and your muscles and joints protest a little louder — and a little longer — than they did back then, often leaving you sore and achy. And an injury can set you back twice as long now as it did when you were a 20-something.

Menopause gets your attention, up front and personal, with less than subtle physical reminders such as hot flashes, weight shifting to your middle, heart palpitations, and the like. You can't help but take notice that your body is changing.

There's another way of looking at menopause, though. Think of menopause as a welcome wake-up call to help you make the most, not just of these important years, but of the rest of your life. It's an opportunity for taking stock, and, if necessary, for making a few critical course corrections. Lower estrogen levels may increase your risk of medical problems such as osteoporosis and cardiovascular disease, but a healthy diet and lifestyle can lower your risk for many of these medical issues, give you more energy, and improve your quality of life. It can also reduce some of the annoying symptoms of menopause, such as hot flashes.

Paying attention to your eating habits — not just *what* you eat, but *how* you eat — is critical at this point in your life. Because your metabolism starts to slow down, and because you may be inclined to decrease your physical activity as you reach middle age, gaining weight is easier and taking it off can be harder than it used to be.

In this chapter, we don't recommend any quick fixes. To stay healthy, you have to develop healthy *habits*. Habits are built on small changes that you can live with — without feeling as though you're making tremendous sacrifices. If you adopt healthier eating habits, you can avoid dieting and feel better. We don't have a miracle program; we just give you some great ways to eat healthier so you can get to a healthy weight, maintain it, and help reduce your risk of many diseases that strike menopausal women.

# Eating to Promote Good Health

"You are what you eat" may sound trite, but it's true. Scientific evidence demonstrates that the foods you ingest affect your health, but you probably have real-life experiences that prove this point. During the major transformation that is menopause, you want maximum energy and protection from disease. A proper diet can help ensure success on both fronts.

How do you promote good health through your diet? By adopting or maintaining healthy eating habits. Many studies link healthy eating habits to good health. *Healthy eating habits* mean eating a balanced diet of foods that keeps your body well nourished and able to fend off disease and environmental toxins.

Studies show that people who eat at least five helpings of fruit and vegetables each day cut their risk of stroke by nearly a third (and they also lessen their risk of cancer and heart disease). Another study found that the single most important factor in keeping the immune system healthy is a balanced diet.

Eating right helps your body fight off illness and protects your blood vessels, your bones, and your heart and other organs from chronic disease. Dieticians recommend that you eat five to ten servings of fruits and vegetables each day. Why? The antioxidants, phytochemicals, and fiber in fruits and vegetables build immunities, lower your blood pressure, and reduce your risk of heart disease, stroke, and many types of cancer.

Eating healthy is easier than you think. You don't have to walk around with a calorie-counting book. You don't have to eliminate all your favorite foods. You don't have to eliminate snacks. And you don't have to live solely on grapefruit juice and tofu. All you have to do is eat the right proportion of carbohydrates, protein, and fats and consume the right number of calories per day. The number of calories you need to maintain your current weight is probably between 1,500 and 2,200 calories each day. Your doctor can help you to figure out the right number for you, which will depend on your height, weight, how active you are, and your body mass index (to figure out your body mass index, or BMI, read the "Finding a healthy weight" sidebar, later in this chapter).

# Sneaking in the vegetables

We admit that some folks aren't crazy about vegetables, or find them bothersome to prepare. If you're one of them, try these easy and painless tips for fitting more vegetables into your diet:

✔ **Add chopped carrots, bell peppers, zucchini, or yellow squash to meatloaf.** These veggies make tasty additions, and vegetable-phobic folks barely notice them.

✔ **Add vegetables to your pasta.** Sauté garlic, onions, and chopped carrots or zucchini in a pan sprayed with vegetable oil. When the pasta is tender, dump it in with the sautéed vegetables.

✔ **Combine a variety of colorful vegetables together.** You can stir-fry (spray vegetable oil on the pan instead of pouring it from the bottle to lower the amount of oil you use), roast (spray with vegetable oil and broil in the oven for 10 minutes), or grill the vegetables outside (forget the vegetable oil altogether) and then arrange them in colorful layers to make them visually appealing.

✔ **Cook vegetables ahead to use all week.** If you're grilling or roasting anyway, toss some sliced onions, zucchini, tomatoes, and peppers with a little vegetable oil and cook them alongside your other food. Stored in zip-top bags, they'll be ready in your fridge to add to pasta or sandwiches, or to top pizzas.

✔ **Add chopped vegetables to rice.** Peas, corn, broccoli, tomatoes, and bell peppers work well, but you can use any of your favorite vegetables.

✔ **Take advantage of convenience.** Snag some bags of pre-sliced or shredded vegetables from your grocer's produce section, or frozen vegetables from the arctic aisle, and you're halfway there.

Here's a quick example of a simple fruit-and-veggie meal plan that provides even more than five of these great foods in one day:

✔ **Breakfast:** Add a handful of raisins and some diced apple to your morning oatmeal, and drink a glass of fruit juice with it.

✔ **Mid-morning snack:** Snack on an orange or a banana.

✔ **Lunch:** Prepare a small green salad or cup of fruit salad with your meal.

✔ **Afternoon snack:** Munch on some raw veggies with low-fat dip or hummus.

✔ **Dinner:** Be sure to have a vegetable and a salad or two vegetables.

✔ **Evening snack:** Enjoy a stem of grapes or another glass of juice.

See how easy that is? Even the most die-hard veggie haters like *something* from the vegetable group, and nearly everyone enjoys fruit, so turning your diet in a healthier direction can be fun and enjoyable.

Trendy diets come and go — and then come back again with a new name. Forget about them. You don't need to follow the advice of some late-night, slick-talking, infomercial guru to eat healthy and achieve or maintain a healthy weight. A well-balanced diet will keep you full, and proper portion sizes along with exercise and planning will keep you at your preferred weight.

We list several great resources for eating healthier and losing weight or keeping it off in Appendix B.

## Getting the right mix of nutrients

People eat for a lot of reasons other than to satisfy hunger. In fact, sometimes people eat even when they're not hungry (we're guilty and bet you are too, sometimes). You may eat for emotional reasons: out of boredom, because you're tired, angry, lonely, sad, happy, anxious — you name the emotion and we've all eaten in the throes of it. Sometimes certain environments trigger eating — you nibble as you clear the table, talk on the phone, or watch TV.

If you want to stay healthy and stick to a healthy weight, you need to eat with a purpose! Think of food like fuel. What do you need to keep your body fueled during the day? (The "fuel" is your blood sugar, which gives you the energy to build muscle, repair cells, and fight illness.) You need to feed your body the right mixture of proteins, complex carbohydrates, and fats to keep your well-tuned machine purring. Table 18-1 shows the breakdown for a healthy, balanced diet.

| Table 18-1 | Balancing the Scales of a Healthy Diet |
|---|---|
| *Nutrient* | *Percent of Daily Calories* |
| Protein | 10–20 |
| Complex carbohydrates | 50–70 |
| Fats | 15–30 |

*Based on American Heart Association dietary guidelines.*

Proteins, carbohydrates, and fats work as a team to keep your energy level high and your body in good repair. Simple carbohydrates (such as sugar) give you quick energy, but it only lasts a few minutes. Complex carbohydrates (such as whole grains, fruits, and vegetables) fuel your body for one to three hours. Proteins provide energy over the course of four or five hours, and fats fuel your body for most of the day (five to six hours). Getting the right combination of foods throughout the day will give you energy and keep you from having sudden cravings or feeling tired, anxious, or sleepy.

*Phytochemicals,* plant nutrients that are still being researched, may protect against heart disease and cancer and build your immune system. They're found in red grapefruit, tomato, watermelon, lemons, and limes.

At any given meal, you don't want to include too much refined sugar (the energy you get only lasts 15 to 20 minutes, and you quickly become tired and hungry) or too much fat (provides lots of calories, but not enough short-term energy). If you get the right combination of protein, complex carbohydrates, and fats you'll feel fully charged for three to five hours.

The best way to approach this nutritional trio is to eat some foods belonging to each category during each meal, but if you can't manage that, make sure you achieve the proper proportion by the end of the day.

In addition to eating right, you need to drink plenty of fluids. Although you'll still hear lots of recommendations to drink eight glasses of water a day, most researchers now say that listening to your body is a better guide. If you're thirsty, drink. If you're exercising, drink a little extra water before, during, and after your workout. If you're increasing the fiber in your diet, you may want to drink a couple more glasses of water each day to help the flushing process. Coffee, tea, sugar-free hot chocolate, and sugar-free soft drinks help you keep your fluids up without tacking on too many extra calories. Don't forget that caffeine has a diuretic effect — it can actually promote the passage of fluids out of the body (more peeing!), and carbonated soft drinks, even the sugar-free kind, inhibit calcium absorption and can also contribute to heartburn, so limit your intake of these.

If you blow it one day, don't stress out. If you find yourself regularly struggling to eat the right amounts of the right foods, try sitting down and planning out your meals for a few days at a time. Paying attention to what you eat helps you control your eating and weight.

### Fine-tuning your carb intake (carbohydrate, not carburetor)

The bulk of your diet should consist of complex carbohydrates, which works out well because fruits and vegetables — the food group you're supposed to eat five servings of each day — generally contain complex carbohydrates.

#### Simple carbohydrates

The quickest way to raise your blood sugar is to eat sugar (soft drinks, candy, jam). It takes very little effort for your body to take sugar and put it into your bloodstream.

These simple sugars give you a quick burst of energy, but your blood sugar drops just as quickly after about 15 minutes. Even athletes find that the quick rush of sugar doesn't do much to enhance their performance, so avoid these.

### Complex carbohydrates

Think of complex carbohydrates as "plant foods" because they include fruits and vegetables as well as whole grains. They are digested more slowly than simple carbohydrates so they provide fuel over a longer period of time — one to three hours.

Choose fresh fruits and vegetables over the canned or processed variety because the fresh versions contain more nutrients and fiber and less sugar and salt. Choose whole-grain products (flours, breads, cereals, and so on) over refined or processed grains because a lot of the vitamins, minerals, and fiber are in the outer layer (the hull) of the grain, which is removed during processing. If you're not a fan of dense and chewy whole wheat products, try some of the "white wheat" products, which are lighter but still provide some of the nutrients of whole wheat.

*Fiber* is a type of complex carbohydrate and is sometimes called *roughage*. Fiber is simply plant material that doesn't break down in the human digestive system.

- ✔ **Soluble fiber** dissolves in water and is found in a variety of berries and other fruits as well as oats, legumes, and potatoes. Because they pass more slowly through your digestive system, you keep a full feeling longer.

- ✔ **Insoluble fibers** are not digested, so they act like brooms sweeping through your digestive system and ushering out those partially digested remnants from yesterday's meal. This type of fiber prevents constipation and improves a number of digestive problems such as spastic colon and hemorrhoids.

You should eat eight or nine servings of high fiber foods everyday. This isn't as tough as it seems if you eat your vegetables and fruits and choose whole grain breads and cereals. If you ever have colon polyps, you'll want to bump up the amount of fiber in your diet.

### Building with proteins

Proteins help build and repair cells, muscles, and tissues.

Meat, fish, and dairy products, as well as peas and beans, are foods high in protein. Most of these foods, with the exception of peas and beans, also contain high levels of fat and cholesterol. (Chapter 5 tells you about the dangers of too much cholesterol.)

So how do you keep your body healthy while getting adequate amounts of protein? By choosing lean cuts of meat over fatty cuts. Put fish or chicken on your plate more often than red meat (fatty fish such as salmon or tuna provide a special nutrient called Omega-3 acids — we'll talk more about these in the next chapter). Place low-fat milk products in your grocery cart instead of their whole-milk cousins, or try soy milk. And limit your daily calories from protein to 10 to 20 percent of your total intake.

Most Americans eat a lot more protein than your body requires. You only need four ounces of protein per day. (A four-ounce serving of meat is about the size of a deck of cards.) A serving of fish or meat and a couple servings of low-fat dairy products will give you enough protein for the day.

### Energizing with fats

Fats supply fatty acids that your body can't produce and help your body absorb the (fat-soluble) vitamins A, D, E, and K.

Per gram, fats give you twice the energy of carbohydrates and proteins, but they also contain *twice* the calories! High-fat foods are packed with calories and help you gain weight more quickly and easily than other foods. Fats also raise your cholesterol levels and increase your risk of cardiovascular disease, cancer, and diabetes.

You need a certain amount of fat in your diet, but you don't have to work to include it. Most Americans get way more fat than they need, which helps explain why the United States is an overweight nation.

Foods high in fats include both plant and animal foods. Here are just a few: fried foods, salad dressings, meats (bacon, roast beef, lamb, pork, hot dogs, and more), dairy products (cream cheese, butter, ice cream, cheese, milk, and so on), pastries, nuts, and many other foods we love! (For more information on the dangers of fats and cholesterol when it comes to your cardiovascular system, please check out Chapter 5.)

The lowdown on the three basic types of fats:

- **Saturated fats:** Found in butter, whole milk, meat, peanut butter, and pastries (among other things), saturated fats elevate your cholesterol and triglyceride levels.

  Avoid eating more than 10 to 20 milligrams of saturated fats a day (less if you can). *Trans-saturated fats* ("trans fats") also raise cholesterol levels. You find these rascals in fried foods, bakery goods, and hard margarines. (Look for margarines that have "No trans fats" printed on their labels. Your heart will thank you.) Packaged foods must now include information on their labels that tell you how much trans fat they contain.

- **Polyunsaturated fats:** These fats usually come from plants. Corn oil, safflower oil, and many soft margarines fall into this category. Polyunsaturated fats lower your bad cholesterol (LDL), but they also lower your good cholesterol (HDL). Limit yourself to one tablespoon of polyunsaturated fats a day.

✔ **Monounsaturated fats:** Although these fats are a bit more helpful than the others, you still need to keep monounsaturated fats under control (between 15 and 25 milligrams per day, which equals about 2 table-spoons of oil). These fats lower your bad LDLs and keep your good HDLs high. You can find monounsaturated fats in peanuts and peanut oil, olives and olive oil, and avocados.

Opt for polyunsaturated and monounsaturated fats over saturated fats and trans fats. And take advantage of the low-fat options that line the aisles of grocery stores. If you keep your consumption of fats down, you can cut your risk of cancer.

## Rethinking how you eat

To maintain a high level of energy and keep yourself charging ahead through-out the day, you have to put the right type of fuel into your tanks and main-tain a continuous flow of fuel to your body.

To maintain your energy level, build muscle, and burn calories, balance your eating over the course of the day. Eat at regular intervals — approximately every three to six hours. If you follow this timetable, snacks actually play a key role in your daylong meal plan. They add the right types of food for bal-ance and keep you from feeling deprived of food. This doesn't mean to add to the overall amount you're consuming every day — just parcel out the meals a little differently.

When it is time to sit down for a full meal, try re-imagining the way you plan your meals and prepare your plates. The American Heart Associations "New American Plate" initiative helps you to make the transition from a mostly meat-based meal to one that's a little lower on the food chain. In this plan, vegetable- and grain-based dishes take center stage while protein and fats play supporting roles. You may already eat a number of meals this way — think of a dinner of pasta with pesto and a little cheese, or a chef salad with lots of veggies and a bit of cheese, ham, and egg, for instance.

Increasing numbers of Americans are identifying themselves as vegetarians, vegans, or "flexitarians," so it's also easier than ever to find mostly plant-based meals, even when you eat out. Ethnic restaurants are often wonderful places to find this kind of eats — consider Greek salad (ask for the dressing on the side), Buddha's Delight at a Chinese restaurant, or vegetarian stews and curries at an Indian restaurant. In our supersized culture, portion sizes in restaurants are still likely to be way too big. As soon as your food arrives, ask for a carryout container and put half or more of your order into it before you even start eating. You won't be tempted to overindulge, you'll have great left-overs for tomorrow, and — eventually — restaurants may get the idea.

Some people eat only once a day. Why? Some folks take up this bad habit in an attempt to lose weight. Others claim that they don't have time to eat throughout the day. Whatever the reason, it's a bad idea. If you only eat once a day, you're more likely to pig out when you do eat and get so stuffed that you feel tired and groggy after the meal. Plus, a once-a-day feeding regimen doesn't give your body the nutrients it needs to burn calories and build muscle and tissue throughout the day.

# Eating to Prevent or Contain Problems

Feeding your body the right foods can help forestall some health problems and diet can be part of a treatment regimen for certain conditions. This section talks about the most helpful nutrients for health maintenance and prevention:

- **Antioxidants:** Ongoing research shows the importance of antioxidants in slowing the aging process. *Antioxidants* eliminate free radicals from your body. *Free radicals* are to your body what rust is to your car: They promote damage to your infrastructure, leading to heart disease, lower immunity, cataracts, diabetes, and cancer. Antioxidants hook up with the free radicals and escort them safely out of your body so they can do no harm. Colorful fruits and vegetables (such as broccoli, berries, grapes, and carrots) are especially high in antioxidants.

- **Fiber:** Fiber pushes food through your digestive system helping protect your body against colon cancer, *diverticulitis* (inflammation of the little pouches inside your colon), spastic colon, other digestive problems, and hemorrhoids. It helps lower your cholesterol levels and stabilizes blood-sugar levels. Fiber also gives you a full feeling and helps you control your weight.

Fiber is found in the skins of vegetables and fruits and the outer layers of grains, so eating the skin of your baked potato and choosing whole grains helps increase the amount of fiber in your diet.

- **Phytoestrogens:** Researchers are just beginning to discover the benefits of *phytoestrogens*, which are sometimes called *isoflavones*. Soy proteins and isoflavones are *phytoestrogens* (plant estrogens), which lower cholesterol and support your immune system. They may protect against breast cancer, heart disease, and osteoporosis. You can find soy in tofu, tempeh, soymilk, and soy yogurt. Flaxseed is another powerful source of phytoestrogens. These miniscule, teardrop-shaped seeds come in brown or golden varieties and contain essential fatty acids, Flax is no Johnny-come-lately seed — its benefits have been touted for centuries and are promoted for their cholesterol-lowering capabilities. Research suggests they may also hold promise as a cancer-fighting food. Flaxseed must be ground to be absorbed by the body and it has a short shelf life. Buy them in small quantities and grind them in a spice mill or coffee grinder, then sprinkle on oatmeal or mix into baked goods such as breads and muffins. Flax oil may also be of benefit but should not be used for cooking; heating destroys its beneficial properties.

A very small percentage of people are allergic to flaxseed. Start with only ½ teaspoonful a day, and call your doctor immediately if you experience allergy symptoms such as a rash or shortness of breath.

A single serving of soy per day is beneficial. Some research indicates that too much soy can negatively impact your hormone balance.

## The joy of soy

Soy isn't just hidden away at the health-food store any more. These days it's found in all kinds of products at the grocery store: tofu is right there on the shelf in the produce department, and crisp green *edamame* — fresh, unfermented soy beans — are making a splash as chichi bar snacks.

There's a good reason why soy is popping up all over. Researchers are increasingly convinced that soy may offer significant benefits to perimenopausal women. Studies have linked it with decreases in breast cancer, heart disease, and osteoporosis.

This beneficial bean contains special proteins and isoflavones (plant estrogens) that lower cholesterol and support your immune system.

Other researchers, however, are concerned about whether the isoflavones in soy could themselves promote the growth of estrogen-sensitive cancers. Your age may make a difference, too. A Dutch study showed that soy's benefits were greater for women who added it to their diets during the perimenopausal period. Women who jumped on the soy bandwagon in their 60s and 70s showed little improvement in

bone density. Here again, prevention is likely to be far more effective than trying to improve your health after it has begun to decline.

Most doctors agree that a single serving of soy per day is beneficial. Here are some easy ways to add it to your diet:

- ✔ Snack on edamame, or toss them into salads. Shelled or still in the pod, these bright green beauties can be found in the frozen food aisle. Follow package directions to cook them and salt lightly.

- ✔ In Asian restaurants, ask for tofu to be added to your vegetable stir-fry or your pad thai.

- ✔ Substitute soy milk (it even comes in chocolate) for regular in your glass or over your breakfast cereal.

- ✔ Don't care for tofu? Try tempeh, another fermented soy product that comes in a variety of flavors, baked or in stir fries.

- ✔ Stir a spoonful of miso into soups and salad dressings. This salty paste adds a subtle savory taste to foods, and keeps for a long time in your refrigerator.

# Strengthening your bones

*Osteoporosis* (brittle bones) is particularly common in women after menopause because long periods of lower estrogen levels promote bone loss. To slow the rate of bone loss, it's important that you have plenty of calcium in your diet and an adequate supply of the vitamins that help your body absorb calcium.

Diet and exercise are two of the best and easiest ways to improve the health of your bones. In the following sections you'll find some great information for bone-healthy eating.

## Feeding your calcium needs

You should ingest between 1,200 to 1,500 milligrams of calcium each day (check out the table in Chapter 4 for your exact dosage). If you want to break that down into an eating plan, you need to eat two cups of dairy products, one cup of juice with added calcium, and two calcium-rich foods each day.

Many foods are naturally high in calcium, including dairy products (try to get the low-fat type) and green, leafy vegetables such as kale and collard greens (green vegetables that are high in oxalic acid, such as spinach, inhibit your body's absorption of calcium). Fish canned with its bones, such as canned tuna or salmon, is also high in calcium. Many juices, breakfast products (such as cereal and frozen waffles), and breads are "calcium-fortified," making it even easier to add calcium to your diet.

Many women, especially those who are lactose intolerant and have trouble digesting dairy products, don't get enough calcium through the foods they eat and find it easier to take calcium supplements. If you're one of these people, take supplements (usually a pill or chewable tablet) throughout the day rather than in one large dose. This way you'll ensure maximum absorption of the calcium.

*Calcium citrate* and *calcium carbonate* are the recommended supplements because they're more easily absorbed than calcium phosphate, calcium lactate, and calcium gluconate, and they're free from contaminants. Avoid using bone meal and dolomite as calcium supplements because they can be contaminated with lead.

Take calcium supplements with a glass of orange juice or tomato juice — the vitamin C helps you absorb the calcium. Taking calcium supplements with milk is also great because the lactose and vitamin D in milk also helps you absorb calcium.

Here are some great tips (if we do say so ourselves) to help you get more calcium into your diet:

- If you eat cereal for breakfast, try the brands that have 400 or 500 milligrams of calcium in each serving. Instant oatmeal is also a good source of calcium but only contains about 100 milligrams of calcium in each packet.

- Add low-fat grated cheese to baked potatoes, salads, toast, or your favorite vegetables.

- Combine fat-free ricotta cheese with fat-free cream cheese and a squeeze of honey for a great bagel spread. You get more calcium and a very satisfying treat.

- Add nonfat, dry, powdered milk to oatmeal, casseroles, pancakes, yogurt, or smoothies to bone up on calcium.

- Citrus juices with added vitamin D and calcium are easy to work into your daily routine and can give you much of the calcium you need each day.

- Some antacids, such as Tums, not only relieve indigestion, they also contain 500 milligrams of calcium. They're worth a chew!

### Absorbing some helper vitamins

You need 400 IU (international units) of vitamin D each day to help your body absorb calcium. That recommendation increases to 600 to 700 IU after your 70th birthday. But don't ever exceed 800 IU of vitamin D a day, because vitamin D is a fat-soluble vitamin and can be toxic if you get too much. Most milk products and cereals are fortified with vitamin D so it's not difficult to meet your daily requirements through a good breakfast.

You can get all the vitamin D you need by getting 10 to 15 minutes of sunshine each day. Sunshine stimulates your skin to produce vitamin D. (Take a walk and kill two birds with one stone! You can get your vitamin D *and* some exercise.) Don't forget to protect your skin, though, by avoiding the midday sun. Take your sunshine early or late in the day.

Vitamin K is also good for your bones and is found in green vegetables such as lettuce, broccoli, cabbage, and spinach.

If you take medications to thin your blood or to prevent blood clots, talk with your doctor before consuming large amounts of green vegetables, as vitamin K can interfere with the effectiveness of these medicines.

Potassium and magnesium are also critical in your quest to maintain bone strength. You can get these nutrients by including greens (as in collard greens, mustard greens and so forth), beans, whole grains, vegetables, and fruits in your meals every day.

## Alcohol and menopause

Recently there's been lots of mixed press about the health effects of alcohol. Some reports indicate that drinking in moderation may actually have benefits for heart health, could raise good cholesterol, and inhibit the formation of blood clots. A cocktail or a glass of wine, however, can trigger and intensify your menopausal symptoms. Alcohol temporarily increases the level of estrogen in your bloodstream, making hot flashes more likely. A drink can also further interfere with your ability to remain asleep at night. There may be even more serious consequences of drinking alcohol if you're taking hormone replacement therapy. Findings from the Nurse's Health Study indicate that for those on HRT, consuming even one and a half drinks a day makes your risk of breast cancer 30 percent higher than it is for women who don't drink alcohol at all. Here are some tips:

- ✔ If you don't drink, this is not a great time to start.

- ✔ If you do drink, moderation's the watchword. Limit your intake to no more than one drink a day.

- ✔ Consider substituting a healthier beverage for booze at least some of the time. Seltzer or club soda, tomato or fruit juice, iced tea, or smoothies are thirst-quenching and can be just as festive — good for your spirits as well as your body.

## *Pumping up your cardiovascular system*

Keeping your cardiovascular system healthy is a matter of keeping your blood lean and your vessels clean. Lean blood (low in LDL cholesterol — "bad cholesterol" — and triglycerides) prevents the fatty deposits that can lead to all sorts of cardiovascular problems from forming in your arteries.

Curbing the fats in your diet and replacing them with fruits, whole grains, and vegetables can help maintain healthy blood, arteries, and heart. The antioxidants, fiber, and other beneficial nutrients found in these plant foods help prevent cholesterol from oxidizing and damaging your arteries and heart.

Fruits and vegetables deliver more fiber and complex carbohydrates and less fat than any other food group, which is critical to maintaining lean and clean blood. Also, the calcium, antioxidants, and other vitamins found in fruits and vegetables keep your blood, blood vessels, and heart healthy. Plus fruits and vegetables are 90 percent water (low in calories) and very filling.

Watch those high-cholesterol foods such as egg yolks, sausage, bacon, ice cream, butter, cheese, pastries, fried foods, and fatty cuts of meat. Not surprisingly, these foods can raise the cholesterol levels in your blood.

Watch your sodium if you're concerned about high blood pressure (and one out of five Americans should be concerned). Avoiding processed foods, smoked meats and fish, salty snack foods, canned vegetables, olives, pickles, and fast food can greatly reduce the sodium in your diet. Choose fresh vegetables and meats and low-sodium alternatives.

# Weighing in on the Weight Issue

You know, we know, everybody knows that being overweight is unhealthy. But did you know that some variations on excess weight are more dangerous than others? Lower estrogen levels at this time not only make gaining weight more likely, but they also trigger redistribution of fat. That curvy pear shape turns into more of an apple shape as fat migrates to your middle. Carrying excess belly fat around in your menopausal years entails greater health risks than fat distributed more evenly around your frame.

The good news is that menopause can provide the perfect opportunity to assess yourself and your goals near the midpoint of your life, and get you started down the road to a new, healthier you.

## How much weight is too much?

Two-thirds of Americans are overweight. Whether you count yourself among them or not, weight is likely to have been of at least middling (no pun intended) concern to you at some point in your life. Here are just some of the reasons why weight has an incredibly important effect on health.

- Overweight women are more likely to suffer heart disease, stroke, diseases of the blood vessels, and certain types of cancer, including breast and colon.

- Overweight women are also more likely to die at a younger age than the average woman.

- Maintaining a healthy weight is kinder to joints and muscles and makes exercising regularly easier and more fun.

- Extra weight increases your risk of high cholesterol and *arteriosclerosis* (hardening of the arteries),

- Overweight women are more likely to die at a younger age than women of normal weight.

## Menopause and diabetes

Adult-onset diabetes can lead to a slew of other medical conditions, such as hypertension, circulation problems, skin ulcers, nerve disorders, stroke, blindness, heart disease, and kidney problems. If you've gained more than 12 pounds since you were 18, you've increased your risk of adult-onset diabetes; if you've gained more than 40 pounds, your risk of diabetes has gone way up, and you don't want that. Women who lose weight can reduce their risk of diabetes dramatically.

If you already have diabetes, the onset of perimenopausal symptoms may throw off all your carefully laid plans to maintain your blood sugar at a healthy level. Even worse, because variation in both blood sugar level and estrogen level can lead to similar symptoms — such as hot flashes and fatigue — you may not know which one to blame. The combination of diabetes and dropping estrogen levels can exacerbate sexual symptoms such as vaginal dryness and yeast infections, too.

More than ever, you need to monitor your blood sugar carefully, follow a healthy diet, and work with your healthcare provider to keep your treatment regimen working for you. The dosages of any medications you are on will probably have to be fine-tuned, and your doctor may recommend a statin or other cholesterol-lowering medication. These drugs are highly effective at reducing bad (LDL) cholesterol levels. This in turn can combat the increased risk of heart disease posed by menopause.

A *healthy weight* is one that is associated with people who have few health problems. You can find your recommended weight by referring to weight tables published by insurance companies. Insurance companies try to figure out the weight ranges for women who live the longest. This is one of the simplest ways to determine a healthy weight.

One of the best ways to help your overall quality of life during and after the change is to maintain a healthy weight.

Body fat (measured by your Body Mass Index — BMI — explained in the "Finding a healthy weight" sidebar) is an even better predictor of your potential for health problems than weight. Studies show that the higher your BMI, the greater your risk of hypertension (high blood pressure). Menopausal women are already more susceptible to hypertension and other cardiovascular diseases (see Chapter 5). The risk of hypertension begins to increase when your BMI gets above 20 and rises steadily as your BMI increases. It's thought that extra weight makes blood vessels constrict. Even a modest weight gain (5 to 10 pounds) after menopause raises your risk of *hypertension* (high blood pressure). The Nurses' Health Study found that women who lost 10 to 20 pounds during the course of the study had a lower risk of hypertension than women who maintained a steady weight.

## Finding a healthy weight

Your very own, personal healthy weight can be fine tuned by evaluating your body fat. Body fat is the real villain in this story, not weight. To measure body fat, visit your physician or health club. Your doc (or a helpful individual at your local club) will use calipers to measure the amount of fat in several places on your body, or if she wants to be really accurate, she'll immerse you in a tub of water to see how much water you displace. A good, general rule of thumb is that healthy women have between 18 and 27 percent body fat.

Another measurement, your *Body Mass Index* (BMI), is based on height and weight, provides a good estimation of body fat, and is easier to calculate. To determine your BMI:

1. Multiply your height (in inches) by itself.

2. Divide your weight (in pounds) by the number you got in step 1.

3. Multiply your answer in step 2 by 705.

This is your BMI. If your score is less than 25, you're in the healthy range. Women with a BMI higher than 30 (or if you're using a weight table — 20 percent more than your recommended weight) are considered obese.

Because of estrogen's role in maintaining healthy blood and vessels, women's risk of cardiovascular problems rise after menopause as estrogen levels fall. In addition, your risk of cardiovascular disease increases even more as your BMI increases.

If you've gained more than 12 pounds since you were 18, you've increased your risk of adult-onset diabetes; if you've gained more than 40 pounds, your risk of diabetes has gone way up, and you don't want that. Women who lose weight can reduce their risk of diabetes dramatically.

## Eating to control body weight

Many of us struggle with controlling our weight, and it's no wonder. If you're like us, you grew up with a parent or grandparent telling you to "clean your plate if you want dessert" and with advertisements claiming that "nothin' says lovin' like somethin' from the oven!" But we're here to tell you that the struggle to control your weight is a worthwhile battle. Achieving or maintaining a healthy weight has a tremendous impact on your overall health.

You don't have to quit eating your favorite foods; just watch the size of your portions. Awareness is the first step.

### Counting calories

To lose weight, you have to reduce the calories you eat and/or burn more calories through exercise. To maintain a healthy weight when you reach that point, you have to strike a balance between the calories you eat and the calories you burn through activity. But remember: you must get the proper nutrients to keep your body healthy and protect it from disease throughout the process. That's the secret to success.

Let's face it, nobody likes to count calories. If you're at a healthy weight and simply want to eat a healthier diet, try eating lower on the food chain (more fruits, veggies and grains, and fewer animal-based products), and making desserts and high-fat snacks an occasional treat, not a part of your everyday diet. You'll have more energy, suffer fewer food cravings, and help your body ward off disease and chronic medical conditions.

If your goal is to eat healthy to shed pounds, you need to become aware of the calories you're eating and the source of those calories. Keep your calories within a healthy range, add a bit of exercise five days a week, and you can shed pounds while you improve your health.

Most people can eliminate lots of empty calories — the calories you eat without a purpose just because they're there. Do you ever finish up the French fries on your child's plate? Do you snack on leftovers as you clear the table? If so, you're falling into the empty-calorie trap.

Here are the calorie recommendations for women:

- ✔ **To maintain your weight:** 1,500 to 1,600 calories a day
- ✔ **To lose weight:** 1,300 to 1,400 calories a day

If you're extremely active (exercising for more than an hour each day), add 100 calories to the recommendations.

Exercise burns up calories, so you can lose weight more easily and keep it off by incorporating exercise into your fitness plan. For some tips on fitting fitness into your daily life, check out Chapter 19.

If you're trying to watch your calories, watch the alcohol. Limit your alcohol intake to no more than three drinks (1½ ounces of liquor, a 4-ounce glass of wine, or 12 ounces of beer) a week. Wine and beer have about 100 to 150 calories. The alcohol in a mixed drink is 100 calories or so, and if you mix it with something sweet, you can consume up to 400 calories per drink.

# Discouraging diets

It seems as if someone is always pushing a new diet that promises to make weight disappear using a secret no one else has discovered. Many of us try one of these "miracle" diets and end up looking for a new one because the weight we lose reappears. The secret to getting to a healthy weight and staying there is to — are you ready for this? — avoid diets. Most diets have you chomping at the bit, waiting for the pounds to come off so you can go back to eating the foods you want. When you go back to your old habits, the weight returns.

Eating healthier can help you lose weight and keep it off because it encourages you to change the way you think about food. You begin to think about food as a fuel, as opposed to a treat that you can't have or a substance that you must eat despite its cardboard-like flavor. You begin to think about what your body needs to stay lean,

build muscle, rejuvenate tissue, and ward off disease.

Beware of unbalanced diets that tell you to completely avoid one of the major nutrients (complex carbohydrates, fats, or protein). By cutting out one of these groups, you may also eliminate fiber, antioxidants, or phytochemicals that protect your body from aging and disease.

Low-carbohydrate and high-protein diets are high in cholesterol and low in fiber, which may increase your risk of heart disease, cancer, and digestive problems.

Liquid diets offer quick weight loss, but you mostly lose muscle. When you lose more muscle than fat, you actually have a higher percent of body fat even though you weigh less. Also, some liquid diets can damage your heart, kidney, and liver and cause an irregular heartbeat and many other health problems.

## Nibbling on little nothings

The following list provides some good nutritional tips that have little or no caloric cost:

- ✔ Lettuce, parsley, radishes, watercress, and celery provide nutrients without the calories.
- ✔ Use butter-flavored sprays when cooking instead of oil to shave off fat and calories.
- ✔ Sugar-free gelatin adds a bit of free dessert to any meal.
- ✔ Hot pepper and picante sauces add a bit of spice without a lot of calories.
- ✔ Low-fat bouillon is a great substitute for butter-based sauces when serving pasta or steamed vegetables.
- ✔ Fat-free cream cheese, mayonnaise, salad dressing, and sour cream are free in terms of fat calories as long as you use only 1 tablespoon.

### *Foregoing fat*

It's really tough. Many of our favorite foods are high in fat. Take away the fat, and they don't seem so good. Believe it or not, we have some tips for eating *satisfying* meals that are a bit less fatty. If you really dislike the low-fat alternatives, go ahead and have the high-fat food, just reduce the portion size, and have it less often. Only eat half of that bratwurst or eat a donut hole instead of the whole donut. Here are some other great tips:

- ✔ Try mixing instant bouillon in hot water and adding a few tablespoons to vegetables, rice, or pasta instead of putting butter or margarine on the food. You get that rich taste without the fat.

- ✔ Similarly, a tiny drizzle of olive oil — one of the "good" fats — provides great flavor without a lot of unhealthy calories.

- ✔ Choose lean cuts of beef (tenderloin instead of rib-eye, for example) — they have less marbling than the fattier cuts.

- ✔ Try putting low-fat yogurt or low-fat cottage cheese on top of your baked potato instead of butter or sour cream. Salsa's great on baked potatoes, too, and adds no fat at all.

- ✔ When you order a salad at a restaurant, get the salad dressing on the side. And, if the restaurant doesn't have a low-fat alternative, try using one tablespoon of a vinaigrette — or even a spoonful of a balsamic vinegar, which has such a rich flavor you probably won't even miss the oil.

- ✔ Eat spicy toppings such as salsa, ginger, or picante sauce instead of cream sauces.

# Chapter 19

# Focusing on Fitness

· · · · · · · · · · · · · · · · · · · · · · · · · · · · · · · · · · · · · · · · · · · ·

· · · · · · · · · · · · · · · · · · · · · · · · · · · · · · · · · · · · · · · · · · · ·

*W*ith all the changes going on with your body, now is a great time to make sure that you're physically fit. Physical activity and exercise during perimenopause and menopause can relieve many of the common physical and mental/emotional symptoms that accompany the change.

We have some good news: You don't need to be an athlete or join a health club to realize tremendous health benefits from exercise. According to several studies, one hour of moderate exercise five times a week improves the quality and duration of your life. In this chapter, we introduce you to exercises that you can do in your home, and show you ways to fit fitness into your busy life.

Maybe you're already physically active, and you want to move your program up a notch. If so, pat yourself on the back. Studies indicate that only 20 percent of American women get 30 minutes of exercise five times a week. Even if you've got a head start on the rest of us, though, we'll offer tips everyone can use to reduce health risks and help control menopausal symptoms.

## Recognizing the Benefits of Exercise

The lower estrogen levels in your body during the change can contribute to a number of medical conditions, memory lapses, and emotional transformations. Physical activity can help you reclaim your grip on life and fight off cardiovascular disease, diabetes, cancer, osteoporosis, and more.

The type of physical activity we're talking about consists of movement that burns calories. Jogging or playing tennis burns lots of calories quickly, but seemingly mundane activities such as vacuuming, gardening, and raking leaves can be beneficial if you do them for a long enough period of time (45 minutes to an hour). The trade-off is simple: Do a vigorous activity for a short period of time or a moderately demanding activity for a longer period of time.

Many terrific studies show that physical activity makes a difference in the health of menopausal women. Exercise puts a positive spin on many of the health concerns women face during and after the change.

## Tweaking your attitude

A variety of studies show that exercise and physical activity improve your ability to cope with stress and depression. One study even shows that running is more effective than psychotherapy for reducing depression, and the results aren't that difficult to believe. The term *runner's high* isn't a joke — physical activity helps your body release *endorphins,* substances that naturally relieve pain and elevate your mood.

You can relieve the perimenopausal symptoms of anxiety, irritability, mood swings, decreased libido, and depression by sticking to a fitness plan that gives you time to build your mental and physical fitness.

Setting aside some time for exercise each day also helps you organize your thoughts and feelings, relieve stress and anxiety, and re-establish your grip on life. If you make the initial effort, you'll begin to look forward to *your* time.

## Flashing less — sleeping more

Only about 1 in 20 women who exercise experience hot flashes. Compare that stat to the ratio of women in the non-exercising crowd who experience hot flashes — about 1 in 4 — and you can quickly see why tying on those sneakers and going for a walk is a good thing. Hot flashes are a pain in their own right, but they can also turn into night sweats and cost you precious dream time. Exercise can lessen this effect and make your sleep more restful.

Exercise also helps women sleep better at night for another reason. Yes, exercise makes you tired, but there's more to the story. Exercise affects the amount of *melatonin* (a hormone that helps regulate sleep) in your body.

Melatonin levels are normally high in young children, but they appear to decline gradually with age in some adults. Exercise keeps the pineal gland producing melatonin at night (when levels are naturally higher), even though melatonin levels actually decline when you exercise.

## Shedding pounds

Women typically gain about one pound a year from their late 30s through their mid-60s. A pound may not sound like much, but it adds up over the years. Weight gain raises your risk of many diseases. Women who incorporate 30 to 60 minutes of physical activity into their lives *every day* can maintain their present weight or lose weight (but exercising an hour each day is the prescription for overall health, not just weight loss).

You can find all kinds of ways to lose weight, but to lose weight and keep it off, walking is one of the most effective physical activities. After studying thousands of dieters, one study found that 49 out of 50 people who lost 30 pounds or more walked for at least half an hour at a brisk pace every day. The bonus: you don't need any equipment or special conditions other than comfortable shoes and personal motivation.

## Keeping your heart healthy

Just because a woman generally has the heart of a man 10 years her junior because of the estrogen her body produces, doesn't mean that heart disease doesn't catch up with the female of the species. Keeping your heart healthy through diet, exercise, and medication, if necessary, should be a priority for your menopausal years.

### Cleaning up with good cholesterol levels

Physically active women tend to have higher levels of the good cholesterol (HDL) than women who aren't so active. If you start exercising today, you can notice higher HDL-cholesterol and lower LDL (bad) cholesterol levels within a few months.

### Listening to a beating heart

Because physical activity improves your cholesterol profile, your blood vessels are less apt to play host to fatty buildup that results in arteriosclerosis. Arteriosclerosis can cause hypertension (high blood pressure), heart disease, and stroke, so getting physical reduces your risk of all three.

The Nurses' Health Study revealed that walking briskly for three hours a week can reduce your risk of heart disease by 40 to 50 percent. The study also showed that even women who just started walking regularly benefited by reducing their risk of heart disease.

The more often you exercise and the longer your workout, the more benefits you gain.

### Keeping a lid on blood pressure

Because exercise improves your cholesterol profile, your risk of high blood pressure goes down too. With a healthier cholesterol profile, your blood vessels are less likely to get clogged with *plaque* (deposits of fat mixed with other substances that are covered with a layer of calcium and found on the walls of your blood vessels). Arteriosclerosis causes your blood vessels to narrow and forces your heart to beat harder to get the blood through, raising the pressure in your blood vessels and resulting in hypertension (high blood pressure).

### Exercising sound judgment

In case you haven't guessed by now, regular exercise seems to cure whatever ails you. This statement is especially true in relation to cardiovascular disease. Moderate exercise, such as walking for 30 minutes five times a week, can improve the health of your body and mind.

Exercise benefits your cardiovascular system in many ways:

- ✔ Improves your circulation
- ✔ Increases your good (HDL) cholesterol levels
- ✔ Reduces total cholesterol, triglycerides, and blood pressure
- ✔ Increases your endurance
- ✔ Reduces anxiety, depression, and emotional stress
- ✔ Increases your metabolism so that you burn more calories, even at rest
- ✔ Builds another support group when you do it with friends

## Shoring up your bones

After menopause, women begin losing bone density. They risk developing *osteoporosis* (brittle bones; check out Chapter 5 for more info) as a result of the loss. People who have osteoporosis are prone to fractures. This tendency forces them to restrict their daily activity, which in turn impacts the quality and longevity of their life. To prevent osteoporosis and fractures, take our advice:

- ✔ Include weight-bearing exercises in your exercise routines to increase bone density (bone strength) and to slow or prevent bone loss. (See "Strengthening bones and toning muscle" later in this chapter.)
- ✔ Improve your balance and flexibility with stretching and core-training exercises that can help you reduce your risk of falling and fracturing your bones. (Jump to the "Flexing through stretching" section later on for more information.)

## Doing without diabetes

Diabetes is a serious health condition that can produce a host of other medical problems ranging from hypertension to blindness. Exercise can reduce your risk of adult-onset diabetes by helping you keep your weight in a safe range and by improving your body's response to insulin. (For more on diabetes, see Chapter 15.)

Even if you're overweight or leading a sedentary lifestyle now, you can reduce your risk of developing diabetes by beginning a fitness program. A small increase in activity will help, but more activity provides more protection against diabetes. In one study, women who walked briskly for three hours a week reduced their risk of diabetes as much as women who worked out vigorously for half that amount of time. Our point? You don't need to train for a marathon to reduce your risk of diabetes.

## Steering clear of colon cancer

In Chapter 14 we discuss the benefits of getting your colon checked regularly. Exercise is another way to protect yourself against colon cancer. Exercise keeps waste (and any carcinogens you may have ingested) moving through your digestive tract and out of your body so the waste doesn't linger in your colon. The level of activity we recommend earlier in this chapter (an hour a day five days a week) offers some protection against colon cancer.

## Sharpening your memory

Staying active as you age has been proven to have a very positive impact on memory and judgment. Getting more blood and oxygen flowing to your brain seems to trigger these positive effects.

## Living long and prospering

Without cracking open a fortune cookie, we can say with some confidence that daily exercise can extend your life. One group of 60- to 80-year-olds cut their death rate in half by walking two miles every day. Not too shabby.

# Focusing on Fitness Fundamentals

Whatever activities you decide to do to improve your physical fitness, make sure that you enjoy them. If you don't like an activity, you won't work it into your daily schedule, and you won't do it for long.

Plan your week out in advance to make sure that you reserve time for your workout. Make your fitness time a priority that you won't give it up whenever things get busy. Planning your exercise in the morning, before other responsibilities throw you off-course, is helpful. People who make exercise a life-long habit are more likely to exercise in the morning. And exercise in the a.m. increases your metabolism and keeps it elevated until you go to sleep — many more hours of increased metabolism.

Whenever you exercise, working physical activity into your day helps you accomplish your primary long-term goal — living a long and healthy life — and it makes you feel pretty good in the short term, too.

## Getting started

If you haven't been getting much exercise, begin your program slowly. For the first few weeks, exercise three times a week for about 20 or 30 minutes per session. Then, when you feel good with that pace and decide you want to bump it up a notch, add a few more days and a little more time to your workout. Another way to move to the next level is to increase the intensity of your workout. If you're walking, go further or faster or walk twice a day on certain days of the week. Or you may want to start jogging instead of walking. The bottom line: You gain more by exercising longer or faster.

Regardless of how you decide to increase the intensity of your workout, make sure that your body gets used to each level before you move on to the next. If you start experiencing any abnormal symptoms (such as chest pain, shortness of breath, and so on) as you increase your exercise intensity, please contact your doctor immediately.

Health clubs or the local YMCA are nice because they offer motivation and instruction as well as an opportunity to form a support group with people who are also trying to stay healthy. But you don't have to join a club to receive these kinds of benefits. Asking a friend from your neighborhood to join in your morning walk or play a set of tennis can also provide the support and motivation you need to stick with it.

If you have any health problems, visit your doctor for a thorough physical before starting a new or more vigorous exercise program.

## Pumping your blood on busy days

Here are five simple ways you can incorporate physical activity into an already busy day.

1. Take the stairs instead of the elevator. Whether you go up or down, you get your blood pumping and your legs working.

2. Walk the dog. Studies show that people who walked their dog five days a week for 20 minutes a day lost an average of 14 pounds in less than a year (and it's good for Fido's health, too).

3. When you go shopping, park your car away from the store and walk briskly to your destination. When you're in a mall, take a lap or two.

4. On your break time at work, climb the stairs or take a walk. Some days, this may be the only time you have to get moving. Remember: Every little bit helps.

## Fitting in fitness

Does anyone have a spare hour (or half-hour) in her day? When someone raises the subject of exercise, you may think, "When do I have time to take a walk or work out?" We know that demanding days leave you with little discretionary time or energy.

But your family and your friends would agree that nothing is more important than your health. Besides, you're going to take time out of your life and away from your family and friends for your health whether you exercise or not. So, either take the time to exercise now or spend some time with the medical professionals taking care of your health later.

## Planning your program

After the onset of perimenopause, you want to keep your hormones balanced, your diet balanced, and yes, your fitness program balanced. You should incorporate three types of activities into your fitness routine: aerobic exercise, flexibility training, and strength training. Don't worry — you don't have to do all three each day, but you should fit all three into your weekly fitness plan.

✔ **Aerobic activity:** Aerobic activity strengthens your cardiovascular system, helps your endurance, and also helps you burn fat. Basically, it's the perfect type of exercise for women of all ages. Whether you perform your aerobic activities in vigorous, relatively short bursts or at a slightly slower pace for longer periods of time, the benefits work out the same. For example, you can burn 200 calories by walking for 30 minutes or by jogging for 18 minutes.

Aerobic exercise benefits your body because it forces your cardiovascular system and muscles to exert themselves. Too little exertion, and you don't gain all the benefits of exercise; too much exertion, and you stress your cardiovascular system (and your muscles).

More vigorous forms of aerobic exercise include jogging, walking, cycling, aerobic dance, martial arts, and jumping rope. Even activities you probably don't think of as exercise can give you a light aerobic workout — walking your dog, golfing, shopping, gardening, or playing with the kids.

✔ **Flexibility training:** This aspect of your workout routine can protect you from injury, improve your balance, and provide muscle flexibility. Stretching is the simplest and easiest way to improve your flexibility and agility. Working with a *fitness ball* can improve your flexibility and balance while strengthening and toning your muscles. Yoga is probably the oldest form of stretching.

✔ **Strength training:** Incorporating strength training into your exercise schedule helps you build muscle tone, endurance, and bone density. Because strength training builds muscle, it speeds up your metabolism so you burn more calories — even when you're resting. (Muscle burns more calories than fat does, so the more muscle you have, the more calories you burn.) Weight training and Pilates both improve muscle strength.

## Scheduling fitness fun time

A total fitness program incorporates aerobic exercise, flexibility training, and strength training in a weekly fitness plan. One example of such a plan includes one easy day and two (non-consecutive) rest days. On the other four days, work out at a steady pace. No time? Working out for three 15 minute periods is as effective as working for one 45 minute stretch.

If you have trouble sticking to your fitness routine, make an appointment. Schedule a standing appointment with yourself to take a brisk walk first thing in the morning or after dinner each day or make an appointment to get up earlier in the morning so you have a focused time to work out — put it on the calendar and stick to it!

Be sure to warm up before each session and cool down afterward. (For more information, see the "Warming up and cooling down" section later in this chapter.) In the fitness programs mentioned here, we fit stretching into the program by doing it as part of our warm-up and cool-down routines, but you can add more stretching to your program or add a yoga class to your schedule. Stretching improves flexibility and keeps your muscles from getting sore.

# Zoning in on your target heart rate

Your target heart rate tells you how much effort you put into an exercise. Here's how you can check your heart rate:

1. Put your index and middle finger on your opposite wrist and find your pulse. (You can also use the carotid artery in your neck, which is under your jawbone.)

2. Count the number of beats for ten seconds (you need a clock with a second hand).

3. Multiply that number (the number of beats in ten seconds) by six. The result is your number of heartbeats per minute — your heart rate.

After you know how to figure out your heart rate, you can figure out your *target heart-rate zone,* which is important when exercising. You should try to keep your heart rate within your target heart-rate zone during exercise to achieve the perfect workout intensity and maximum benefits.

1. Subtract your age from 220, which is the maximum heart rate (a heart rate you don't want to even approach).

2. Multiply your answer from Step 1 by 0.6. The resulting number is the lower limit of your target heart-rate zone.

3. Multiply your answer from Step 1 by 0.85. The resulting number is the upper limit of your target heart-rate zone.

✔ **Day 1:** Start off with a warm-up. Then move onto 20 to 30 minutes of aerobic activity followed by 20 minutes of strength training (see the "Strengthening bones and toning muscle" section later in this chapter). End your workout with a cool-down that includes at least 5 to 10 minutes of stretching.

✔ **Day 2:** Do 20 to 30 minutes of aerobic exercise but at a lower intensity than your Day 1 workout. Remember your warm-up and cool-down time.

✔ **Day 3:** Do the Day 1 routine — warm-up, aerobic exercise, strength training, and then a cool-down with some good stretching. Your intensity should be the same as that of Day 1.

✔ **Day 4:** Take a day off to rest and restore your muscles. Resting is also important for your body.

✔ **Day 5:** Follow the same workout as Days 1 and 3.

✔ **Day 6:** This is ladies' choice day. Do something different for your aerobic exercise, something a bit lighter — gardening, dancing, yard work, swimming with the kids, or golfing — but do it for 45 minutes rather than a half-hour.

✔ **Day 7:** Take the day to rest and relax to restore your muscles.

Talk to your doctor about your fitness plan first, especially if you haven't exercised in a long time, you have heart disease, you're overweight, or you have any other medical condition. After you get the okay from your doctor, consider using a certified personal trainer to guide you.

## Flexing through stretching

What's so tough about stretching? You probably did it back when you were taking grade-school gym class, doing ballet, or running track, right? Well, things have changed a bit. In the past few years, medical and exercise experts have come a long way in understanding the physics behind stretching. Some of the old stretching exercises actually hurt your body more than they helped it. Be sure to follow this good advice about stretching while performing the great stretching routine found in the section, "Warming up and cooling down," later in this chapter (see Figures 19-1 through 19-6):

- ✔ Stretch during your warm-up and cool-down periods.

- ✔ Don't bounce. Stretch slowly until you feel some tension, not pain.

- ✔ When warming up, hold the position for 10 to 30 seconds, relax, and then stretch again.

- ✔ When cooling down, hold the position 30 seconds, relax, and then stretch again. If you're working on flexibility, try doing each stretch twice during the cool-down and stretch a bit further the second time.

  If you increase your stretching intensity during the cool-down period when your muscles are already warm, you can increase your range of motion and get more out of your stretch. Stretching when your muscles are warm helps you build flexibility much more quickly because warm muscles stretch better than cold ones, and elastic and stretched muscles are flexible muscles.

- ✔ Never stretch a muscle if you've had a recent muscle, ligament, tendon, joint, or bone injury or if you feel a sharp pain. If you feel a sharp pain — as opposed to the dull ache of well-exercised muscles — consult your doctor before continuing with your stretching routine.

If you're interested in additional information on stretching, take a look at the resources in Appendix B.

Yoga and Pilates are both terrific activities if you really want to work on your flexibility, balance, and core strength. Yoga consists of three main components: exercise, breathing, and meditation, and Pilates offers exercises derived from yoga, dance, and other areas. With either, start at the beginning and be patient with yourself. If you're interested in finding out more, check out *Power Yoga For Dummies* (Doug Swenson, Wiley Publishing, Inc.) and *Pilates for Dummies* (Ellie Herman, Wiley Publishing, Inc.).

# Warming up and cooling down

Be sure to start *each workout* with an easy warm-up period and end each session with a cool-down period. Warming up puts your muscles and cardiovascular system on alert that they're about to go to work. Cooling down gives them a chance to relax after a satisfying workout. You can do the same activities for both your warm-up and cool-down sessions.

Warming up and cooling down can be as simple as walking or cycling for 5 to 10 minutes and then doing some *light, gentle* stretching for another 15 minutes.

Never stretch cold muscles — you can damage them. That's why you start your warm-up session with a bit of walking or cycling. Also, don't bounce or pull hard as you stretch during your warm-up, a time when your muscles are still pretty cold.

If you're worried about time, you may be inclined to skip your warm-up and jump right into your routine. Not a good idea. Warming up prevents injury and helps you ease into your workout without straining your muscles. Starting slowly actually lets you exercise longer.

The six simple stretches shown in Figures 19-1 through 19-6 stretch each of your major muscle groups. Try holding each stretch for 10 to 30 seconds. Over time, you may want to try to stretch further, which is great, but don't strain your muscles and be sure to stop when you feel tightness — don't stretch until you feel pain. If you stretch until you hurt, your muscles actually begin to contract, and you don't accomplish anything except hurting your muscles.

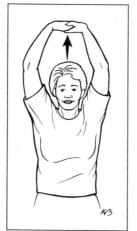

**Figure 19-1:**
Stretching
your upper
torso and
arms.

1. Clasp your hands above your head, interlocking your fingers.
2. Push your palms upward.
3. Stretch until you feel tightness and hold.

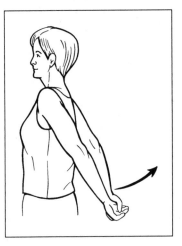

**Figure 19-2:**
Stretching
your chest
and
shoulders.

1. Clasp you hands behind your back.
2. Slowly and carefully lift your arms.
3. Stretch until you feel tightness and hold.

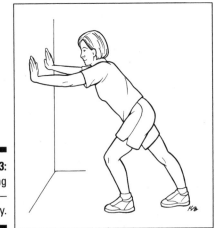

**Figure 19-3:**
Stretching
your legs —
all the way.

1. Stand close to a wall with one leg forward.
2. Bend your front leg at the knee and keep your back leg straight.

3. Steady yourself by putting your hands on the wall.

4. Stretch forward keeping your back foot (including your heel) flat on the floor.

5. Switch legs and repeat Steps 1 through 4.

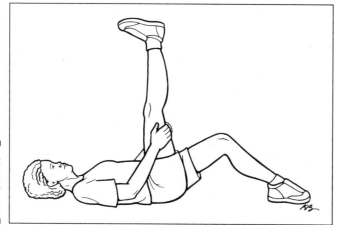

**Figure 19-4:**
Stretching
more of your
legs.

1. Lie flat on your back.

2. Stick one leg up in the air.

3. Grab your thigh below your knee.

4. Slightly bend the leg that is on the floor at the knee.

5. Gently pull your leg toward your chest keeping this leg straight.

6. Repeat Steps 1 though 5 with the opposite leg.

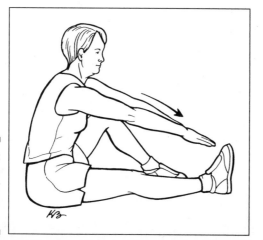

**Figure 19-5:**
Stretching
your lower
back and
buttocks.

1. Sit on the floor with both legs extended straight out in front of you.

2. Bend one leg so that your knee touches your chest.

3. Lean forward, reach out, and touch your toes.

    If you can't touch your toes, stretch as far as possible without experiencing pain. With time, you'll be able to get closer and closer.

4. Repeat Steps 1 through 3 with the opposite leg.

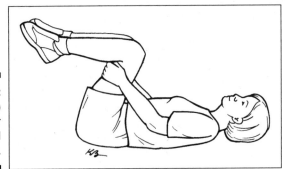

**Figure 19-6:**
Warming up your lower back and upper legs.

1. Lie on your back.

2. Raise your legs in the air and bend them at the knee.

3. Grab both legs behind and below the knee.

4. While keeping your back as flat to the floor as possible, pull your thighs in toward your chest.

A lot of people tend to cheat at the end of their workout, but definitely do some light stretching as part of your cool down — it's terrific for your flexibility, and can minimize soreness later.

# Exercises for Women with Osteoporosis

The best exercises to prevent or slow down osteoporosis are *weight-bearing exercises* — exercises, such as walking and strength training, that include gravity and tension on your muscles. Stress builds bone (see, stress is good for something), and putting weight on your bones provides the stress your bones need to grow in strength. Weight-bearing exercise promotes bone growth, which is critical for women of any age. During and after the change, when your estrogen levels are lower, weight-bearing exercise can keep bones strong and healthy by increasing bone density.

Although you move your muscles when you swim or cycle, these aren't the best exercises for building bone. The water (in swimming) and the bicycle seat (in cycling) take a lot of the load off your bones.

If you have osteoporosis, your bones may be more liable to break. Weight-bearing exercises are great for strengthening bone, but increasing your flexibility and balance can also help you avoid osteoporosis-related complications by reducing your risk of falling and breaking bones in the first place. You can improve your flexibility by including stretching in your fitness routine (check out the two preceding sections). And you can improve your balance through exercise as well.

## Strengthening bones and toning muscle

Walking is a great way to fight osteoporosis, but a combination of walking and strength training is even better for building bone. You may choose to do both of these weight-bearing exercise routines on the same day or split them up during the course of the week. Weight-bearing exercises strengthen only the bones that you work, so walking strengthens your legs, but it won't help your other bones. You need to introduce strength-training exercises into your fitness program to accomplish that feat.

The best strength-training program is one that includes all your major muscle groups. This type of program improves your bone density in important areas, but it also improves your balance, which is important in avoiding falls that can cause fractures.

Start your strength-training regimen with a good, all-around strength-training routine using the seven exercises shown in Figures 19-7 through 19-13. These exercises strengthen your chest, arm, shoulder, leg, abdominal, and back muscles. You can start with three to five repetitions of each exercise and increase the number as your interest and endurance dictates. If you want to vary this routine or try some more advanced strength-training exercises, check out Appendix B for additional resources.

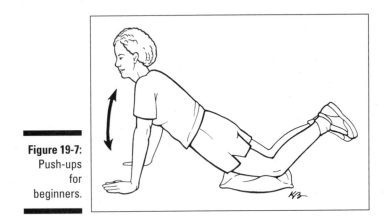

1. Kneel on the floor.

2. Place your hands a little wider than shoulder-width apart on the floor in front of you.

3. Keeping your knees on the floor (or on a cushion on the floor), raise your feet a bit.

4. Lower your upper body by bending your elbows.

5. Push back up and straighten your elbows.

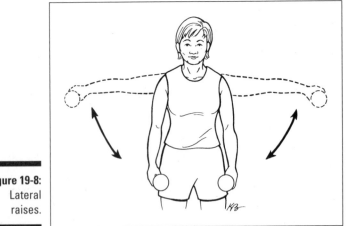

1. Stand up straight with your chest out and knees slightly bent.

2. Hold a two-pound weight in each hand with your arms down at your side.

3. With your elbows slightly bent, raise your hands to shoulder level. (Don't raise them higher than shoulder level.)

4. Slowly lower your hands until the weights are back at your side.

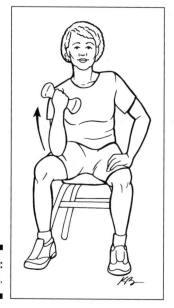

**Figure 19-9:**
Bicep curls.

1. Sit on the edge of a chair with your back straight and your legs slightly apart.

2. Lean forward (keeping your back straight).

3. Bend your elbow toward your chest and place it on the corresponding thigh while holding a two-pound weight. (You can increase the weight as you get stronger.)

4. Slowly lower your arm by straightening out your elbow. (The palm of your hand should be facing up at the end of the motion.)

5. Bring the weight back toward your chest.

6. Repeat Steps 1 through 5 with your other arm.

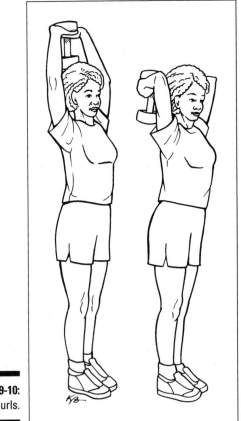

**Figure 19-10:**
Tricep curls.

1. Stand up straight with your knees bent slightly.

2. Hold a two-pound weight with both hands and raise it over your head.

3. Keeping your arms close to your head, lower the weight behind your head by bending your elbows.

4. When your forearm touches your upper arm, slowly raise the weight back up.

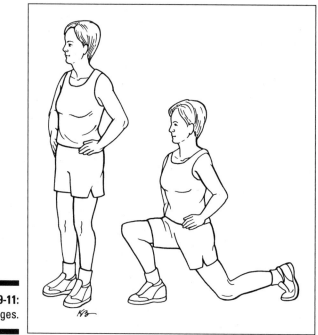

**Figure 19-11:**
Lunges.

1. Stand up straight with your hands on your hips.

2. Step forward with your right leg, keeping your back, neck, and head straight.

3. As your front heel hits the ground, bend both knees so that your left knee almost touches the floor (or go as low as you can).

4. Step back to the starting position.

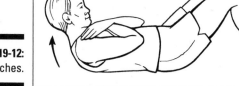

**Figure 19-12:**
Crunches.

1. Lie on your back with your arms crossed over your chest and both legs bent so that your shoes rest flat on the floor.

2. Slowly lift your upper body until your back is flat on the floor.

   Don't just lift your head or you'll exercise your neck instead of your abdomen. And don't strain to pull your upper body further up — just pull until your back is flat on the floor.

3. Relax and slowly lower yourself back to the floor.

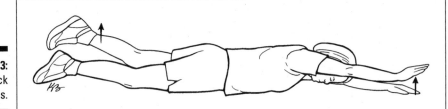

**Figure 19-13:** Back extensions.

1. Lie face down on the floor with both legs straight out behind you and both arms straight out over your head with your palms facing down.

2. Keeping your knees and elbows as straight as you can and your hips, tummy, and forehead flat on the floor, slowly lift your right arm and your left leg at the same time.

   Don't laugh. It's not as easy as you may think.

3. Switch sides and lift your left arm and right leg at the same time.

## Adding balance to your routine

To avoid falling and possibly breaking a bone, spend some time working on balance. You can challenge the muscles that keep you balanced in many fun ways, and you can tone your muscles at the same time. Talk to a personal trainer to find out more about the following exercise aids:

✔ **Fitness balls:** Sometimes called Swiss balls or exercise balls, fitness balls are becoming very popular because they help you strengthen the *core balancing muscles* (abdominal, back, and hip muscles) that you use in many everyday activities.

   If you're up for a challenge, sit on one of these balls and try to lift your feet; you can work up a sweat, exercise your abdominal muscles, and feel like a seal in a sideshow all at the same time. There are a million ways to use these balls to improve your balance, as well as your muscle tone.

✔ **Balance boards:** Stepping on this board feels like jumping on a moving surfboard after drinking three glasses of wine. Essentially, a ball is attached to the bottom of the board to challenge your balance (to say the least). As you strengthen your "balance" muscles with this contraption, you improve your overall sense of balance and your muscle tone.

✔ **Exercise tubing:** If your friends or family members see you with this one, they'll think that you're playing with a giant rubberband, so you may want to use this exercise aid in private. Exercise tubing is used in conjunction with stretching to increase flexibility.

All of these props can help you improve your balance, flexibility, and strength. They can be used at home or in a health club.

# Exercises to Protect Your Heart

A balanced fitness plan will keep you stay healthy after menopause. Aerobic exercises, which are the core of a good cardiovascular workout, increase your blood circulation, strengthen your heart muscles, and improve your cholesterol profile.

## Working on and working up to heart health

You can choose from any number of great aerobic sports or activities to improve your fitness. Cycling, jogging, swimming, and stair climbing are few examples. If you want to vary your workout, try an aerobic activity other than walking or check out the resources in Appendix B that have more information on beginning a fitness plan.

Exercise is the best gift you can give your cardiovascular system. Just 30 minutes of walking five or more times a week can effectively improve your cardiovascular health. All you need for walking is a comfortable pair of shoes and 30 minutes. If you need to break your workout up into two 15-minute sessions or three 10-minute sessions during the day, don't worry; it still works!

As you improve your cardiovascular fitness, you'll feel less tired when you workout even though you're doing the same amount of exercise. You'll also notice that your heart rate will gradually decrease, both during exercise and when at rest.

Build your endurance and stamina slowly. Don't over do it when you first begin an exercise program. Be sure to stay within your *target heart range* (see the "Zoning in on your target heart rate" sidebar earlier in this chapter). If you're a beginner, keep to the lower end of your target range until you establish a comfortable workout plan. You can lower your risk of heart problems associated with exercise if you monitor your heart rate. To get the most out of your aerobic exercise, exercise at your target heart rate for at least 20 minutes.

A simple way to check whether your workout intensity is appropriate is what we call the *walk-and-talk test*. If you're exerting yourself but you can still carry on a conversation while you exercise, you're probably exercising at the right pace.

If you want to continue to build your cardiovascular fitness, increase the intensity of your workout by increasing the

✔ Distance you run, walk, swim, or jog

✔ Speed at which you move

✔ Time you spend doing the activity

✔ Number of days you exercise

✔ Level of difficulty of your course. (If you're a walker or cyclist, find a hilly course; if you use a treadmill, increase the incline or spend some time on a stair-climbing machine.)

As you increase the intensity of your workout, your cardiovascular fitness will improve and you will burn more calories. But when you make your workout more challenging, do it slowly and take one step at a time. For example, you may choose to exercise at the same pace but add another ½ mile to your walk.

## Walking for fun and fitness

Walking is perhaps the easiest way to begin a fitness program. You don't need a bunch of equipment; all you need is the will to get moving. But before you put your feet to the pavement, you have to map out a route you'll follow on you daily trek. Here are some pointers:

✔ Measure out a 2-mile course that you can easily expand to a 3-mile course when you want to increase the length of your walk.

✔ Pick a pretty area in your neighborhood, around your workplace, or at a local park. Or maybe your neighborhood park or school has a track you can use (though circling a track can get monotonous).

✔ Make sure that your route is conveniently located. You don't want to give yourself the "it takes too long to get there" excuse.

For the first two weeks of your new walking regimen, walk the 2 miles three times a week and time yourself. Your pace should be brisk enough to get your heart pumping, but not so fast that you can't talk and breathe at the same time. A good pace for many folks is to walk 2 miles in about 35 minutes. During Weeks 3 and 4, you can step up your program a bit. Walk four times a week instead of three. And try to increase your pace — do your 2 miles in a half-hour.

At this point in your exercise progression, you need to check yourself and see how you feel. How easy was the transition from Weeks 1 and 2 to Weeks 3 and 4? Do you feel like you can do more or are you comfortable with your current routine? Depending on your age and your health, you may want to stick with this walking schedule for a while. When you feel your body getting stronger and your outlook is ready for another challenge, you can move along to the next level. (For the sake of simplicity, we use a weekly progression to outline this entire schedule. But remember that your Week 5 doesn't have to begin until you are ready for it.)

During the course of the next four weeks, your goal should be to walk 3 miles five times a week. Work up to this goal slowly. Add ½ mile to your distance during Week 5. At that point you're walking 2.5 miles four times during the week. Then, for Week 6, walk 2.5 miles again but try to walk five times this week instead of four times. Keep your pace brisk.

If you're ready to go on after Week 6, charge ahead and add another half mile to your distance and walk five times this week. By Weeks 7 and 8, you've reached your goal of walking 3 miles five times a week. But just because you've reached this goal doesn't mean you can't aim higher. The important thing is that you find your comfort level. Many people are fine with this workout level for the rest of their lives — it can boost your spirits and your health.

Want to take your program further? You've got the idea by now — simply add distance, go faster, or make the course harder (try gentle hills). If you miss a workout, don't beat yourself up about it — just start again the next day — good habits are hard to break!

It may take you three or four months to reach the goal of 3 miles five times a week — and that's fine. It's not a contest. You're doing this for yourself and your health. Your only opponent is inactivity.

# Chapter 20

# Enjoying a New Lease on Life

· · · · · · · · · · · · · · · · · · · · · · · · · · · · · · · · · · · · · · · · · · · · ·

## In This Chapter

▶ Staying on top of your health

▶ Interacting with everyone in your life

▶ Making decisions about work

▶ Finding your passion, honoring your spirit

▶ Getting the most out of your life

· · · · · · · · · · · · · · · · · · · · · · · · · · · · · · · · · · · · · · · · · · · · ·

*E*ventually, perimenopause turns into real menopause. One of these mornings you'll take a look at your calendar and realize that your last period was a full 12 months ago. It may occur to you that you haven't had a hot flash in ages, and that your moods are smooth and steady. Or you may already be beyond that magic 12-month marker.

Congratulations: You're post-menopausal! At 16 or 30 or 45 you might not have thought of this as a positive milestone. After all, women in their second half century are *old*. Dried up. Sexless. Crones. Past their sell-by date. Yeah, right. Tell that to Tina Turner. Lauren Bacall. Gloria Steinem. Astronaut Sally Ride. Billie Jean King. Television Journalist Diane Sawyer. Dolly Parton. In fact, try telling that to any number of your friends, relations, and co-workers who are active, healthy, lively women of — as they used to say — *a certain age.*

You've seen the joke cards and birthday cake inscriptions: "Life begins at 40." Many menopausal women will tell you that, for them, life began at *menopause.* In this chapter we talk about why, far from being the end of the line, lots of women find that reaching menopause marks the beginning of the best stage of life. We'll also talk more about the context of your whole life and all that goes into it, not just about specific health issues.

# Going from Menopause to Infinity

Sure, there are health issues to stay on top of after you reach menopause. Throughout this book we talk about the fact that changes in your body's production of hormones are linked to an increase in your risk for a number of potential health problems, including

- Cardiovascular disease (look back to Chapters 6, 12, and 16 for more on heart disease)
- Osteoporosis (bone up in Chapters 5, 15, and 16)
- Hypertension (more in Chapters 5 and 16)
- Weight gain (check Chapter 18 for the skinny on diet and weight)
- Memory loss (wait, wait — oh, yeah, remember to look in Chapters 10 and 15)

But you can take advantage of a couple of ways to make this part of life just as enjoyable, or even more so, than it always has been:

- **Make healthy lifestyle choices.** The best lifestyle choices can help to minimize health risks. Sticking to a healthy diet and a regular exercise plan that you love enough to make it a part of your life can go a long way toward keeping you young — at heart and everywhere else (see Chapters 18 and 19).

- **See your healthcare provider regularly.** It's important to have a doctor who views this stage of your life as being promising and full of potential. When you were a young girl and got your first period, you may have felt like this was a good time to see a new doctor (maybe a specialist in adolescent medicine, and maybe a woman, if you had been seeing a man up to this point).

In many ways, this time of life is a lot like that one. Menopause is just as much a marker as adolescence was that you've reached a new stage in your development. If you're happy with your healthcare situation, consider yourself fortunate and stay with the providers you're seeing now. If you're not, though, this is a good time to shop around for a doctor's or physician's associate with whom you feel more simpatico. It seems ironic to quote the tagline from a cigarette ad campaign when we're talking about good health, but here goes. You've come a long way, baby. Make sure your health advisors aren't stuck back in the 1960s in the way they view women at midlife and beyond.

Here are some tips when searching for a new doctor:

- Look for a healthcare provider who sees you as a whole person, not just a medical history or a bearer of symptoms.

- Help your doctor to avoid stereotypes about aging.

- Look for a doctor who advises you to be as active as possible (then follow the advice).

- Listen to the way your doctor talks about you and your health. Is he or she concerned not just with helping you to stay free of disease, but with your overall wellness and happiness?

# Working and Playing Well with Others

Menopause and the changes in your life at this time can affect the people around you in various ways. This is certainly true of your husband or partner (who, don't forget, is also aging). It's true of your children, your friends, your boss, your co-workers, and everyone else.

## Managing a family

Menopause can be a funny time for women with families, especially if you still have children at home. You may have spent the past few years wondering whether your periods would stop before your daughter's began. Or wondering whether you could have just one more baby. Or living in *fear* of having one more baby. Whether this makes your life easier or harder, menopause cuts off some of your choices in this regard. Unless you plan to adopt, or fate fixes you up with a partner who comes with ready-made kids, you aren't going to have more children.

Of course, you may have children still at home. This can be a wonderful time with your children. You may have more patience than ever and more of a sense of perspective on life's ups and downs. Reaching midlife also seems to make the clock and the calendar pages turn faster. Suddenly the years of parenthood seem foreshortened — the years of childhood slip away faster, and your kids reach new life stages of their own, even as you have. Watching them make this transition brings a host of competing feelings: delight for them, worry, envy at their chance to explore new activities and roles, sorrow at their impending absence, pride at the job you've done raising them, or just plain relief.

The other side of this coin is that watching your children grow up may bring you a sense of sadness that these young years have passed for you. Some women find this especially true of watching their adolescent daughters reach their sexual maturity. Envy of youth isn't pretty, but it happens to all of us to one degree or another. Try not to beat yourself up about it.

## Looking back, looking forward

Progress doesn't always proceed in a straight line. Sometimes it's two steps forward, four steps backward, and a couple of baby steps forward again. The first medical text on menopause, published in 1837, offered women reassurance that what they were going through was perfectly normal, that menopause was not a disease, and didn't have to be a big deal to get through: menopause was described as "a temporary inconvenience" was how the enlightened (male) author described the change of life.

Now try this one on. Almost 100 years after this enlightened (male!) author spoke so sensibly of menopause, medical journals took a giant step backward, and began using phrases such as "sheer misery," "hatred between husband and wife," and "cow-like passivity and disinterest" when describing menopause and what couples and women could expect from these years.

Do yourself and other women a favor, and refuse to be part of the stereotype, or to put yourself in the care of any healthcare providers who foster this kind of attitude.

## *You and your partner*

When you married or started living together, or when your children were born, the dynamic between you and your husband or partner probably changed dramatically. Instead of going through life face-to-face, concerned mostly with each other, parenthood repositioned you. Your chief (shared) responsibility became your child or children. You began to travel through life side-by-side, facing outward to take care of children, jobs, a home, and all the responsibilities of adult life.

When the last child moves out, the dynamic will change again. By now you both probably have too much going on to re-create those intense, face-to-face, me-and-you-against-the-world days, and you might not want to anyway. In addition to shared interests outside of the home, the members of most couples also have interests of their own.

More than a million older women are abused in a relationship every year. Few shelters have specific programs for older women, but your need for safety and security is the same as everyone else's. If you need help, call the national domestic violence hotline at any time of day or night: 1-800-799-SAFE (7233).

There are no rules for how a couple should behave at this stage of life together. Many find that this is a time of renewed togetherness and discovery of the changed and developed people you both are. Sadly, others find that the mutual changes in your respective goals, values, and outlook have led to irreconcilable incompatibilities. We can't tell you what to expect, except to advise that change is almost inevitable during this part of your lives together.

This can be scary as you search for new footing together. This period can also be exciting and wonderful, but it almost always takes some hard work, dedication, and commitment. Find what works for the two of you.

If you find that, for either or both of you, this period is simply agonizing, seek help from a professional counselor. You might benefit from couples' (or individual) counseling if:

✔ One or both of you feels angry and resentful.

✔ One or both of you feels bored and stuck in a rut.

✔ There are unresolved issues over an infidelity.

✔ The relationship is physically or emotionally abusive.

If either or both of you are concerned, don't wait until counseling becomes a last resort, and don't assume that the need for counseling means the relationship is over. Think of it instead as an opportunity for course correction and renewal. Neither of you is the person you were when you got together, so it's unrealistic to expect the relationship to be the same. It's perfectly reasonable, though, to expect that it can be something new, and something better.

## *Caring for aging parents*

You're a part of the "sandwich generation." As our parents live longer and many of our children stay home longer or return to the nest after leaving, we're in the middle, taking care of members of both a younger and an older generation. Even as you may be offering loving and supportive good-byes to all the baby birds in your nest and looking forward to having some more room and time and resources for yourself, or yourself and your partner, new nest-mates may come to roost in your home.

---

### Sandwiched in between

If you're taking care of both your kids and one or more of your parents, you're not alone:

✔ Close to half of all Americans between 45 and 55 have dependent children and living parents.

✔ The American Association of Retired People (AARP) says that 22 million Americans take responsibility for caring for aging parents or other relatives.

✔ Most of these caregivers are women (bet you're not surprised).

✔ Most women caring for older parents are also still employed either full- or part-time.

If you're one of these people, we know that *you* know that bearing this much responsibility — for one or more children, a spouse or partner, one or both parents, a job, a house, and other responsibilities in the community may become so great that just having a guest for dinner or having to feed the cat when your kids forgot to do it can put you right over the top. This kind of stress can get so bad that your health may begin to suffer.

Be kind to yourself. Take steps to get some help:

- ✔ Enlist the assistance of siblings and other family members (including those kids).
- ✔ Call on professional help. Ask your or your parents' physicians for local resources, or call your state's office on aging (look in the blue pages in your phone book).
- ✔ Get some exercise nearly every day, and try to eat right.
- ✔ Get a little respite by spending time with friends or engaging in hobbies.
- ✔ Investigate adult daycare centers in your area. Even the occasional use of centers or respite caregivers can give both you and your parents a break.
- ✔ Ask your employer if your company's Employee Assistance program has resources for adult caregivers.

# Retiring Gracefully (or Not)

Being menopausal at home is one thing. For many women, dealing with menopausal symptoms at work can be altogether different. In the United States, women make up roughly half of all the workers in the paid labor force. Most of these women plan to continue working up until they reach retirement age. This makes it likely that you'll go through menopause while you're still working.

## Taking care of your body on the job

When it comes to workplace issues, some nations are a few steps ahead of others. In the United Kingdom and Australia, for instance, meeting the workplace needs of menopausal women is actually an issue that's being discussed and worked on.

If you're pregnant, laws in the United States and other countries protect your job. You can't, for instance, be fired for being pregnant. And if your pregnant body aches when you stand up all day, the law says they have to give you a chair — or change your duties, or protect you from potential workplace hazards. We think it would be nice if employment law made basic, compassionate allowances for things such as:

- Making sure perimenopausal women with unpredictable, Niagara-style periods have access to decent, private bathrooms, and permission to use them whenever they need to. Ever try teaching a classroom full of 4th graders all morning without being given 10 minutes to change a tampon?

- Ensuring that a little fresh air actually enters the workplace of women whose internal thermostats are likely to set themselves, without warning, to thermonuclear. Nobody loves a workplace princess who hijacks the air conditioning, but is it too much to ask that the powers-that-be let you cool off for a few minutes to keep you from passing out?

- Advice, support, and informed personnel in the company health office.

- Time off for medical appointments.

- While we're at it, how about fewer menopause jokes from the guys in the boardroom about hot flashes, and more offers of support?

If you're dealing with menopausal symptoms on the job, try these tips:

- Plagued by hot flashes? Keep cool water or iced tea in the office fridge.

- Dress in layers — say, a cardigan or jacket over a shell — so you can remove one or two without your co-workers think you're initiating a game of strip poker.

- Exhausted after a night of insomnia? In the best of all possible worlds, call in and say you'll be working from home today. Don't work in the best of all possible worlds? Perk yourself up with a brisk walk on your lunch break.

## Looking before you leap

How does the notion of changing jobs ("At *your* age?") make you feel? Terrified? Amused? Excited and wistful? If you fall into the latter group, it may be just the right time to think of making the leap to something new. Many women find that, after they've weathered the emotional and bodily changes that come with menopause, they feel braver and more able to take on lifestyle changes. The hard truth of knowing that probably a little less than half of your lifespan lies ahead of you may make you view your time as something that's more precious than ever. This can make you less patient with a job that makes you unhappy.

Don't let anyone hand you any baloney about old dogs and new tricks. Before you hand in your two-week notice, however, ask yourself some important questions:

- ✔ What skills do you have to bring to a new job? What kind of work environment do you enjoy? If you can envision your dream job, what does it look like?

- ✔ Do you want a new job because you want a new job, or because you think it will fix other problems in your life?

- ✔ What kind of work environment makes you happy? How busy do you like to be? Do you enjoy having people around, or do you like to work by yourself?

- ✔ How long can you afford to be unemployed while you look for or create another job for yourself?

- ✔ How will changing jobs affect your health insurance?

# Finding Your Spirit in Whatever You Do

So you've come out — or will soon come out — on the other side of menopause. Gone are the periods (which, we admit, may be a source of regret for some). Gone are the hot flashes. Gone are the "menopause moments" — those brief episodes of frustrating and embarrassing forgetfulness. In exchange, you get back your sense of emotional well being, your equanimity, and your even temper.

## Appreciating the upside

Many women find that getting through menopause brings them unexpected physical, psychological, and emotional gifts:

- ✔ **Freedom from worrying about an unwanted pregnancy:** This can contribute to a freer, richer, more spontaneous sex life, as well as to a sense of closure with respect to your reproductive years.

- ✔ **A larger sense of freedom:** We don't just mean freedom from worrying about whether there's a maxipad in your purse or a tampon in your pocket. We mean a broader sense of freedom from worry about whether you can take care of yourself and your life, and from worry about what others will think of you if you speak your mind or do what you want to do.

✔ **More energy:** Lots of women talk about not just needing less sleep after menopause, but of having a greater sense of energy, power, and possibility.

✔ **Less concern with living according to the expectations of others:** In this way, as in others, menopause mirrors adolescence, giving you a sense of play and exploration, an open space in which to reinvent yourself.

✔ **Less tolerance for putting up with things that annoy you or waste your time, and less tolerance for people who don't treat you well:** Because (we hope) this is coupled with a diminished likelihood to let anger take center stage in your emotional life, you probably won't need to blow anyone out of the water with your displeasure. At the same time, you may feel completely comfortable asking an intimidating maître d' for a better table, explaining sweetly to your insurance company why they're in the wrong to reject one of your claims, or turning down a lunch date with someone who makes you feel inferior.

✔ **A reassessment of what's important in your life.** Maybe vacuuming the living room can wait while you take the dogs for a walk or write in your journal. Perhaps this is the year to turn the chairmanship of the community center bazaar over to someone else so you have time to paint every morning. Maybe you need to get away by yourself for a weekend once in a while, just to walk in the woods or meditate or go a whole day without talking. Or maybe you and your sweet baboo will finally quit putting off that trip to Paris.

## Seeing things in a new light

Midlife and the onset of your post-menopausal years are busy and sometimes hectic. Still, we find that this is a good place to stop and rest for a moment. You may find yourself wanting to take stock at this point and ask yourself some of the big questions:

✔ Am I happy?

✔ Am I achieving what I want to be achieving?

✔ Am I making a positive difference in the lives of the people I love?

✔ What do I want to do with the rest of my life?

## Facing the Silver Screen

At the video store, do you ever have the urge to ask the clerk to direct you to the section of films starring people who were alive during the Eisenhower administration? Pop some popcorn and invite a few friends over for your very own Menopause Madness Film Festival.

✔ **The African Queen:** Katherine Hepburn steers a steamboat down the rapids, wins the battle for the Allies, finds true love with a reprobate steam boat captain, and never loses her handkerchief — or her cool.

✔ **Bread and Tulips:** When bored, neglected wife and mother Rosalba is accidentally left behind by her son and her philandering husband at a vacation rest stop, she takes control of her own life, with charming results. Get the Italian original.

✔ **Calendar Girls:** Helen Mirren and the members of the Rylstone Women's Institute of North Yorkshire reveal themselves to be innovative fundraisers.

✔ **Fried Green Tomatoes:** We love watching Kathy Bates's repressed Evelyn Crouch as she transforms herself.

✔ **The Grass Harp:** From a story by Truman Capote. The critics thought this was a coming-of-age story about a young man in the south. *We* think the real coming-of-age story revolves around the young man's timid aunt, Dolly (Piper Laurie), who finally learns to stand up for what she believes.

✔ **Mrs. Henderson Presents:** Who doesn't want to grow up to be Dame Judi Dench?

✔ **Prime Suspect:** Helen Mirren again (what can we say?), starring this time as Detective Chief Inspector Jane Tennison in the gritty British television crime drama series.

✔ **Shirley Valentine:** Pauline Collins finally gets the vacation she's always wanted — and more.

✔ **Something's Gotta Give:** Let's see . . . Jack Nicholson or Keanu Reeves? Who says older women don't have choices?

Some women, at this stage in their lives, report feeling a sense of spirituality and connectedness with others that they had never experienced before. You may have had to deal with the deaths of one or more relatives or friends. You may even be coping with the death of a spouse or lover. Many women at this age have faced health scares of their own. In short, while old age is still pretty far up the road, having to deal with issues of mortality may change the way you look at life. Sadness is normal in the face of unavoidable crises of this sort, but so is a bittersweet new sense of perspective on life from beginning to end.

If you find yourself really unable to move on after the death or illness of a loved one, or a health crisis of your own, seek counseling.

It's quite possible, though, that becoming intimately aware of the transient nature of life will just make every moment of it more precious. Take care of your life and the lives of those around you. Live every moment as if it is important — it is.

# Living Happily Ever After

Your experience of menopause — and of the many years ahead — will be shaped by lots of different things:

- ✔ Your health
- ✔ Your expectations for this time and the expectations of those around you
- ✔ The way the other women in your family view menopause and midlife
- ✔ The opportunities available to you in your work and your life

When you were a child, people would ask you what you wanted to be when you grew up. Throughout your life you've had to make decisions that have helped to shape the answer to this question. A handful of choices you've made along the way — about education, romance, employment, where to live — have gotten you where you are today. We hope that's a good place.

Menopause can be viewed in lots of ways: as a journey, a milestone, a process, a path. We especially like to think of it as a ride that takes you places you've never been before and opens new and unexpected doors in your life. Most of all, we like to think we've helped you not only to survive this little milestone in your life but to relax and enjoy the ride.

Now it's your turn to help the women in your life who are just starting down the perimenopausal path. Encourage them to stay informed, to take charge of their own health, and their own lives, and to expect the best (or at least to *not* expect the worst) of these years.

Finally, we wish you the best of health and all the happiness in the world. Most of all, we hope you never stop asking, "Where do I go from here?"

# Part V
# The Part of Tens

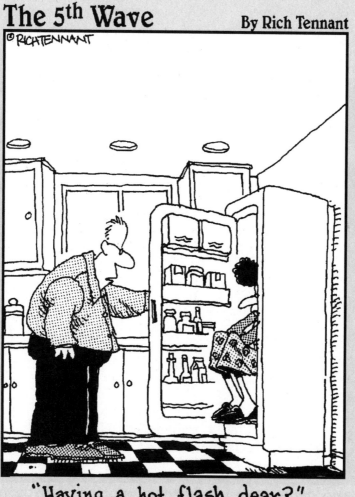

The 5th Wave          By Rich Tennant

"Having a hot flash, dear?"

## In this part . . .

This just wouldn't be a *For Dummies* book without a yellow and black cover and a Part of Tens. We like to think of the Part of Tens as the icing on the cake — better yet, the fat-free whipped topping on the bowl of fruit. If you like top-ten lists, you've come to the right part of the book. In this part, we expose myths about menopause, and give you the scoop on medical tests that you may run into. We also outline some great ideas and programs that you can use to kick-start or jazz up your exercise routine, and we tempt you with some fabulous foods that prove that healthy eating doesn't have to be boring.

# Chapter 21

# Ten Menopause Myths Exposed

*O*ne survey we recently came across shows that half of all women going through menopause feel unprepared and uninformed to face the change. Check out these common menopause myths and see how many of them you've heard — and how many you bought into! Because menopause and misconceptions go hand and hand so often, we couldn't limit ourselves to ten myths in this Part of Tens chapter.

## You're Too Young to Be Menopausal in Your 30s and 40s

*Not really.* Even though most women begin menopause sometime between 45 and 55 years of age (and the average age is 51), going through menopause earlier isn't impossible or unheard of. Making the situation seem even less cut and dry are those annoying symptoms, such as hot flashes, crying jags, mood swings, and interrupted sleep, that usually occur years before you actually quit having periods (official menopause). Those physical changes that characterize what most people refer to as the change are really more characteristic of *perimenopause* (the period of fluctuating hormone levels leading up to menopause). You can experience perimenopausal symptoms for a decade before the onset of menopause. So having hot flashes and fertility issues pop up when you're in your late 30s and early 40s is perfectly normal.

But keep your gynecologist informed about your periods because skipping periods during your late 30s or early 40s can also indicate medical problems. For some women, certain conditions and medical treatments cause the early onset of menopause, for example:

- Chemotherapy or radiation treatment may cause your ovaries to shut down early, depending on the type of treatments used.

- If you have both of your ovaries removed, you immediately experience *surgical menopause*. The ovaries, once responsible for producing the active form of estrogen that serves many bodily functions, are gone, and menopause begins.

- *Prolonged anorexia* can cause you to stop menstruating. If the problem isn't addressed in time, anorexia can lead to early — and irreversible — menopause.

- *Autoimmune disorders* (diseases of your immune system) and thyroid problems can result in *premature menopause*. (Chapter 3 can tell you more about menopause before age 40.)

If you go through menopause earlier than most women, you may also increase your risk of developing menopause-related medical conditions, such as osteoporosis and cardiovascular disease, earlier. So talk to your doctor about ways you can prevent these conditions.

# Menopause Is a Medical Condition That Must Be Treated with Medicine

*Not exactly.* Remember puberty? Well menopause is puberty in reverse, with all the accompanying physical and emotional changes. (Sounds like a lot of fun when we put it that way, huh?) Menopause is not a medical condition in that it is not a disorder. It's a natural passage from your reproductive years to the rest of your life.

Menopause isn't a condition that requires medical attention any more than puberty requires medical attention. (The same degree of patience, however — along with a good dose of humor — is required.) The changes that take place are normal and natural. The care given to women on their journey through menopause is meant to alleviate discomfort and prevent disease rather than to interfere with the natural process. Many women don't experience any symptoms at all — they have no discomfort associated with the change, so there's nothing to treat. Other women find that herbs or a healthy lifestyle are effective in relieving symptoms. (We discuss the herbal route in Chapter 17, and Chapters 18 and 19 provide some great information on diet, nutrition, and exercise.) As it turns out, eating healthy and staying fit go a long way toward keeping your body and mind healthy without the estrogen they used to rely on.

Sometimes you need an extra biological boost, which can come in the forms of food supplements (calcium, for example) and hormone replacement therapy (HRT).

Because lower levels of estrogen over prolonged periods of time can result in other medical problems, work with your doctor to weigh up the risks and benefits, consider your own concerns and health history, and find therapies that are appropriate for you.

Keep in mind that it's tempting to attribute all symptoms during your perimenopausal and menopausal years to menopause. During this time you're still as susceptible to the same illnesses and diseases as anyone else, so don't be shy about bringing troublesome symptoms to the attention of your doctor.

# Menopause Isn't a Disease, So There's No Need to See a Doctor

*Think again.* Menopause isn't a medical condition, but that fact doesn't mean you can ignore it. Your doctor should be aware of any new symptoms you experience or new medical issues that arise as you enter perimenopause and menopause.

Night sweats, fuzzy thinking, interrupted sleep, hot flashes, mood swings, fatigue, and irritability are recognized (and annoying) symptoms of perimenopause. But these symptoms can also signal more serious medical problems such as anemia, Epstein-Barr virus, thyroid problems, and other issues. You want to rule out the more serious medical issues before you assume that you're experiencing perimenopause symptoms. So keep track of your symptoms: Write down when, how often, and for how long you experience them, and then share this information with your gynecologist or primary-care physician.

You may think that the main purpose of a visit to your doctor is to *assess* your current health and *fix* the related problems. But as you reach the point in your life at which most women enter perimenopause and menopause, your doctor will spend a greater amount of time trying to *prevent* the development of serious conditions including breast cancer, cervical cancer, hypertension, cardiovascular disease, high blood-cholesterol levels, and more.

# You Lose the Urge to Have Sex after the Change

*Hardly.* Nearly half of menopausal women are satisfied with their sex life. If you do your own poll of your premenopausal friends (or tune into a daytime talk show), you'll probably find that the percentages are pretty comparable. Some women actually find sex more enjoyable and feel sexier than ever. You don't have to worry about getting pregnant, you and your partner have some experience under your belts (so you know how to enjoy yourselves and your relationship), and you and your special someone may have more time to spend together.

That said, some women find intercourse to be painful because of vaginal dryness or vaginal atrophy. If this is a problem for you, you can find some great remedies at the pharmacy or the grocery store. Vaginal moisturizers and vaginal estrogen pills or creams can be used regularly to treat vaginal dryness. Lubricants can be used during foreplay to eliminate painful intercourse.

Sexual stimulation begets sexual lubrication. In other words, the more you use it, the slower you lose it. Don't forget that masturbation can help you stay in shape, too — orgasms are good for you, no matter how you have them. In fact, that famous sex doctor, Alfred Kinsey, found that even though marital intercourse declined as women got older, solitary sexual activity didn't decline until women were well past 60. Another study found that even though women's overall lubrication and sexual activity declined *slightly* after menopause, the frequency and pleasure of orgasm did not. For more about the change and your sex life (and making changes to your sex life), check out Chapter 9.

# Irregular Vaginal Bleeding Always Means Cancer

*Not exactly.* Almost all perimenopausal women experience irregular menstrual cycles. In some months, you go 25 days between cycles; in others, you go 38 days. Some months are heavy, and others are light. Or you may even skip a month or two. These menstrual irregularities are generally caused by fluctuating hormones that get out of balance during perimenopause.

If you go through a super-absorbent pad or tampon every couple of hours, experience bleeding after intercourse, or experience bleeding more often than every three weeks, see your gynecologist to find out what's happening. Sometimes this type of irregular bleeding can signal more serious problems. Also, if you're bleeding between your menses or you bleed after you've gone even six months without a period; please consult your gynecologist right away.

# Humps Accompany Old Age — End of Story

*No way.* Women don't automatically turn into camels as they age. Vertebrae only collapse and result in spinal humps in some cases of *osteoporosis* (brittle bone disease).

If you don't want to acquire a hump, though, you need to begin strengthening your bones early in life by getting lots of calcium in your diet and exercise in your day. Osteoporosis is largely treatable with medicine and can often be prevented with the help of good nutrition, exercise, and calcium substitutes.

If your bones are in bad shape as you approach menopause, several drugs that can slow bone deterioration are on the market. The estrogen in hormone therapy is also very effective at slowing the rate of bone loss. A non-pharmaceutical approach to avoiding a hump is to add some regular strength-building exercises to your week.

# Only HRT Can Relieve the Symptoms

*False.* Although hormone replacement therapy is a very effective way to eliminate many annoying menopausal symptoms, it's not the only way. But before we get to the matter at hand, we want to remind you that less than half of all women experience the symptoms we so often associate with menopause (or perimenopause). So you may get lucky and avoid these symptoms without any type of intervention. Also, remember that the symptoms, such as hot flashes, interrupted sleep, fuzzy thinking, mental lapses, and so on, are temporary and may eventually go away in their own time.

Now, if these symptoms are making your life miserable, you can try a number of different remedies. Start out by adopting a healthier lifestyle. Here are a few quick ideas (for more info, check out Chapters 18 and 19):

- Cut down on fats and junk foods.
- Eat only moderate amounts of meat and protein.
- Fill your plate with vegetables and fruits.
- Keep an eye on your alcohol intake. (Don't drink more than three to five alcoholic drinks a week.)
- Exercise at least three to five days a week for a half-hour each day.

You may also want to try an herbal remedy (such as black cohosh) or include some soy in your diet. Edamame (a type of large-seed soybean) and tofu are excellent sources of soy. (For more information on alternative ways to deal with the change, turn to Chapter 17.)

# Women Don't Need to Worry about Heart Attacks

*Wrong.* Heart disease kills many more women each year than cancer does. In fact, the odds are that one out of two women will die of a heart attack or stroke. Estrogen seems to provide some protection to your cardiovascular system, so women generally have a lower risk of heart attack than men. After menopause, when you no longer produce estrogen, your risk of heart attack and stroke rises. A healthy diet and regular exercise can help lower your risk of cardiovascular disease.

# Most Women Get Really Depressed During Menopause

*False.* Actually, women tend to get more depressed during the "procreation" years than during menopause. However, your emotions can take a tumble during perimenopause. Irritability, mood swings, and interrupted sleep can take a toll on your emotions. (For more information on the mental and emotional issues tied to menopause, peruse Chapter 10.) But you can find ways to alleviate these symptoms. A healthy diet and a regular exercise program help many women alleviate symptoms. Also a slew of pharmaceutical and herbal therapies can help resolve mental and emotional symptoms. (Take a look at Chapter 16.)

If you fought bouts of depression earlier in life, you may see a return of the symptoms during perimenopause, but remember that perimenopausal symptoms are transient and will go away in time. If you experience symptoms or signs of depression, talk to your doctor.

# You'll Break a Bone If You Exercise Too Hard

*Nope. Weight-bearing exercise* (exercise that puts stress on your bones) is one of the best ways to help your body build bone. If you have osteoporosis or your bone density is getting low, the combination of weight-bearing exercise and calcium supplements (with vitamins D and K and magnesium) will prevent further bone loss.

If you've been living a sedentary lifestyle with little or no regular exercise (or you want to change your exercise regimen), discuss your exercise plan with a physician before you begin moving that body. Combining exercises that help your flexibility and balance with a walking program is a good way to get started. Flexibility and balance exercises can help you avoid falling and fractures. After you have that body moving, try adding some weight-bearing exercises to the routine. (Check out Chapter 19 for some terrific suggestions.)

# A Blood Test Can Determine Whether You're Going Through Menopause

*Well, here's the deal:* Many gynecologists will test your levels of *follicle stimulating hormone (FSH)* to determine whether you're going through menopause. FSH is the hormone that tells the ovaries to get a follicle ready — this message kicks off your menstrual cycle. As your ovaries slow down, your brain tries to keep things moving at the regular pace, so it shoots out lots of FSH. Also, your brain doesn't see much estrogen coming back that says, "Alright already, the follicles are on their way," so FSH keeps on coming. Consistently high levels of FSH indicate the onset of menopause to the medical community.

But here's the catch: FSH levels will tell you when your ovaries are pretty close to shutting down follicle production, but they won't tell you if your hormones are in the wild state of fluctuation typical of the perimenopausal years. Unfortunately, most women are most interested in finding out what's going on with their bodies when they just start experiencing weird things such as hot flashes, mood swings, and heart palpitations. By the time their FSH levels remain high, they've already figured the puzzle out — periods have pretty much stopped and the test just confirms the logical deduction that menopause is indeed near.

# Chapter 22

# Ten Medical Tests for Menopausal Women

*T*his chapter lists some basic health tests that help doctors identify diseases and other problems in their early stages — when they're more treatable. (We must confess that we include more than ten tests in this chapter, which kind of goes against the letter, but not the spirit, of the Part of Tens law.) *Early detection* is the key to successful treatment of nearly every disease that affects menopausal women. Avoiding the tests doesn't mean that you can avoid the related diseases, so visit your doctors regularly and follow through with their recommendations.

## Pelvic Exam and Pap Smear

No one likes to put their feet in the stirrups and their privates in the saddle every year, but doing so sure helps you avoid some nasty problems down the line. You should have an annual gynecological exam. The gynecologist will check your female organs including your breasts, your vaginal tissue, your cervix, and your uterus. Your gynecologist will also perform a *Pap smear* to test for cervical cancer every year.

If you've had a complete hysterectomy for benign reasons, you should have a pelvic exam and Pap smear (to check for noncancerous medical issues) every year for three years, and then, the Pap can be done every three years. However, you still need a breast and pelvic exam every year.

# Rectal Exam

Everyone squirms when this exam is the subject at hand. Everybody hates it, but the risks of postponing a rectal exam can be quite devastating to you and your loved ones. Regular rectal exams can help detect problems early — when they can be easily and painlessly treated. Part of this test is a *digital exam* in which the doctor checks your organs for signs of disease. The doctor inserts a gloved finger into your rectum to evaluate the health of your tissues. Keep in mind that the long-term benefits greatly outweigh the short-term unpleasantness of the procedure. And also remember that your doctor *chose* this field of medicine.

The other part of this exam is a *fecal occult test,* which enables doctors to check whether you have blood in your stool. This part of the test is necessary because the presence of blood can be an indication of problems, such as cancer, in your colon.

You should have a rectal exam once a year during your annual gynecological physical, especially after age 50.

# Colonoscopy

Colon cancer is a form of cancer that progresses very slowly and is readily treatable. But it's the third leading cause of cancer deaths among American women. No one likes the test — it's that simple. And women avoid discussing the issue until they have symptoms. The problem is that patients very often don't experience any symptoms until the disease is in an advanced stage — a point when successful treatment is much more difficult.

While performing a colonoscopy, your doctor can find and remove precancerous polyps (doctors know them as *adenomatous polyps*) before they have a chance of becoming cancerous. The night before your colonoscopy, you drink a potion that helps clean out your colon. While you're under the influence of a light sedative, the doctor inserts a flexible scope into your colon that allows her to view the colon walls in search of polyps or other unhealthy tissue. If she finds a polyp, she can remove it and send it to the lab for analysis. Lab analysis determines if the polyp is benign or precancerous.

Want to cut your risk of colon cancer by one-third? All you have to do is regularly schedule (and go through with) a colonoscopy. If you're over 50, have a colonoscopy every five years — more often if you have polyps, or if you have a family history of either colon cancer or polyps.

# Bone-Density Screening

If you have strong risk factors for osteoporosis (such as a history of anorexia or many family members who have had bone density problems), your doctor may recommend that you get a baseline bone-density screening at around 40. The results provide your doctors with something to compare future screenings to. If you show signs of bone loss in this or subsequent tests, you'll have bone screenings every two years.

If you've never had a bone screening, you're over 40, and you have no specific factors that put you at especially high risk, talk to your doctor about whether you need a bone screening, and if so, when.

# Mammogram

Early detection is the key to reducing your risk of breast cancer, so you should begin getting annual mammograms when you're 40 years old with a baseline taken at age 35. If your mother or sister has had breast cancer, get your first mammogram even earlier, when you're 30.

The American Cancer Society recommends that you get a mammogram every one to two years after age 40 and every year after you turn 50. Other groups advise less frequent mammograms. In our opinion, annual mammograms are your best bet even if scientists are still debating the merits of a yearly regimen.

# Cholesterol Screening

A cholesterol screening checks your total cholesterol, *LDL cholesterol* (bad cholesterol), *HDL cholesterol* (good cholesterol), and *triglycerides* (another form of fat found in your blood) and computes your cholesterol ratio. Take this simple blood test every five years. You should take it when you're fasting — nothing to eat or drink for 12 hours before the test. If your doctor identifies problems with your cholesterol or triglyceride levels or you have a history of high blood pressure, diabetes, thyroid problems, or obesity, your doctor may want to screen you more frequently.

If you have diabetes, make sure you have a complete cholesterol screening every year.

# Fasting Blood-Glucose Test

Adult-onset diabetes can lead to coronary heart disease, so you want to diagnose this problem early. Begin having your blood sugar (*glucose*) tested when you're 20 and repeat the test every three to five years — more frequently if you experience problems. The blood-glucose test is a simple blood test administered after you've had nothing to eat or drink for 12 hours (that's where the *fasting* part of the name comes from). You can also screen for diabetes by checking for sugar in your urine.

# Thyroid Screening

The symptoms of thyroid problems and the symptoms of menopause can be quite similar. Get your first thyroid screening at age 35. The screening measures your levels of thyroid-stimulating hormone (THS) and thyroid antibodies.

# Ovarian Hormone Screening

Out of necessity, the standard practice for prescribing hormone therapy is a method of trial and error — a "try this regimen and let me know how you feel" kind of approach. Everybody processes hormones differently, so the amount of hormone in a medication isn't the amount that reaches your bloodstream. For example, the same form of estrogen may affect two women differently. And your body may respond better to some estrogens than others.

The key to what "works" and what doesn't is the amount of *estradiol* (the active form of estrogen) your body produces in response to the estrogen you're taking. The only accurate way to know how much estradiol you're churning out is to draw blood and analyze it for hormone levels. (Saliva tests are available, but they're less accurate.)

That said, the majority of doctors stick with the standard dosing formulas and do the trial-and-error thing until you tell them you're feeling better. You do have the option of having a hormone screening to find out whether you're in menopause, or how far along you are on the road toward it, but not many doctors recommend it. Estradiol levels below 90 pg/ml result in the typical hot flashes, interrupted sleep, mood swings, and other annoying perimenopausal symptoms. If your estradiol level is closer to 20 or 30 pg/ml, you are almost certainly in menopause.

That said, ovarian hormone screening is far from perfect. For starters, estrogen levels fluctuate quite a bit during your cycle. Secondly, if you're perimenopausal, your cycles are not as reliable as they used to be, so it's hard to tell exactly where you are at any given time. The symptoms you're experiencing are likely to tell you as much — you're perimenopausal — as a blood test will.

# Stress Test

You may think that your life has been one big stress test, but actually, a stress test is a legitimate medical procedure. A stress test is basically an electrocardiogram (EKG) that a technician performs while you walk on a treadmill. You may have had an EKG in the past to qualify for life insurance or as part of an annual exam. The purpose of the test is to see how your heart responds to the stress of exercise. If you're overweight, have high blood pressure, or experience chest pain or shortness of breath with mild exertion, your doctor may suggest a stress test. Your doctor may also perform a stress test to check out your heart before you begin a new exercise program.

The procedure is simple. A technician sticks some electrical wires on your chest to record the electrical activity in your heart. This information tells the doctor if your heart is getting enough oxygen or if it's been damaged. To stress your heart, you walk on a special treadmill while you're plugged into the EKG.

## Chapter 23

# Ten Terrific Fitness Programs for Menopausal Women

*In This Chapter*
▶ Walking your way to better health
▶ Swimming for shore
▶ Developing a hankering for yoga

**N**eed help getting your fitness program off the ground? In this chapter, we provide some great suggestions to help you clear the runway.

Many women dread the thought of a workout, because to them, the concept implies sweat, finding time that they don't have, and too much effort. If this description fits you, think again. You can find a workout that fits your schedule and your desired level of energy output. (If you hate to sweat, check out the water-based workouts we include in this chapter.)

Be sure to warm up and cool down for five to ten minutes before and after you workout. If you have trouble with your heart, blood pressure, cholesterol, or diabetes; if you suffer from a respiratory condition; if you're overweight; if you smoke; or if you've been a couch potato for more years than you can remember, discuss your physical-fitness plans with your doctor before getting started. And think of your weekly fitness routine as a buffet. Include a little of everything on your plate — aerobic training, strength training, and flexibility and balance-building exercises.

## Core Strength Training

Core-stability training and weight training are great ways to improve your balance and flexibility, reduce your risk of injury, and lessen your amount of soreness associated with performing daily activities. Core stability training is basically strength training that targets the muscle groups that make up the core of your body — the abdominal, lower-back, hip, and pelvic muscles are the primary focus. Strengthening your core muscles allows them to do their job (maintaining your body's stability and balance) better. Adding weight training to your workout maintains strength, raises your metabolism, and is great for your bones. (For more on safely working with weights, check out *Weight Training For Dummies,* by Liz Neporent, Suzanne Schlosberg, and Shirley Archer, and *Ten Minute Tone-Ups For Dummies,* by Cindy Targosz, both published by Wiley.)

These muscles are the foundation of support for just about any activity your body does. The everyday aches and pains that many women feel are often the result of weakened core-muscle groups. Your body tries to compensate for these weak muscles, which can lead to pain in your lower back and arm and leg joints.

Here's how core strength training works: You incorporate exercises that challenge your abdominal, lower-back, hip, pelvic, and oblique muscles. You can strengthen these muscles with traditional exercises and callisthenic-type movements. (Chapter 19 is full of great exercises to help you strengthen these muscles, and we include even more resources in Appendix B.)

Some additional toys are available that can add variety and fun to your workout and make your workout more effective. Equipment such as balance balls, stability boards, and old-fashioned medicine balls makes targeting the muscles that help maintain your stability and balance easier. Strengthening these muscles can also improve your posture.

## Walking

Walking is an inexpensive and convenient way to relieve stress, improve your fitness, and build muscle tone. However, only 6 percent of people who get all their exercise from walking meet the U.S. Surgeon General's guidelines for fitness. To make sure that your efforts bring you good health, walk

- ✔ At least 30 minutes per session
- ✔ At least four times a week
- ✔ At a moderately intense pace. You should cover about 3½ miles in an hour (or 1¾ miles in a half hour). For more on how hard to work when you work out, see "Zoning in on your target heart rate" in Chapter 19.

Chapter 19 has a whole section on how to design a walking program.

# Elliptical Training

The elliptical-training machine is a terrific way to get aerobic exercise without hurting your joints with high-impact workouts. An elliptical trainer looks like a combination of a treadmill and a climber that grew arms! The machine is called an elliptical trainer because your feet move in the shape of an oval during the workout instead of back and forth like they do on a treadmill or up and down like they move on a climber. Because your feet follow an oval path, the exercise is low impact but still provides a full range of motion for your legs. The arms on the machine go back and forth while you stride, so you get a total body workout.

# Running

Running reduces your risk for developing heart disease, high blood pressure, adult-onset diabetes, and several types of cancer. It also increases the levels of good (HDL) cholesterol in your blood, which helps you get rid of the bad (LDL) cholesterol. (For more information on cholesterol levels, see Chapter 5.) Running also improves your cardiovascular and respiratory systems and can help you control your weight. (Some people lose up to 12 pounds the first year they start running without reducing the calories they eat.)

Getting started on a running regimen is easy; all you need to do is chart out a course (in a safe area) and get a pair of good running shoes. If you're a beginner, try running a mile. If you can't do a mile, try alternating between running and walking until you can cover the entire mile without the walking part. Then add a little distance at a time. Initially schedule about 30 minutes of running time and build up the duration as you go.

# Swimming

Swimming is easy on your joints and helps build muscle strength equally on both sides of your body. In fact, swimming forces you to use all of your muscles. Now that's what we call a workout! It's a great exercise for people looking to increase their overall physical fitness and endurance or recover from an injury.

If you've had a hip or knee replaced or you suffer from arthritis, swimming is an excellent way to maintain aerobic conditioning through low-impact exercise.

# Cycling

Perhaps walking and running are too slow for you, and you're not really a water person. Taking up cycling, whether in the gym or on the road, may be for you. Cycling is a great aerobic workout that improves your cardiovascular health, muscle tone, and stamina.

If you're just getting started, you may want to try a stationary bike at your local YMCA or health club. Try riding for six minutes at 15 miles per hour (or 55 revolutions per minute), five times a week. Gradually work up to 20 to 25 minutes, five times a week, at the same speed. As you become accustomed to cycling, you can build your aerobic fitness even more by increasing your speed.

After spending some time in the saddle, you may want to try a spinning class. A *spin class* is a group indoor-cycling class that can really help you build your aerobic fitness. You can find spin classes at many YMCA locations, community colleges, and health clubs across the country. An instructor guides each class and makes your "ride" on a special stationary bike as challenging as you like.

If you're more of the outdoor type, get that bicycle out of the garage, check the brakes and tires, and take it out for a ride. Don't forget about safety: Always wear a helmet and choose a course in a safe neighborhood that has little traffic and contains few hills.

Start by riding for ten minutes on a relatively flat course (preferably away from traffic) five times a week. Add two minutes to your workout each week (riding five times a week) so that by the end of Week 11 you're riding for 30 minutes five times a week.

# Yoga

Yoga is a great way to improve your health. Studies have shown that yoga can reduce stress, lower blood pressure, relieve arthritis, and build strength and flexibility. The breathing techniques used during a yoga workout help increase the oxygen levels in your blood.

Some styles of yoga focus more on spiritual aspects, such as meditation or chanting, and are great for stress reduction and relaxation. Other forms focus on body alignment and challenging workouts that improve muscle tone, balance, and flexibility. All forms of yoga use poses and breathing techniques to heighten the mind-body connection. You can pull out your copy of *Yoga For Dummies* (Georg Feuerstein, Wiley Publishing, Inc.) for more information. What? Don't have one? You may want to check it out.

# T'ai Chi

T'ai chi helps stretch and tone muscles, relieve stress, and improve balance and circulation. It may even lower your blood pressure. This ancient, Chinese form of exercise, meditation, and self-defense involves controlled movements done slowly and continuously. The forms are similar to those used in other martial arts. If t'ai chi sounds like it may be up your alley, *T'ai Chi For Dummies* (Therese Iknoian with Manny Fuentes, Wiley Publishing, Inc.) is one place to start.

# Pilates

Even though Pilates (puh-*lah*-teez) entered fitness centers fairly recently, its roots actually date back to the 1920s. You can think of Pilates as a combination of yoga, stretching, and calisthenics all rolled up into one set of exercises.

These exercises work on many of the same muscle groups as a core-stability-training program (check out our "Core Strength Training" section earlier in this chapter) and offer many of the same advantages. In Pilates, you perform slow, extremely focused movements that work the muscles in your abdomen, lower back, and buttocks. And yes, there's a snazzy yellow-and-black covered book on this subject too — *Pilates For Dummies* (Ellie Herman, Wiley Publishing, Inc.).

# Water Aerobics

Here's a great exercise for women who feel out of place jumping around in an aerobics class in front of a bunch of other people. Why's it so great? Your legs are under water — if you miss a step or have to take a breather, no one's the wiser. Water aerobics helps you work your cardiovascular system, arm muscles, and leg muscles. It's less stressful on your joints than a lot of exercise programs, which makes it a great exercise for people with arthritis, and it improves your balance and coordination. Many health clubs and YMCA locations offer classes led by professional trainers. Water aerobics is a great way to have fun, stay cool, and get active.

# Chapter 24

# Ten Powerhouse Foods for Menopausal Women

● ● ● ● ● ● ● ● ● ● ● ● ● ● ● ● ● ● ● ● ● ● ● ● ● ● ● ● ● ● ● ● ● ● ● ● ● ● ● ● ● ● ● ● ● ●

### In This Chapter

▶ Ten foods for a healthier lifestyle

▶ Tips for buying, storing, and preparing them

● ● ● ● ● ● ● ● ● ● ● ● ● ● ● ● ● ● ● ● ● ● ● ● ● ● ● ● ● ● ● ● ● ● ● ● ● ● ● ● ● ● ● ● ● ●

*T*here are thousands of healthy, delicious foods out there that are great for women at any age and have special nutritional benefits during your menopausal years (and beyond). These are some of the stars of this lineup.

## Soy Joy

Soy is the queen of powerhouse foods. Researchers believe that soy offers benefits to perimenopausal women in the form of reduced menopausal symptoms (such as hot flashes). Soybeans and their derivatives contain proteins and isoflavones (plant estrogens) that may lower cholesterol. Some researchers, however, are concerned that plant estrogens may have some of the same effects as regular estrogens, and that too much soy may even promote the growth of estrogen-sensitive cancers.

Most doctors agree that a serving a day of soy products is probably safe. Tofu and other soy products are excellent sources of protein, iron, and calcium, making them a staple for vegans, vegetarians, and those who want to limit their consumption of animal fats.

 In addition to the salt, sweet, bitter and sour tastes we all recognize, gastronomes have identified a fifth basic flavor called *umami* (sometimes spelled *umame*). Umami is described as savory and meaty. Cheeses, mushrooms, seaweed, fish sauce, nuts, and soy products have this flavor.

Soy crumbles, a kind of textured vegetable protein, can stand in for ground meats in soups, chili, or pizza. Soymilk doesn't taste much like cow's milk, but can be a reasonable substitute if you're a vegan or lactose intolerant. You can eat edamame (green soy beans) as a snack, or sprinkle them into salads or pasta dishes. Tempeh, a solid form of soy with a chicken-like texture, can be grilled or roasted. Tofu in its different forms can be blended, stir-fried, grilled, or drained and crumbled. Miso, a smooth, salty, savory soy paste, adds that delicious *umami* hit to many foods — stir a spoonful into salad dressing or soup.

# Nuts to You

It's true, nuts are a fatty food, but their fats are largely unsaturated. Besides, we're not suggesting you eat ounces and ounces of them every day. Nuts such as walnuts and almonds contain linoleic and alpha-linoleic fatty acids (good-for-you fats), antioxidants, magnesium, vitamin E, selenium, and other nutrients. They've been touted for their beneficial effects fighting blood clots and osteoporosis.

Think of nuts as accessory foods — the gold belt on your little black dress. Chop and add to salads, pasta, stir-fries, fruit dishes, and desserts, or just grab a few whenever you're struck by the urge to munch something crunchy.

# Catch of the Day

One: fish is really good for your heart and cardiovascular system. Two: fish can be a source of unhealthy toxins. Which is true? Both. But because fish really *is* a very heart-healthy food, adding 1 or 2 servings a week to your diet is a great way to take care of yourself *and* treat yourself. At the same time, doing what you can to minimize your risk of exposure to the mercury fish around the world have picked up through exposure to environmental pollution is important.

Fish is delicious and versatile, and the tastiest ways to prepare it tends to be quick and simple. But we also love fish because it's high in protein and contains heart-healthy omega-3 fatty acids, the kind that lower bad LDL cholesterol and raise healthy HDL cholesterol. A diet rich in fish may also help to protect you from blood clots, inflammation, osteoporosis (especially fish canned with the bones), arthritis, and certain cancers.

Keep your mercury exposure low while you enjoy the benefits of fish. The Environmental Working Group's online calculator (`http://www.ewg.org/ issues/mercury/20031209/calculator.php`) uses your weight to determine how much tuna you can safely eat every week. Some fish markets now buy their fish from merchants who test and certify their products as being mercury-free — ask your fishmonger for more information.

The sky (or the sea) is the limit when it comes to cooking fish. Grill it, broil it, bake it, steam it, just don't slather it with mayonnaise or bread it and fry it.

# I Yam What I Yam

Are those yams or sweet potatoes at the grocery store? Both are terrific for you and easy to prepare, but yams have an edge over sweet potatoes when it comes to nutrition. Yams are yummy, inexpensive, and a great source of antioxidants, vitamin C, potassium, magnesium, vitamin B6, and fiber. Eating them regularly has been linked to a decrease in hot flashes.

Select yams that are firm, without cracks or blemishes. Bake, mash, or steam them, or cut into small pieces and add them to vegetable stir-fries. Store yams in a cool spot (not the fridge, and never in plastic bags) out of direct sunlight, and use within 10 days of purchase.

# The Berry Blues

Okay, we admit it, we're partial to blueberries, but we can sneak in lots of other berries under the same heading and still stay within our "Ten Powerhouse Foods" limit. When your mom said to eat your fruits and vegetables, she might as well have said, "eat your colors," because deeply colored fruits and veggies tend to have the most nutrients.

Berries are delicious and fun to pick. Blueberries are high in vitamin C and fiber, and they pack a whopping 38 percent more antioxidants than other berries. But cranberries also offer up a healthy helping of vitamin C, and are well-known fighters of urinary-tract infections. Raspberries have similar benefits, and a serving of strawberries has even more vitamin C than your recommended daily allowance. Eat them by the handful, toss them onto cereal or oatmeal, fold them into muffins, or mix them together for an all-berry fruit salad.

# Flax Flying

Flaxseeds, like soy products, are a great source of phytoestrogens. Flax packs a lot of nutrition into its tiny, teardrop-shaped seeds. The oil hidden within the seed contains essential fatty acids that have been associated with lowered cholesterol. Flaxseed may also be valuable for its cancer-fighting properties.

A very small percentage of people are allergic to flaxseed. Start with only ¼ teaspoonful a day, and call your doctor immediately if you experience allergy symptoms such as a rash or shortness of breath.

Flaxseed must be ground (in a mill rather like a pepper mill) in order for your body to absorb its nutrients. Because the oils spoil rapidly, only grind what you're going to use within a few days and refrigerate what you don't use immediately. Sprinkle over cereals, salads, and soups, or mix into breads and muffins. Bottled flax oil can also be used, but heating destroys its benefit, so don't cook with it.

# Orange You Glad . . .

. . . we didn't say bananas? Yeah, bananas are great for you, too (the fiber! the potassium!), but oranges have their own appeal (ouch).

With only about 60 calories in a medium orange and a boatload of vitamin C, fiber, antioxidants, and other beneficial nutrients, oranges are associated with a decreased risk of stomach and other cancers, and have anti-inflammatory properties that promote healing. Eaten (or drunk the form of orange juice) when you take your iron supplement, oranges promote absorption of iron. Eat them plain, drink their juice, or slice them and add to salads, stir-fries, and Asian dishes. Even orange zest (the bright orange part of the orange peel) contains nutrients — add it to salads, drinks, and savory stews.

If you and milk are no longer friends, look for calcium-enriched orange juice. Sadly, there is still no rhyme for "orange."

# Tea for You

Tea's just so darned *civilized* that if we were stranded on a desert island we'd probably be okay as long as we'd brought some along. Besides being delicious and somehow both calming and stimulating, both green and black teas are terrific for you. Tea contains the most powerful antioxidant polyphenols of any food, making it effective at fighting the cell damage associated with inflammation and heart disease. Tea also has cancer-fighting properties. Drinking tea — hot or iced — is still the most common way to take it. Some Asian recipes also incorporate tea leaves into stir-fries and marinades. Tea ice cream is increasingly widely available.

Green tea is made from tea leaves that haven't been fermented like black tea. Herb teas, while sometimes delicious and nutritious, are not true teas at all. Only leaves from the *Camellia Sinensis* plant are true tea leaves.

# It's Easy Eating Greens

It was too hard to select just one leafy green — here's the whole group. We may not have loved them when we were little kids, but we do now. Leafy, green vegetables such as kale, spinach, bok choy, Swiss chard, mustard greens, turnip greens, collard greens, and all their friends and relations have earned a place at our tables. Leafy greens all differ a little from each other, but in general they're marvelous sources of iron, fiber, vitamin C, manganese, calcium, copper, B vitamins, and antioxidants.

With greens, the less cooking the better. Some are best gently steamed or stir-fried, some are happy to be eaten raw in salads. Store greens, unwashed and wrapped gently in paper towels and placed in a plastic bag, in the refrigerator. Before using, rinse well, drain or pat dry, and chop or tear into the right-sized pieces for your recipe.

# Yo! Yogurt!

Even if you're not a huge fan of dairy foods, or if you're lactose intolerant and have trouble digesting lactose (the sugar in milk and milk-based foods), you can still be friends with yogurt. Periodically there are reports of people in various parts of the world who claim that yogurt helps members of their culture (no pun intended) to live to be 120 years old or more. Although we can't vouch for that, we can confirm that yogurt's a fabulous source of calcium, perfect for helping you to stave off osteoporosis.

If your doctor prescribes antibiotics, eating yogurt every day while you're taking the medicine can help to prevent the stomach upsets that can accompany antibiotics. It can also help to ward off another unfortunate consequence of antibiotic use: vaginal yeast infections. Be sure to look for yogurt that contains live *Lactobacillus acidophilus* cultures.

Is frozen yogurt better for you than ice cream? There's no easy answer to this one. On average, frozen yogurt has less fat than ice cream, but depending on the brand and the flavor, frozen yogurt may have plenty of sugar and almost as many calories as ice cream. To be safe, treat frozen yogurt as an occasional treat, and read the label to be sure of what you're getting.

Yogurt's great straight from the carton, but it's also wonderful spooned over granola or other cereals, or mixed with fruit salad. Try to avoid heavily sweetened varieties, and choose low-fat or fat-free over whole milk yogurt. If you'd rather not eat it plain, mix in a little fresh fruit or a spoonful of fruit spread. Yogurt can also take the place of some or all of the mayonnaise or sour cream in salad dressings to lighten them up. When buying yogurt, look for the words "active yogurt cultures" or "Contains *Lactobacillus acidophilus* cultures" on the label.

# Part VI
# Appendixes

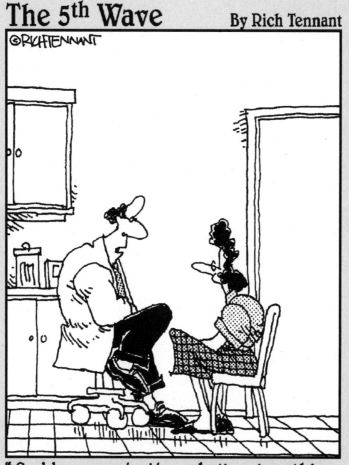

The 5th Wave          By Rich Tennant

"Sudden perspiration, shallow breathing, and rapid heart rate are all signs of menopause. The fact that those symptoms only occur when the pool boy is working in your backyard, however, raises some questions."

# In this part . . .

Literature on menopause is often filled with a dazzling array of medical terms, jargon, and other overstuffed phrases. We, of course, try to simplify this state of affairs. But, in case you run across a word that you need a quick definition for, whether it's in this book or other literature about menopause, we include a glossary of terms — Appendix A. In Appendix B, we provide you with a bunch of additional sources of information — from books to Web sites —that do a great job covering menopause and other health-related issues of interest to women.

# Appendix A

# Glossary

● ● ● ● ● ● ● ● ● ● ● ● ● ● ● ● ● ● ● ● ● ● ● ● ● ● ● ● ● ● ● ● ● ● ● ● ● ● ● ● ● ● ●

**Adenomatous polyp:** Pre-cancerous polyp in the lining of the colon.

**Amenorrhea:** Condition in which menstrual periods cease because of some congenital defect, malnutrition, hormone imbalance, or other cause (including normal ones such as pregnancy).

**Androgens:** Hormones that produce masculine effects on the body, such as a deep voice and facial hair. Both men and women produce androgens, although women produce them in much smaller amounts.

**Angina:** Pain in the chest, arm, or neck caused by lack of blood flow to the heart. Angina is often a symptom of *coronary artery disease.*

**Antioxidant:** A substance, such as vitamins A, C, E, or beta-carotene, that protects cells from damaging *oxidation,* which appears to encourage aging and certain diseases.

**Aromatase inhibitors:** A class of drugs which decrease the amount of estrogen your body produces after menopause.

**Arteriosclerosis:** See *atherosclerosis.*

**Atherosclerosis:** A type of arteriosclerosis in which *cholesterol* and other fatty substances build up in the walls of blood vessels, causing narrowing of the blood vessels. Sometimes referred to as *hardening of the arteries.* It can lead to *coronary artery disease.*

**Atrophy:** See *vaginal atrophy.*

**Bisphosphonates:** A group of medications used to treat *osteoporosis* that stimulate bone growth and slow down bone destruction.

**Body Mass Index (BMI):** A formula for estimating body fat using a weight-to-height ratio. For weight in pounds and height in inches, BMI = Weight/Height$^2 \times 704.5$.

**BRCA1:** A gene responsible for controlling cell growth. Inheritance of an abnormal version of this gene increases your risk of developing breast cancer.

**BRCA2:** A gene responsible for controlling cell growth. As with BRCA1, inheritance of an abnormal version of this gene raises your risk of developing breast cancer, but BRCA2 also increases your risk of ovarian cancer.

**Carcinoma *in situ*:** Condition in which abnormal cancer cells are contained within a specific location within the body and haven't spread to other areas. At this stage, most cancers can be successfully treated.

**Cardiovascular disease (CVD):** Disease that affects the heart, arteries, veins, and capillaries.

**Cholesterol:** A fat-like substance that comprises an important part of the body's cells. At normal levels, cholesterol performs important functions involving certain hormones and nutrients. In excess, cholesterol is associated with an increased risk of cardiovascular disease. Three forms of cholesterol are found in blood: high-density lipids (*HDL*), low-density lipids (*LDL*), and very-low-density lipids (VLDL). Found in all foods made from animals.

**Combination therapy:** A type of hormone therapy that includes both *estrogen* and *progesterone.*

**Conjugated estrogens:** A mixture of estrogens sometimes used in *hormone therapy.* They're chemically different from human *estrogen* and can come from either plants or horses.

**Continuous combination therapy:** A type of hormone therapy regimen in which a woman takes *estrogen* and *progestogen* together throughout the month.

**Coronary artery disease (CAD):** A disease in which the blood vessels that feed the heart become narrow and restrict blood flow to the heart. *Atherosclerosis* is the process that leads to coronary artery disease.

**Coronary heart disease (CHD):** Damage to the heart resulting from *coronary artery disease.* Because the terms are so similar, many people use them interchangeably.

**Corpus luteum:** A yellow sac formed from the remains of the *follicle* after the follicle releases an egg. The corpus luteum produces *progesterone* if the egg is fertilized.

**Cyclic combination therapy:** A type of hormone therapy regimen in which a woman takes estrogen by itself for several days of the month, followed by a period in which she takes *estrogen* and *progestogen.*

**Deep vein thrombosis (DVT):** Blood clots in the veins near the bones that are surrounded by muscle (usually the upper arm, thigh, or pelvic areas). These veins lie deeper under the skin than surface veins and return more blood to the heart. A clot in one of these veins can be fatal if not detected and treated.

**DEXA:** Abbreviation for *dual-energy x-ray absorptiometry* — a method of measuring bone-mineral density. Used to screen for *osteoporosis.*

**DHEA:** Abbreviation for *dehydroepiandrosterone,* a male hormone produced in a woman's adrenal glands and *ovaries.*

**Dowager's hump:** A slang term for the appearance of a hump in the back associated with osteoporosis. Caused by the collapse of vertebrae in the spine due to porous, brittle bones. The term comes from the outdated idea that osteoporosis is a condition that only strikes postmenopausal women (little old ladies, or dowagers).

**Endometrium:** The lining of the uterus.

**Estradiol:** The active form of *estrogen* made in the *ovaries* prior to *menopause.* The most potent form of estrogen in humans. Plays a role in many bodily functions.

**Estriol:** Form of *estrogen* only produced during pregnancy.

**Estrogen:** A female hormone produced in the *ovaries* and in the adrenal glands.

**Estrogen receptor:** A "docking station" on a cell that allows that particular body part to make use of *estrogen.* Estrogen receptors are located all over a woman's body but are highly concentrated in estrogen-sensitive tissues such as uterus and breast tissue.

**Estrone:** A type of *estrogen* made by the *ovaries,* adrenal glands, and body fat before *menopause.* After menopause, body fat makes estrone; therefore, estrone is the only type of estrogen in good supply after menopause. Estrone is less active than *estradiol* estrogen.

**Fibrinogen:** A type of protein that helps blood clot.

**Follicle:** A little sac created from an *oocyte* (seed) in the ovary. The follicle produces estrogen in the ovary. At least one of these little guys releases an egg each month during a woman's reproductive years. After the egg is released, the follicle is called a ***corpus luteum.***

**Follicle-stimulating hormone (FSH):** A hormone produced in the brain that promotes ovulation by triggering the ***ovaries*** to begin developing ***follicles.*** Doctors consider continued high levels of FSH to be an indication of ***menopause.*** The FSH keeps trying to stimulate follicle production when the cupboard is bare — the ovary can no longer crank out follicles — which is a sign that the ovary is entering retirement and you're entering menopause.

**HDL:** Abbreviation for high-density lipid. HDL is "good" cholesterol because it can carry fat from the body cells back to the liver for excretion. *Lipids* are made up of protein and fat. Lipids with more protein than fat are called high-density lipids; lipids with more fat than protein are called low-density lipids ***(LDL).***

**Hormone:** Chemicals produced in organs that travel through the body to activate or moderate functions in other parts of the body.

**Hormone-receptor site:** A "docking station" on a cell where hormones can connect to cells to manipulate them.

**Hormone replacement therapy (HRT):** See ***hormone therapy.***

**Hormone therapy (HT):** Treatment designed to adjust hormone levels using synthetic or natural female hormones. Doctors generally administer this treatment to women going through ***perimenopause*** and/or ***menopause.***

**Hypertension:** Another name for high blood pressure.

**Hysterectomy:** Surgical removal of the uterus. A *simple hysterectomy* removes only the uterus. A *complete hysterectomy* removes the uterus and the ***ovaries.*** A complete hysterectomy causes ***surgical menopause.***

**Incontinence:** The inability to "hold it" or keep from urinating.

**Interstitial cystitis (IC):** A bladder condition that's hard to diagnose, but the symptoms include mild discomfort, pressure, tenderness, or intense pain in the bladder and surrounding pelvic area. Symptoms may include an urgent need to urinate (*urgency*), a frequent need to urinate (*frequency*), or a combination of these symptoms.

**Isoflavone:** See ***phytoestrogen.***

**Labia:** The lips of the vaginal opening. See also *vulva.*

**LDL:** Abbreviation for low-density lipids. LDLs are found in the bloodstream and are thought to carry cholesterol from the liver to body cells. Eating a diet high in saturated fats and cholesterol will raise your LDL levels. The higher the LDL level, the greater the incidence of heart attack or *coronary artery disease.*

**Libido:** Sex drive.

**Lobules:** Milk-producing glands in the breast. Cancer sometimes starts in the lobules.

**Luteinizing hormone (LH):** A hormone made in the pituitary gland. In women, it triggers *ovulation.*

**Menarche:** The onset of menstrual periods, which signals the beginning of a woman's reproductive maturation.

**Menopause:** The technical meaning is the end of menstruation — no *menses* for 12 months. Because periods are so irregular in the months leading up to menopause, the medical community generally doesn't consider you to be officially menopausal until 12 months after your last period. Strictly speaking, *menopause* should only refer to the time after periods have stopped, but it's often used loosely to refer to all stages of menopause including *perimenopause,* menopause, and *postmenopause.*

**Menses:** This word is derived from the Latin word for *month.* The term refers to your period — the periodic flow of blood from the uterus.

**Oophorectomy:** Surgical removal of one or both ovaries.

**Osteoblast:** Cells that build new bone.

**Osteoclast:** Cells that break down bone during the bone-maintenance process.

**Osteopenia:** Loss of bone density that isn't sufficiently severe enough to be called *osteoporosis.* If action isn't taken to better maintain the bone, this condition will turn into osteoporosis over time.

**Osteoporosis:** Loss of bone density. Makes bones brittle, porous, and weak.

**Ovaries:** Female sex organs that store "seeds" (*oocytes*), some of which develop into *follicles.* You're born with two ovaries. They produce the hormones *estrogen* and *progesterone* as well as a small amount of *testosterone.*

**Ovulation:** The process by which the egg is released from the *follicle.*

**Oxidation:** Technically, this term refers to the process through which oxygen combines with another substance — as when metal turns to rust. So what does this have to do with menopause? Unstable oxygen molecules, *free radicals* in med speak, are produced as your body's cells go about their daily chores. Because they're unstable, free radicals react with other molecules as they move through your body. Oxidation does some good things, but it also damages healthy cells, which can lead to cancer, heart disease, and other ailments common to menopausal women.

**Palpitation:** In this book, we use this term to refer to a rapid heartbeat.

**Pap test:** Papanicolaou test. A routine test performed at your annual visit to the gynecologist, in which a sample of cells is taken from your cervix to check for abnormal and potentially cancerous cells. Sometimes called a pap smear.

**Perimenopause:** Time frame prior to *menopause* when hormones fluctuate radically, periods may be irregular, and women may experience physical and emotional symptoms (such as hot flashes, heart palpitations, mood swings, irritability, and crying jags). Perimenopause may begin ten years prior to menopause but more typically begins four to six years prior to menopause and continues through the first year after menstrual periods stop.

**Phytoestrogen:** *Estrogen* produced by plants (such as the soybean plant) that binds with human *estrogen receptors* and results in estrogen-like actions. Sometimes called *isoflavone.*

**POF:** See *premature ovarian failure.*

**Polyp:** A growth, usually non-cancerous, that protrudes from tissues, usually in a mucous membrane similar to those in the digestive tract. In this book, we discuss colon polyps.

**Postmenopause:** The years after *menopause* when the ovaries have stopped functioning. This is the time when health conditions associated with long periods of low *estrogen* (*osteoporosis* and *cardiovascular disease*) are your top concern.

**Premature menopause:** Experiencing menopause at an unusually early age (such as in your 30s). Premature menopause leaves you at risk of osteoporosis and higher cholesterol fairly early in life.

**Premature ovarian failure (POF):** Failure of the ovaries to perform their normal function, usually because of disease, hormone imbalance, and medical treatments such as radiation or chemotherapy. In some cases of POF, the cause is never determined.

**Premenopausal:** Term associated with women who haven't yet gone through *menopause.*

**Progesterone:** A female hormone produced by the *ovaries* after *ovulation* to prepare the uterus for fertilization.

**Progestin:** Synthetic form of the natural hormone *progesterone.*

**Progestogen:** Any hormone, natural or synthetic, which has the same effect on the body as *progesterone.*

**Pulmonary embolism:** Blockage of an artery in the lungs by a blood clot.

**Sequential combination therapy:** A type of hormone therapy regimen in which a woman takes estrogen, followed by progestogen, followed by a period in which no hormones are taken.

**SERMs:** Abbreviation for *selective estrogen receptor modulators* — special "designer hormones" used in *hormone therapy.* They can activate *estrogen receptors* in some parts of the body while blocking estrogen receptors in other parts of the body. SERMs are particularly useful for women who want the benefits of HT but don't want to increase their risk for breast cancer.

**Serotonin:** A brain chemical that regulates sleep, mood, *libido,* pain, and more.

**Surgical menopause:** *Menopause* that is the result of the surgical removal of the ovaries.

**Testosterone:** A male hormone produced by the *ovaries* in low levels. Helps maintain muscle mass, bone, and *libido* in women.

**Transdermal:** A method of delivering medication in which the medication is absorbed through the skin and goes directly into the bloodstream.

**Triglyceride:** A chemical form of the fats that circulate in the bloodstream and are used by the body to make *cholesterol.*

**Unopposed estrogen:** A type of hormone therapy regimen in which a woman uses *estrogen* without *progestogen* to balance it.

**Urethra:** The little canal through which you urinate.

**Urinary-tract infection (UTI):** An infection that affects the bladder, *urethra,* or kidneys.

**Vaginal atrophy:** Thinning and drying of vaginal tissue often experienced during *perimenopause* and *menopause.*

**Vulva:** Collective term for the external genital organs that are visible between a woman's thighs consisting of the *mons* (fleshy, rounded area covered by pubic hair), *labia* (lips or folds of the vagina), *hymen* (thin mucous membrane that keeps the vagina partially closed), *clitoris* (a woman's pleasure spot), and some glands, including those involved in keeping the vaginal area lubricated.

# Appendix B

# Resources

· · · · · · · · · · · · · · · · · · · · · · · · · · · · · · · · · · · · · · · · · · · · · · ·

*I*f you're interested in finding more information about menopause, hormones, and related conditions, here's a quick guide to some terrific resources.

## *Fabulous Books about Menopause, Health, Fitness, and Related Issues*

These are some of our favorite reference books. They contain some good information, and the authors wrote them with the layperson in mind. You can find these books at your local library or bookstore.

*Better Than I Ever Expected: Straight Talk about Sex after Sixty*, by Joan Price (Seal Press, 2006). Just as the title promises, Price helps you keep the home fires burning (even better than before) through perimenopause to menopause and far, far beyond.

*Bob Greene's Total Body Makeover: An Accelerated Program of Exercise and Nutrition for Maximum Results in Minimum Time,* by Bob Greene (Simon & Schuster, 2004). What has Oprah got that you haven't got? Personal trainer Bob Greene. In this book, Greene offers you a challenging 12-week program of exercise (be prepared to sweat) and appealing, healthy food. Greene knows that you don't live in a vacuum, too — he'll help you out with the emotional aspects of neglecting your fitness and nutrition.

*Caring for Yourself While Caring for Your Aging Parents, Third Edition: How to Help, How to Survive,* by Claire Berman (Owl Books, 2005). At the same time that you're taking care of yourself as you enter menopause, you may still be taking care of your children. More and more women in the middle of their lives are also juggling the care of aging parents. If you're in this group, Berman's advice is invaluable, compassionate, wise, and down to earth.

*Dr. Susan Love's Hormone Book: Making Informed Choices,* by Susan Love and Karen Lindsey (Three Rivers Press, 2003). This updated edition of Love's original book on dealing with the symptoms of menopause and taking care of your health in the years to come presents a balanced approach to menopause and hormone therapy.

*Healthy Women, Healthy Lives,* by Susan E. Hankinson, Graham A. Colditz, JoAnn E. Manson, and Frank E. Speizer (Simon & Schuster, 2002). With that many authors, it has to be good. This updated edition of *Healthy Women, Healthy Lives* offers important lessons about reducing your risk for many chronic diseases and several forms of cancer. Using results from one of the largest studies of women in the world, the Nurses' Health Study, this resource can help you make better-informed personal-health choices. It's informative, yet very easy to read and understand.

*Kathy Smith's Moving Through Menopause: The Complete Program for Exercise, Nutrition, and Total Wellness*, by Kathy Smith and Robert Miller (Warner, 2002). This one has been out for a few years, but the advice Smith offers is still right on target for those of us facing what she calls "the half-time bell." Although the main focus is on exercise (including yoga and Pilates), Smith offers her workout advice in the context of taking care of every aspect of your life.

*Menopause and Perimenopause*, by Mary Jane Minkin (Yale University Press, 2004). Distilled from years of study, practice, and women out there in the hot flash zone, Minkin's book offers clear explanations of what's causing your symptoms, how to manage them, and how to take care of your health in the decades to come.

*Menopause Before 40: Coping with Premature Ovarian Failure*, by Karin Banerd (Trafford Publishing, 2004). Although this is a good general reference on menopause, if you're going through or have gone through premature menopause, you'll find answers to your specific questions about why this is happening to you, and how you can cope with the rush job your body's giving you. Best of all, you get the benefit of the wisdom of other women who've gone through the same thing, and their tips about how best to take care of yourself in the years to come.

*The Okinawa Program: How the World's Longest-Lived People Achieve Everlasting Health — And How You Can Too*, by Bradley J. Willcox, D. Craig Willcox, and Makoto Suzuki (Three Rivers Press, 2002). Yeah, okay, this one's been around for a while, but that's because it's an enduring classic. And, yeah, it's a *long* enduring classic — but there's gold in them there 496 pages. Why do those folks on Okinawa live such long, such healthy, such *happy* lives? Find out.

*Prime Time: The African American Woman's Complete Guide to Midlife Health and Wellness,* by Gayle K. Porter, M.D., and Marilyn Gaston, Ph.D. (One World/Ballantine, 2003). Health information for African American women in the prime of life, including menopause, diabetes, hypertension, and dealing with the healthcare system.

*What You Wear Can Change Your Life*, by Trinny Woodall and Susannah Constantine (Riverhead Trade, 2005). Menopause changes your body in almost every aspect. Why shouldn't your outsides get a makeover, too — one you can control? BBC Television's Trinny and Susannah will help the brand new you to look . . . well, like the brand new you, only with better clothes. Look better, feel better.

*The Wisdom of Menopause: Creating Physical and Emotional Health and Healing During the Change*, by Christiane Northrup, MD (Bantam Books, 2006). Respected holistic physician Cristiane Northrup lived it before she wrote it, and emphasizes not only mental and physical health aspects of menopause, but also the grace and strength to be found in this period of your life.

*Younger Next Year for Women*, by Chris Crowley and Henry S. Lodge (Workman Publishing, 2005). The same straightforward health and lifestyle information that made their earlier books so popular, but with women's issues in mine. Our favorite no-nonsense advice: "Don't eat crap."

# Wonderful Web Sites for Women

If you have access to the Internet, the world of health and nutrition is literally at your fingertips. In this section, we list some of our favorite Web sites. These sites have our personal seal of approval because they have tons of up-to-date information and provide links to lots of other Web sites.

## American Herbalist Guild

www.americanherbalistsguild.com

If you're interested in finding an herbalist in the United States, check out this site. It gives you the organization's code of ethics as well as links to the Web sites of its members. Those of you interested in learning more about herbs will also enjoy the educational programs listed and online courses provided on this page.

## Yoga.com

www.yoga.com

Find an instructor, take a free class, or learn more about the history of yoga. This site is a great place to visit for people just getting interested in yoga and for yoga vets who want more information.

## Dietary Guidelines for Americans

http://www.healthierus.gov/dietaryguidelines/index.html

Here's a Web site that gives you the latest on diet and fitness recommendations from the U.S. Department of Health and Human Services. It's quick and gets right to the point.

## FitDay.com

www.fitday.com

This site bills itself as "Your online diet and fitness journal," and it's the handiest little site on the Internet if you're trying to eat healthier or lose weight. It lets you type in the foods you eat, and it tells you the calories and nutrients found in each. You can also keep track of your food consumption after every meal (or even plan your calories ahead of time). Because the site also keeps track of nutrients, you can make sure your diet is balanced. For women trying to lose weight, FitDay.com has some nice planners and exercise trackers so you can see if you're going to lose weight with your current eating and exercise routines. And the best part? It's all free!

## National Center for Complementary and Alternative Medicine Clearinghouse

www.nccam.nih.gov

This site provides information on alternative medical therapies not commonly used or previously accepted in conventional Western medicine. We particularly like the "Health Information" page because it has links to alerts and advisories that warn you of any harmful therapies on the market. You can also search for information on the particular therapy or condition that interests you.

# National Osteoporosis Foundation

www.nof.org

You can find lots of information on osteoporosis (some of it in Spanish) on this Web site. Because osteoporosis is such a big concern for women after menopause, you may want to refer to this page often. The site features news about osteoporosis, prevention, and treatment, a find-a-doctor feature, and the opportunity to sign up for a weekly newsletter. NOF also offers information about insurance and Medicare benefits for osteoporosis treatment.

# National Women's Health Information Center

www.4woman.gov

This site is provided by the U.S. Department of Health and Human Services to offer information about all aspects of women's health and health care, including menopause and hormone therapy. The information is nicely organized, and you can get right to the issues that concern you. Links to a variety of government and medical groups of interest to women after menopause are also included.

# North American Menopause Society

www.menopause.org

This Web site is dedicated to promoting women's health during midlife and beyond through an understanding of menopause. It contains tons of information on perimenopause, early menopause, menopausal symptoms, long-term health effects of estrogen loss, and a wide variety of therapies to enhance your health.

# Third Age

http://www.thirdage.com/

Third Age has a lively and absorbing Web site on all aspects of life, health, diet, fitness, relationships, sex, beauty, and life-long learning for folks in their 40s, 50s, 60s, and beyond.

## WebMD

www.webmd.com

Now here's a terrific site to find out about what ails you (or what you think might ail you). It has a powerful search engine. You can type in the name of a medical condition or medication and get a list of articles that may be helpful to you. Nearly all the information is user friendly and written for the average person who isn't a medical expert. All the articles are kept current and accurate. Be sure to check out their Menopause Health Center at http://www.webmd.com/diseases_and_conditions/menopause.htm.

## Women and Cardiovascular Disease

www.women.americanheart.org

Don't let the name scare you. The information here can help you *prevent* cardiovascular disease. This Web address takes you to the part of the American Heart Association's site devoted to women. You can find information on women's risks of heart disease, cardiovascular problems, and stroke. This site is full of up-to-the-minute, heart-healthy information and includes links to other cardiovascular-related Web sites.

## Women's Cancer Network

www.wcn.org

The Women's Cancer Network, which can answer many of your questions about gynecologic cancer, is hosted by the Society of Gynecologic Oncologists. You can find everything from the most recent research results to physician referrals here.

# The Study Sites

Throughout this book we've drawn heavily from the findings of a few crucial women's health studies for the information and advice we've passed on to you. Just in case you'd like to read more about some of these studies (and stay up to date on their findings), here are some places to start.

# Women's Health Initiative

http://www.nhlbi.nih.gov/whi/index.html

http://www.whi.org/index.php

Consider this listing a two-for-one bonus. The first address is for the main page of the Women's Health Initiative. The second is a site that was set up for participants in the study, but it has some terrific information on the study's results that have already been published. Also, the section concerning HRT in the news is great because it provides links to all the media coverage of the study's already-published results concerning hormone therapy.

# The Nurses' Health Study

http://www.channing.harvard.edu/nhs/index.html

Since 1979, the Nurses' Health Study (and its second stage, named, appropriately enough, the Nurses' Health Study II) has shed light on what women do to take care of their health — especially with respect to the use of hormone therapy — and how it's working out for them.

# Kronos Early Estrogen Prevention Study

http://www.kronosinstitute.org/keeps.html

This is one to watch — an ongoing study that may provide the answers to some of our — and your — questions about the effects of hormone therapy in women at the younger end of the normal perimenopause spectrum, and about different ways of administering hormones.

# The Framingham Heart Study

http://www.nhlbi.nih.gov/about/framingham/

The good people of Framingham, Massachusetts, near Boston, have opened their hearts (and their medical files) for more than half a decade in the service of improving the health of people everywhere. Check it out — in addition to being an important chapter in American medicine, it's a wonderful human interest story.

# Index

## • *C* •

## • F •

# Notes

# BUSINESS, CAREERS & PERSONAL FINANCE

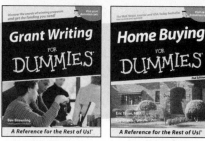

0-7645-5307-0

0-7645-5331-3 *†

**Also available:**

- Accounting For Dummies †
  0-7645-5314-3
- Business Plans Kit For Dummies †
  0-7645-5365-8
- Cover Letters For Dummies
  0-7645-5224-4
- Frugal Living For Dummies
  0-7645-5403-4
- Leadership For Dummies
  0-7645-5176-0
- Managing For Dummies
  0-7645-1771-6

- Marketing For Dummies
  0-7645-5600-2
- Personal Finance For Dummies *
  0-7645-2590-5
- Project Management For Dummies
  0-7645-5283-X
- Resumes For Dummies †
  0-7645-5471-9
- Selling For Dummies
  0-7645-5363-1
- Small Business Kit For Dummies *†
  0-7645-5093-4

# HOME & BUSINESS COMPUTER BASICS

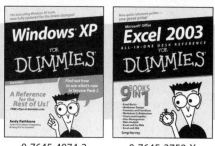

0-7645-4074-2

0-7645-3758-X

**Also available:**

- ACT! 6 For Dummies
  0-7645-2645-6
- iLife '04 All-in-One Desk Reference
  For Dummies
  0-7645-7347-0
- iPAQ For Dummies
  0-7645-6769-1
- Mac OS X Panther Timesaving
  Techniques For Dummies
  0-7645-5812-9
- Macs For Dummies
  0-7645-5656-8

- Microsoft Money 2004 For Dummies
  0-7645-4195-1
- Office 2003 All-in-One Desk Reference
  For Dummies
  0-7645-3883-7
- Outlook 2003 For Dummies
  0-7645-3759-8
- PCs For Dummies
  0-7645-4074-2
- TiVo For Dummies
  0-7645-6923-6
- Upgrading and Fixing PCs For Dummies
  0-7645-1665-5
- Windows XP Timesaving Techniques
  For Dummies
  0-7645-3748-2

# FOOD, HOME, GARDEN, HOBBIES, MUSIC & PETS

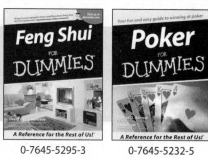

0-7645-5295-3

0-7645-5232-5

**Also available:**

- Bass Guitar For Dummies
  0-7645-2487-9
- Diabetes Cookbook For Dummies
  0-7645-5230-9
- Gardening For Dummies *
  0-7645-5130-2
- Guitar For Dummies
  0-7645-5106-X
- Holiday Decorating For Dummies
  0-7645-2570-0
- Home Improvement All-in-One
  For Dummies
  0-7645-5680-0

- Knitting For Dummies
  0-7645-5395-X
- Piano For Dummies
  0-7645-5105-1
- Puppies For Dummies
  0-7645-5255-4
- Scrapbooking For Dummies
  0-7645-7208-3
- Senior Dogs For Dummies
  0-7645-5818-8
- Singing For Dummies
  0-7645-2475-5
- 30-Minute Meals For Dummies
  0-7645-2589-1

# INTERNET & DIGITAL MEDIA

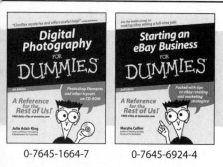

0-7645-1664-7

0-7645-6924-4

**Also available:**

- 2005 Online Shopping Directory
  For Dummies
  0-7645-7495-7
- CD & DVD Recording For Dummies
  0-7645-5956-7
- eBay For Dummies
  0-7645-5654-1
- Fighting Spam For Dummies
  0-7645-5965-6
- Genealogy Online For Dummies
  0-7645-5964-8
- Google For Dummies
  0-7645-4420-9

- Home Recording For Musicians
  For Dummies
  0-7645-1634-5
- The Internet For Dummies
  0-7645-4173-0
- iPod & iTunes For Dummies
  0-7645-7772-7
- Preventing Identity Theft For Dummies
  0-7645-7336-5
- Pro Tools All-in-One Desk Reference
  For Dummies
  0-7645-5714-9
- Roxio Easy Media Creator For Dummies
  0-7645-7131-1

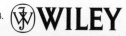

## SPORTS, FITNESS, PARENTING, RELIGION & SPIRITUALITY

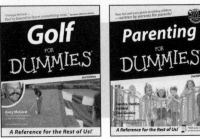

0-7645-5146-9

0-7645-5418-2

**Also available:**
- Adoption For Dummies
  0-7645-5488-3
- Basketball For Dummies
  0-7645-5248-1
- The Bible For Dummies
  0-7645-5296-1
- Buddhism For Dummies
  0-7645-5359-3
- Catholicism For Dummies
  0-7645-5391-7
- Hockey For Dummies
  0-7645-5228-7

- Judaism For Dummies
  0-7645-5299-6
- Martial Arts For Dummies
  0-7645-5358-5
- Pilates For Dummies
  0-7645-5397-6
- Religion For Dummies
  0-7645-5264-3
- Teaching Kids to Read For Dummies
  0-7645-4043-2
- Weight Training For Dummies
  0-7645-5168-X
- Yoga For Dummies
  0-7645-5117-5

## TRAVEL

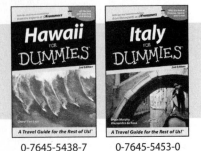

0-7645-5438-7

0-7645-5453-0

**Also available:**
- Alaska For Dummies
  0-7645-1761-9
- Arizona For Dummies
  0-7645-6938-4
- Cancún and the Yucatán For Dummies
  0-7645-2437-2
- Cruise Vacations For Dummies
  0-7645-6941-4
- Europe For Dummies
  0-7645-5456-5
- Ireland For Dummies
  0-7645-5455-7

- Las Vegas For Dummies
  0-7645-5448-4
- London For Dummies
  0-7645-4277-X
- New York City For Dummies
  0-7645-6945-7
- Paris For Dummies
  0-7645-5494-8
- RV Vacations For Dummies
  0-7645-5443-3
- Walt Disney World & Orlando For Dummies
  0-7645-6943-0

## GRAPHICS, DESIGN & WEB DEVELOPMENT

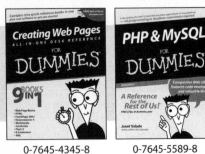

0-7645-4345-8

0-7645-5589-8

**Also available:**
- Adobe Acrobat 6 PDF For Dummies
  0-7645-3760-1
- Building a Web Site For Dummies
  0-7645-7144-3
- Dreamweaver MX 2004 For Dummies
  0-7645-4342-3
- FrontPage 2003 For Dummies
  0-7645-3882-9
- HTML 4 For Dummies
  0-7645-1995-6
- Illustrator CS For Dummies
  0-7645-4084-X

- Macromedia Flash MX 2004 For Dummies
  0-7645-4358-X
- Photoshop 7 All-in-One Desk Reference For Dummies
  0-7645-1667-1
- Photoshop CS Timesaving Techniques For Dummies
  0-7645-6782-9
- PHP 5 For Dummies
  0-7645-4166-8
- PowerPoint 2003 For Dummies
  0-7645-3908-6
- QuarkXPress 6 For Dummies
  0-7645-2593-X

## NETWORKING, SECURITY, PROGRAMMING & DATABASES

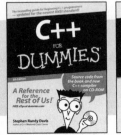
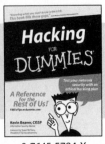

0-7645-6852-3

0-7645-5784-X

**Also available:**
- A+ Certification For Dummies
  0-7645-4187-0
- Access 2003 All-in-One Desk Reference For Dummies
  0-7645-3988-4
- Beginning Programming For Dummies
  0-7645-4997-9
- C For Dummies
  0-7645-7068-4
- Firewalls For Dummies
  0-7645-4048-3
- Home Networking For Dummies
  0-7645-42796

- Network Security For Dummies
  0-7645-1679-5
- Networking For Dummies
  0-7645-1677-9
- TCP/IP For Dummies
  0-7645-1760-0
- VBA For Dummies
  0-7645-3989-2
- Wireless All In-One Desk Reference For Dummies
  0-7645-7496-5
- Wireless Home Networking For Dummies
  0-7645-3910-8

## HEALTH & SELF-HELP

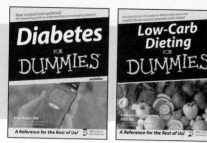

0-7645-6820-5 *†

0-7645-2566-2

**Also available:**

Alzheimer's For Dummies
0-7645-3899-3

Asthma For Dummies
0-7645-4233-8

Controlling Cholesterol For Dummies
0-7645-5440-9

Depression For Dummies
0-7645-3900-0

Dieting For Dummies
0-7645-4149-8

Fertility For Dummies
0-7645-2549-2

Fibromyalgia For Dummies
0-7645-5441-7

Improving Your Memory For Dummies
0-7645-5435-2

Pregnancy For Dummies †
0-7645-4483-7

Quitting Smoking For Dummies
0-7645-2629-4

Relationships For Dummies
0-7645-5384-4

Thyroid For Dummies
0-7645-5385-2

## EDUCATION, HISTORY, REFERENCE & TEST PREPARATION

0-7645-5194-9

0-7645-4186-2

**Also available:**

Algebra For Dummies
0-7645-5325-9

British History For Dummies
0-7645-7021-8

Calculus For Dummies
0-7645-2498-4

English Grammar For Dummies
0-7645-5322-4

Forensics For Dummies
0-7645-5580-4

The GMAT For Dummies
0-7645-5251-1

Inglés Para Dummies
0-7645-5427-1

Italian For Dummies
0-7645-5196-5

Latin For Dummies
0-7645-5431-X

Lewis & Clark For Dummies
0-7645-2545-X

Research Papers For Dummies
0-7645-5426-3

The SAT I For Dummies
0-7645-7193-1

Science Fair Projects For Dummies
0-7645-5460-3

U.S. History For Dummies
0-7645-5249-X

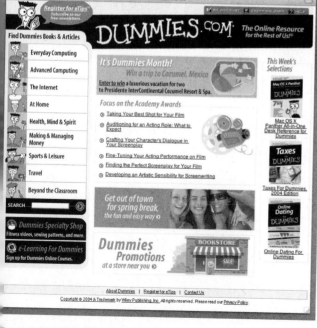

# Get smart @ dummies.com®

- **Find a full list of Dummies titles**
- **Look into loads of FREE on-site articles**
- **Sign up for FREE eTips e-mailed to you weekly**
- **See what other products carry the Dummies name**
- **Shop directly from the Dummies bookstore**
- **Enter to win new prizes every month!**

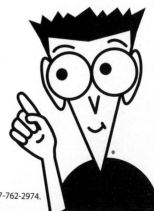

Separate Canadian edition also available
Separate U.K. edition also available

ailable wherever books are sold. For more information or to order direct: U.S. customers visit www.dummies.com or call 1-877-762-2974.
K. customers visit www.wileyeurope.com or call 0800 243407. Canadian customers visit www.wiley.ca or call 1-800-567-4797.

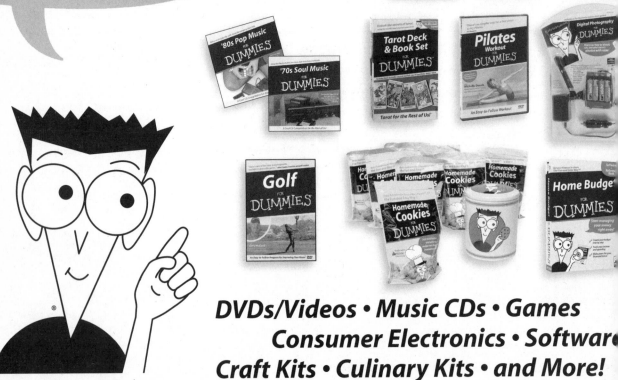